Clinical Alzheimer
Rehabilitation

Prem P. Gogia, DPT, PhD, has more than 30 years of experience in the health care delivery systems. He received a Doctor of Physical Therapy from Drexel University, Philadelphia, Pennsylvania, and a Doctor of Philosophy in physical therapy from Texas Woman's University, Houston, Texas. Dr. Gogia also earned a Master of Health Science degree in physical therapy from Washington University, St. Louis, Missouri. He also holds a Master of Business Administration in Management from Southern Illinois University, Edwardsville, Illinois. Dr. Gogia has published 22 research and special interest papers in professional journals. In addition to contributing a few chapters to books, he is the author of two books titled *Clinical Orthopedic Tests* and *Clinical Wound Management.* Prior to joining PRS Health System, Inc., as president and CEO, he held various positions including Clinical Director of Rehabilitation Services and Wound Clinic at Park Plaza Hospital in Houston, and served as an Adjunct Assistant Professor in the Department of Physical Therapy at the University of Texas Medical Branch in Galveston. Dr. Gogia has extensive management experience in rehabilitation, home health, durable medical equipment, and assisted living facilities.

Nirek Rastogi, MD, graduated from Rutgers College with a Bachelor's degree in biology with honors and a minor in psychology. He attended medical school at Ross University School of Medicine where he graduated with high honors. Dr. Rastogi did his residency training in family medicine at Overlook Hospital in Summit, New Jersey, and served as chief resident during his final year of training. Currently, Dr. Rastogi is working as a private-practice clinician in Phoenix, Arizona. He is a board certified family physician who holds licenses to practice medicine in New Jersey and Arizona. He is a member of the American Academy of Family Physicians and Arizona Academy of Family Physicians.

Clinical Alzheimer Rehabilitation

PREM P. GOGIA, DPT, PhD
NIREK RASTOGI, MD

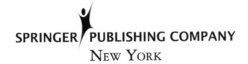

SPRINGER PUBLISHING COMPANY
NEW YORK

Springer Publishing Company, LLC
11 West 42nd Street
New York, NY 10036
www.springerpub.com

Acquisitions Editor: Sheri W. Sussman
Production Editor: Julia Rosen
Cover design: Mimi Flow
Composition: Apex CoVantage

08 09 10 11 12/ 5 4 3 2 1

Library of Congress Cataloging-in-Publication Data

Gogia, Prem P., 1953–
    Clinical Alzheimer rehabilitation / Prem P. Gogia, Nirek Rastogi.
        p. ; cm.
    Includes bibliographical references and index.
    ISBN 978-0-8261-1707-6 (alk. paper)
    1. Alzheimer's disease—Patients—Rehabilitation.   I. Rastogi, Nirek.   II. Title.
    [DNLM: 1. Alzheimer Disease.   2. Alzheimer Disease—rehabilitation.
WT 155 G613c 2008]
    RC523.G63   2008
    616.8'31—dc22   2008016043

Printed in the United States of America by Bang Printing.

This book is dedicated to my father, the late Mr. J. R. Gogia, whose suffering from Alzheimer's disease inspired me to study and to share my experiences with my professional colleagues.
—Prem P. Gogia, DPT, PhD

Contents

Foreword

The aging of baby boomers is a frequent news topic because of the impact on the social-support systems this large group of people reaching age 65 will have. What is clear is that with the increasing numbers of individuals living longer the greater the number of people are suffering from Alzheimer's disease. As discussed in this book, the incidence of Alzheimer's disease is 18% in those age 75–85 and then increases to about 47% in people age 85 and older. Our improved health care has resulted in a large population of people age 75 and older. These figures speak to the cost, both emotional and financial, to all of us as the number of individuals with Alzheimer's disease increases. Society must find effective ways to slow the progression of Alzheimer's and develop effective and efficient strategies to meet the needs of those with this challenging disease. Support of research aimed at preventing the disease should have the highest priority in government funding but that has not materialized. The lack of a cure and an effective form of treatment means that every possible means of slowing the disease and its manifestations must be utilized.

As a physical therapist for 50 years involved in the care of individuals with dementia as well as my firsthand experience with family and friends with Alzheimer's disease, I am acutely aware of the challenging aspects of this disease. Drs. Gogia and Rastogi have provided here a valuable resource to all those involved with individuals with Alzheimer's disease. This book provides a very thorough coverage of all aspects of the disease and is written in a way that meets the needs of the general public as well as health care professionals.

One of the appealing aspects of the book is that one of the authors is a physical therapist. At the time of this writing, one of the most effective forms of treatment for slowing the progression of Alzheimer's disease is 30 minutes of aerobic exercise 3 times per week. Yet in the age group experiencing the disease, being able to exercise has many considerations. Older individuals often have musculoskeletal problems such as degenerative disease of the spine, hips, knees, and feet in addition to the sarcopenia that is present with aging and inactivity. Thus, designing an effective exercise program becomes a particular challenge. The chapter on rehabilitation emphasizes and has useful suggestions about maintaining patients with Alzheimer's disease, which includes exercising regularly and participating in as much activity as possible. The use of medication is certainly an easier treatment route but as with many health care problems, the benefits of exercise are many and the side effects are few, particularly if the program is designed by a therapist.

Although this book incorporates a wide variety of strategies and resources for treatment, the realistic approach to long-term care and the end-of-life issues is particularly well done. Reading this book will enable health care providers and family caregivers to be well prepared for what to expect for the entire course of the disease. If knowledge and preparation are the best defense and offense for being able to manage challenges, then this book is an excellent way to obtain those tools. I highly recommend this very readable and invaluable book.

Shirley Sahrmann, PT, PhD, FAPTA
Professor of Physical Therapy, Neurology,
Cell Biology, and Physiology
Washington University School of
Medicine–St. Louis, MO

Preface

Alzheimer's disease, the most common form of dementia, is a progressive and degenerative brain disorder that results in symptoms such as loss of memory, impaired judgment and reasoning, difficulty with day-to-day functioning, and changes in mood and behavior. As the population ages, the number of people diagnosed with Alzheimer's disease will increase dramatically, as will the cost of care for people with Alzheimer's. Rehabilitation is a vital part of management of this challenging disease. Current research on physical rehabilitation in people with Alzheimer's disease is very limited. In addition, researchers are reluctant to conduct clinical trials with Alzheimer's simply because of communication difficulties, logistical problems, ethical difficulties, and methodological challenges. Furthermore, investigators also believe that the indicators of success are difficult to measure. It is important to remember that, although any skills lost will not be regained, rehabilitation gives special consideration to quality of life for people with Alzheimer's disease. This comprehensive book is written to act as an up-to-date resource for those clinicians and caregivers who are involved in the care of people affected by Alzheimer's disease, either directly or indirectly. Particular attention has been paid to the rehabilitation aspect of management for this challenging population. All that we know about Alzheimer's disease is not being practiced. There are "tools of the trained"—caregiving and diagnostic tools—that have been proven to help arrest Alzheimer's disease. Illustrations and tables are included as needed to enhance the clarity of the text. We hope this book, which is based on these tools and on the newest developments in Alzheimer's research, can serve as the first complete resource for clinicians and caregivers.

Acknowledgments

We wish to thank the following colleagues for their support in reviewing the manuscript and for providing valuable suggestions:

Dr. MaryBeth Brown, Professor, School of Health Professions, Physical Therapy, University of Missouri, Columbia, for reviewing the chapter "Caring at Home for People With Alzheimer's Disease."

Dr. Sharon Olson, Professor and Director of the School of Physical Therapy, Texas Woman's University, Houston, Texas, for reviewing the chapter "Long-Term Care of People With Alzheimer's Disease."

Dr. Elizabeth Protas, Interim Dean and Professor, The School of Allied Health Sciences, University of Texas Medical Branch, Galveston, Texas, for reviewing the chapter "Rehabilitation Challenges of People With Alzheimer's Disease."

The authors also extend special thanks and undying gratitude to Ms. Rashi Mehra for her editorial support throughout the development of this manuscript. Without her valuable input, this manuscript would never have reached its final stages.

Our special thanks to Ms. Sheri W. Sussman and the staff at Springer Publishing for their patience and support in bringing this book to completion.

1 Introduction

Over the next century, experts estimate that Alzheimer's disease will
be more prevalent than AIDS, cancer, and all cardiovascular diseases.
World Health Organization

In 1994, former President Ronald Reagan made a public announcement that touched the hearts of millions of Americans. The President and Mrs. Reagan, each of whom had already survived cancer, were up against their next challenge: "I have recently been told that I am one of the millions of Americans who will be afflicted with Alzheimer's disease," President Reagan said in a handwritten letter to the American people (Reagan, 1994). "Upon learning this news, Nancy and I had to decide whether, as private citizens, we would keep this a private matter or whether we would make this news known in a public way."

The President's announcement was a bold one. At the time, just over a decade ago, Alzheimer's disease (AD) was clouded in mystery—an alarming diagnosis that was best kept behind closed doors. Medical research on Alzheimer's had gained momentum, but the number of undiagnosed cases remained high. Reagan, who was an active partner of the Alzheimer's Association until he passed away in 2004, understood the value of shedding light on the disease: "In opening our hearts, we hope this might promote greater awareness of this condition. Perhaps it will encourage a clear understanding of the individuals and families who are affected by it."

President Reagan wasn't alone in his plight. In 1995, a year after he disclosed his diagnosis, an estimated 377,000 new cases of AD were reported in the United States (Hebert, Beckett, Scherr, & Evans, 2001). Alzheimer's disease afflicts 1 in 10 people over the age of 65 and nearly half of all people age 85 and over (Mintzer & Targum, 2003). People with Alzheimer's live an average of 8 years, although some live up to 20 years or more after the first onset of symptoms (Hingley, 1998). With an average lifetime cost-of-care per patient of $174,000, it is the third most expensive disease in America, following only heart disease and cancer (Ernst & Hay, 1994). Today, approximately 4.5 million Americans have the disease and are learning to live with its inevitable effects (Hebert, Scherr, Bienias, Bennett, & Evans, 2003)

UNDERSTANDING ALZHEIMER'S DISEASE

Alzheimer's disease, the most common cause of dementia, is a progressive, irreversible neurologic disorder that develops over a period of years. It is age related and is characterized by changes in behavior, personality, judgment, and the ability to perform usual activities. The classic triad for patients with AD is memory impairment, visuospatial defects, and language changes. These changes occur in the absence of confusion, mental retardation, or other neurologic disorders and represent a considerable decline from a patient's usual level of functioning.

The course of AD varies from person to person, as does the rate of decline. In most people with AD, symptoms first appear after age 65. The risk of developing AD increases with age, but AD and dementia symptoms are not a part of normal aging.

Normal Aging Versus Alzheimer's Disease

Alzheimer's disease is a complex illness that is still not completely understood by the medical world. As a result, many myths and misconceptions prevail about AD. It is not only laypeople but some physicians, too, who lack a proper understanding of this disease.

One thing is certain: AD causes dementia. Alzheimer's disease effects are gradual, resulting from the slow death of nerve cells in the brain that are vital for memory and other functions, such as speaking, comprehending, reading, abstract thinking, and calculating (Kuhn, 1999). Martin Rossor (2003) offered a simple way to understand the relationship between AD and dementia. Dementia is a syndrome that is associated with many different underlying diseases. "In a sense, it is similar to heartburn or headache, which is caused by many different things, and could require many different treatments," said Rossor. Alzheimer's disease is the most common cause of dementia.

Both AD and dementia are discussed in more detail in chapter 2. For now, it is important to understand that neither AD nor dementia is a natural process of aging.

To distinguish a person undergoing the natural aging process from one with AD, let's compare symptoms of each.

Scenario 1: Forgetfulness

Most elderly persons have occasional lapses in memory. But how can one differentiate symptoms of dementia from normal signs of aging? Consider this example: it is normal for people, as they get older, to forget things like where they put their glasses or where they last placed their keys, but, given a medical test on memory and thinking, they would most likely perform very well (Kuhn, 1999).

Changes in memory and mental ability with normal aging are quite mild and do not continue to get worse over time, nor should they interfere with a person's day-to-day functioning. Normal age-related changes consist primarily of slight changes in memory and learning and processing information a bit more slowly.

The key difference between dementia and what's happening with the "forgetful old man" is that dementia involves loss of memory functions and at least one other domain of cognitive impairment (i.e., language, thinking, or perception) (Rossor, 2003).

In contrast, patients with dementia suffer from worsening memory loss and demonstrate difficulty in other daily functions, which can appear as forgetfulness to an outside observer. People with AD may present the following symptoms:

- Confusion
- Difficulties with language (e.g., not being able to find the right words for things)
- Difficulty with concentration and reasoning

- Problems with complex tasks like paying bills or balancing a checkbook
- Problems with orientation or spatial ability (e.g., getting lost in a familiar place)

Often, it is the patient's family that speaks to the physician about a continuing decline of mental abilities, particularly problems remembering recent information, since patients with actual dementia may be unaware or at least do not complain of problems.

Scenario 2: Senility

Another incorrect belief equates AD with "madness" or senility. As AD progresses, the decline in cognition continues, and personality and behavioral symptoms are more likely to appear. These are a few symptoms of AD that an outside observer may mistake for senility:

- Increased anger, hostility, and/or suspicion
- Aggression and physical violence
- Hallucinations
- Delusions
- Wandering
- Increased number of physical accidents

Although some AD patients have abnormal behavioral symptoms, caregivers must understand that these are an integral part of the disease process. The patients are unable to control their behavior, and therefore, appropriate treatment is necessary.

Often, caregivers of the elderly assume that since old age cannot be reversed, it is futile to seek medical help when a loved one is demonstrating signs of "senility." Under no circumstances should such behavior be considered "madness." The fact is, AD is *not* "normal old age." Every elderly individual does not have nor will not have this disease. It is important to be aware of the signs and symptoms that may suggest this disease and to consult a qualified medical practitioner to assess the person professionally. Table 1.1 present differences between normal signs of aging and dementia.

We have also included several excellent sources for learning more about other brain disorders at the end of this book (see Additional Resources).

Table 1.1

DIFFERENCES BETWEEN NORMAL SIGNS OF AGING AND DEMENTIA

NORMAL	DEMENTIA

Early signs of Alzheimer's disease
Memory and concentration

NORMAL	DEMENTIA
■ Periodic minor memory lapses or forgetfulness of part of an experience. ■ Occasional lapses in attention or lapses in attention or concentration.	■ Misplacement of important items. ■ Confusion about how to perform simple tasks. ■ Trouble with simple arithmetic problems. ■ Difficulty making routine decisions. ■ Confusion about month or season.

Mood and behavior

NORMAL	DEMENTIA
■ Temporary sadness or anxiety based on appropriate and specific cause. ■ Changing interests. ■ Increasingly cautious behavior.	■ Unpredictable mood changes. ■ Increasing loss of outside interests. ■ Depression, anger, or confusion in response to change. ■ Denial of symptoms.

Later signs of Alzheimer's disease
Language and speech

NORMAL	DEMENTIA
■ Unimpaired language skills.	■ Difficulty completing sentences or finding the right words. ■ Inability to understand the meaning of words. ■ Reduced and/or irrelevant conversation.

Movement coordination

NORMAL	DEMENTIA
■ Increasing caution in movement. ■ Slower reaction times.	■ Visibly impaired movement or coordination, including slowing of movements, halting gait, and reduced sense of balance.

Other symptoms

NORMAL	DEMENTIA
■ Normal sense of smell. No abnormal weight changes in either men or women.	■ Impaired sense of smell. Severe weight loss, particularly in female patients.

Source (Most Data): Alzheimer's Disease: Early Warning Signs and Diagnostic Resources, by The Junior League of New York City, 1988. Retrieved April 2007, from http://www.searo.who.int/en/Section1174/Section1199/Section1567/Section1823_8057.htm

Alzheimer's Disease: A Silent Disease

Since AD and dementia are so intertwined, the perception of a person with Alzheimer's tends to be distorted. It is a common belief that everyone with AD suffers from severe loss of orientation and is unable to function on his own—but these characteristics are associated with the disease's later stages. The truth is that most people with AD have a mild form of the disease and usually die from another ailment before it progresses to more advanced stages. The subtlety of the disease is yet another reason it is often overlooked and misdiagnosed as old age.

There is no doubt that, at its worst, AD can forever alter the lives of those affected. People with Alzheimer's who do survive to the disease's later stages require constant supervision, which often places tremendous emotional and financial stress on the loved ones who must care for them. Watching a parent or spouse lose his or her independence is already a painful experience, but adjusting to a new role as caregiver can be equally taxing.

It is important to know the simple truths behind AD. Currently there is no cure, but a diagnosis is certainly not the end. Dr. David A. Bennett (1999), Director of Rush Alzheimer's Disease Center, puts it best: "You do not wake up in the morning with Alzheimer's disease, as would be the case with a stroke or heart attack. Alzheimer's is an insidious disease." Since the disease emerges gradually, people can take steps to prepare themselves and their families for the challenges that lie ahead.

The Race Against Time

Perhaps it is fear that keeps many heads turned away when the topic of AD arises. But no one should remain blind to the staggering facts: AD is a universal threat. It is predicted that by 2020, 30 million people in the world will be affected by the disease and that by the year 2050 the number could increase to 45 million around the world (Rishton, 2005). Right now in the United States alone, one in every three families is affected by AD (American Health Assistance Foundation, 2006). Without a cure, the chance that a person will have to deal with the condition is only increasing as time goes on. Figure 1.1 demonstrates the dramatic increase in the number of new AD cases that is expected up to the year 2050.

Where is this sharp increase coming from? Many believe it is a combination of two key trends. First is the aging of the baby boom

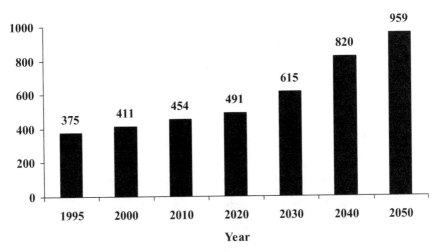

Figure 1.1 Projected increase in new Alzheimer's disease cases through 2050 (number in thousands).
Source: "Annual Incidence of Alzheimer's Disease in the United States Projected to the Years 2000 through 2050," by L. E. Hebert, P. A. Scherr, L. A. Beckett, and D. A. Evans, 2001, *Alzheimer Disease and Associated Disorder, 15*(4), pp. 169–173. Reprinted with permission from Lippincott Williams & Wilkins.

generation—the 77 million Americans born between 1946 and 1964 who make up approximately 28.6% of the U.S. population (Metlife Mature Market Institute, 2005). The baby boomers have reached or are close to reaching their 60s, and this "age wave" has been a hot topic of discussion among policymakers in the employment and health care sectors. Second is the advancement of medicine. The likelihood that an American who reaches the age of 65 will survive to the age of 90 has nearly doubled over the past 40 years—from just 14% of 65-year-olds in 1960 to 25% as of this writing, in 2008. By 2050, 40% of 65-year-olds are likely to reach age 90 (Civic Ventures, 2006). While these trends should give us reason to celebrate, they also give rise to some major concerns, especially in the context of AD. The *Journal of the American Medical Association* (Table 1.2) presents estimated prevalence of Americans diagnosed with AD.

What this means is that the "age wave" is a double-edged sword. As more Americans survive well after their 60s, their chances of developing AD continually increase. It is predicted that 14 million Americans may have AD by the year 2050, and if this trend continues, one out of every two baby boomers may develop Alzheimer's as they reach their senior years (American Health Assistance Foundation, 2006). Figure 1.2 and Figure 1.3 demonstrate the significance of this trend.

Table 1.2

ESTIMATED PREVALENCE OF AMERICANS DIAGNOSED WITH ALZHEIMER'S DISEASE

AGE GROUP	ESTIMATED PREVALENCE
65–74	3.0%
75–85	18.7%
85+	47.2%

Data Source: "Prevalence of Alzheimer's Disease in a Community Population of Older Persons: Higher Than Previously Reported," by D. A. Evans et al., 1989, *Journal of the American Medical Association, 262,* pp. 2551–2556.

All of these statistics point to one thing: we are looking at a time crunch when it comes to finding a cure for AD. People in their 50s are the fastest growing population segment; every 7 seconds, someone in America turns 50 (Solovitch, 2008). This race against time is real. In the words of Daniel Kuhn (1999), "Alzheimer's disease may well become the most pressing health problem of the baby boomers and their offspring."

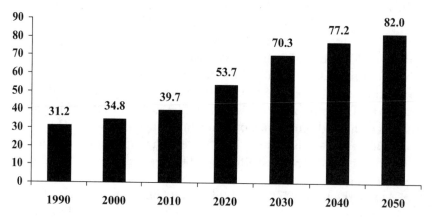

Figure 1.2 U.S. population 65 and older: 1990–2050 (number in millions).
Source: Methodology and Assumptions for the Population Projections of the United States: 1999 to 2100, by U.S. Census Bureau, Department of Commerce, January 13, 2000, Washington, D.C.

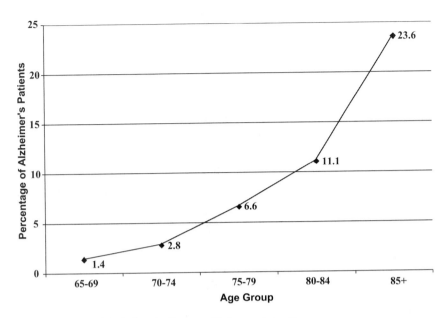

Figure 1.3 Risk of Alzheimer's disease with increasing age.
Source: "The Prevalence of Dementia," Alzheimer's Disease International, Factsheet 3, April 1999. Reprinted with permission from Alzheimer's Disease International.

The financial cost of AD is already a cause for concern. Not only do people with AD have to pay out of pocket for long-term care and prescription drugs, but Medicare covers the cost of basic health care for them and their caregivers, who often suffer from more health problems than their peers (Charity Wire, 2004). Presently, the national direct and indirect costs of caring for individuals with AD are at least $100 billion (Ernest & Hays, 1994). American businesses are losing $61 billion every year, $24.6 of which covers AD health care and $36.5 billion of which covers costs related to caregivers due to lost productivity, absenteeism, and worker replacement (Koppel, 2002).

Stephen McConnell, Vice President of the Alzheimer's Association, has said, "This imminent epidemic of Alzheimer's disease threatens to bankrupt Medicare and Medicaid." McConnell's concern was based on a study prepared by the Lewin Group, which predicted that the Medicare costs of AD treatment will soar from $31.9 billion in year 2000 to $49.3 billion in 2010 (Tarapchak, 1998). As scary as these numbers are, they can also help us measure the impact of increased funding for Alzheimer's research.

Research and Funding Can Make Difference

Without medical and social advancements, AD will become an enormous public health problem. Medical interventions that could delay disease onset even modestly would have a major public health impact.

According to McConnell (Tarapchak, 1998), if every person with AD could delay nursing home placement by just 1 month, it would save the nation $1 billion a year. "By delaying the onset of AD for even 5 years, we can keep half of the baby boomers who are now at risk from even suffering the devastating effects of the disease," said McConnell.

Researchers (Brookmeyer, Gray, & Kawas, 1998) have reported that if interventions could delay onset of the disease by 2 years, after 50 years there would be nearly 2 million fewer cases than projected; if onset could be delayed by 1 year, there would be nearly 800,000 fewer prevalent cases (Figure 1.4). If onset could be delayed by 5 years, it would decrease prevalence in 2050 by nearly 44%. Even a 6-month delay would reduce prevalence in 2050 by 6%.

As these projections indicate, the impact of AD research is tremendous because every bit of new knowledge is a milestone. Since 1982, the Alzheimer's Association has been the largest private funder, awarding $150 million in research grants in the hope of learning more about the disease. As more people have come forward to advocate support of

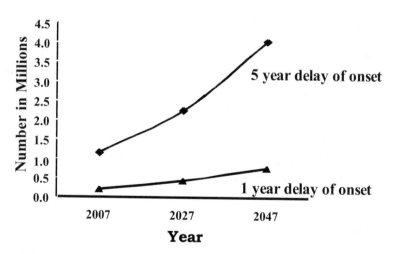

Figure 1.4 Potential impact of interventions to delay Alzheimer's disease onset.
Data Source: "Projections of Alzheimer's Disease in the United States and the Public Health Impact of Delaying Disease Onset," by R. Brookmeyer, S. Gray, and C. Kawas, 1998, *American Journal of Public Health, 88*, pp. 1337–1342.

Alzheimer's research, more dollars have been allocated to discover its causes, best treatment, and an eventual cure. In 2003, the federal government reported spending $640 million on AD research—quite a jump from the 12 grants that were awarded in 1975, which totaled $700,000 (Coste, 2004). Progress is clearly being made on all fronts when it comes to slowing down the effects of AD.

Knowledge Is Power

Scientists have made significant progress in terms of prevention, diagnosis, and treatment of AD. Many new medications have been released to mitigate some symptoms of AD, and many others are still pending approval. Here are just a few examples of the new research areas on AD (note that findings are under development and have not been conclusive as of yet):

- The National Institute on Aging (2002) announced that people with AD often have low amounts of folic acid, so adjusting the diet to include more folic acid might be a first step in prevention.
- Researchers at Case Western Reserve University (2000) found that people who were less active were three times more likely to have AD than people who were more active.
- Studies done at the Salk Institute (2002) showed that neurogenesis—the creation of neurons—is possible in humans. If scientists could restore neurons lost to AD, reversing the disease could be possible.

With continued research, it is possible that one day Alzheimer's will no longer be a threat to our future. A cure for AD, or a treatment that will slow down its progression, might be just around the corner.

Education is essential. The more we all understand AD, the better able we'll be to provide proper care and treatment and ultimately improve life for everyone affected by AD.

WHAT THIS BOOK CAN OFFER

Even though there are resources available for those living with AD, the extensive research being conducted in the field makes it difficult for clinicians and caregivers to stay abreast of new developments, which is where this book comes in.

This book is written to act as an up-to-date resource for those clinicians and caregivers who are involved in the care of people affected by AD and dementia, either directly or indirectly. Particular attention has been paid to the rehabilitation aspect of management for this challenging population.

There are many books and articles that have been written to raise public awareness and share personal experiences of people living with AD. This book is a compilation of facts from these excellent guides, which we hope will reinforce awareness and shed light on new advancements that might not be familiar to many people. This book will also help caregivers and family members who take care of patients with AD and dementia at home or in long-term-care facilities.

All that we know about AD is not being practiced. There are "tools of the trained"—caregiving and diagnostic tools—that have been proven to help arrest AD. We hope this book, which is based on these tools and on the newest developments in Alzheimer's research, can serve as the first complete resource for clinicians and caregivers.

The Underlying Philosophy: Diagnosis and Treatment Tools

Care of people with AD is a challenging task but—according to medical organizations that met in 2002 to discuss strengths and potential pitfalls in the diagnosis and treatment of AD—treatment can be improved. The foundation of this book is composed of key principles that have been agreed upon by clinicians, researchers, and medical organizations that provide services to Alzheimer's patients and their families.

Seven organizations—the American Academy of Neurology, the Alzheimer's Association, the American Medical Association, the American Association of Geriatric Psychiatry, the American Geriatric Society, the American Medical Directors Association, and the World Federation of Neurology—determined that more than two dozen practice guidelines exist to provide guidance to clinicians, yet many caregivers may not be taking advantage of the guidelines available. The following important principles in caring for people with AD were emphasized:

1 **Our Alzheimer's I.Q.**
   Alzheimer's disease is recognizable and can be differentiated from normal aging by clinicians.

2 First Family First

Symptoms are usually first identified by family members and should be reported to the family physician.

3 Alzheimer's Accuracy

Alzheimer's can be diagnosed with 95% accuracy, the same as appendicitis.

4 Elder Care Full

Effective care options exist and can improve the quality of life for patients and their caregivers.

5 From These Resources Come Unity

Resources exist in the community for people with dementia and their caregivers and are important elements to quality care.

According to Catherine Rydell (2002) of the American Academy of Neurology, "Clinicians may make a difference in the quality of life of patients with AD if they follow guideline recommendations." But the first step in making a difference is to inform the public, especially the clinicians who care for people with AD, about these guidelines.

We are optimistic about the future of those who may face and are already facing AD. We believe that adhering to the five basic principles just stated can improve the life of those living with AD. And here's what we consider the best part yet: research findings suggest that it is never too late to get started.

How to Use This Book

In order to understand the changes that take place in a person with AD, a solid understanding of the biological processes that cause the disease is essential. Chapter 2 explains different types of dementia, including AD, and chapter 3 details the medical causes and risk factors for AD, while providing some historical background on how the disease was discovered and where we are currently in terms of understanding AD. Chapter 4 highlights definite symptoms of AD. Chapter 5 outlines new methods of diagnosis. Chapter 6 relays the progression of AD to give an idea of what to expect once a diagnosis has been made, and chapter 7 discusses prevention and treatments, both those that are available and those whose approval is pending. The final four chapters offer a step-by-step guide to caring for persons with Alzheimer's. To conclude, we offer a list of resources to tap into that can facilitate readers efforts and increase their knowledge of Alzheimer's.

This book offers direction based on our understanding and experience as health care providers and on the experiences of other physicians and caregivers who work with people with AD. But from time to time, people will need to consult competent professionals for specific advice about medical, legal, and financial matters. Also remember that a local Alzheimer's Association chapter or area agency on aging should be able to offer a referral to professionals with a proven track record.

Our hope is that people will use this book as a reliable resource as they care for a patient or a loved one. AD has many challenges, but, with a positive outlook and the tools advanced in this book, there is promise of a brighter future.

2 Dementia Syndrome

An estimated 25–29 million people in the world suffer from dementia…vascular dementia and Alzheimer's disease constitutes the vast majority of cases.

World Health Organization

WHAT IS DEMENTIA?

Dementia is a disorder that is characterized by impairment of memory and at least one other cognitive domain (i.e., aphasia, apraxia, agnosia, executive function). According to the *Diagnostic and Statistical Manual of Mental Disorders (DSM–IV)*, diagnosis of dementia is made when a patient presents with a decline from a previous level of functioning that is severe enough to interfere with daily function and independence (American Psychiatric Association, 1994). In Latin, *dementia* means irrationality. In a sense, this is true—people with dementia exhibit emotional and behavioral problems, which include depression, anxiety, hallucinations, paranoia, and inappropriate social behaviors, such as cursing, wandering, hoarding items, and experiencing disrupted sleep patterns. On a cognitive level, people affected by dementia have difficulty with decision making, judgment, memory, spatial orientation, thinking, reasoning, and verbal communication. Dementia is a disruption in the way the brain works and is reflected by memory loss and the inability to perform daily activities.

Sometimes older people have emotional problems that can be mistaken for dementia. As people age and face retirement or cope with the death of a family member or a peer, it is common for them to feel sad, lonely, worried, or bored. These changes can leave some individuals feeling confused or forgetful. Emotional problems of this nature can be relieved by supportive friends and family or by professional help from a physician or counselor. It is imperative that anyone suffering from memory loss or other impairments in functioning undergoes a thorough medical and clinical evaluation to identify any treatable conditions. This way, if a diagnosis of dementia is confirmed, both the individual and his or her family can take the next steps to prepare for proper treatment.

How often is a diagnosis of dementia positive? The U.S. Congress Office of Technology Assessment (1990) estimates that 1.8 million Americans have severe dementia and another 1 to 5 million Americans have mild to moderate dementia. Dementia occurs predominantly in the second half of a person's life. As the life span of individuals continues to increase, so does the probability that they will suffer from dementia. The frequency of dementia rises with age. Of all persons over age 65, 5%–8% are demented (Brynes, 2007). This percentage increases considerably with age. Of people over age 85, 25%–50% are affected (Table 2.1). Every third person over 90 years of age suffers from moderate to severe dementia (Bickel, 1996).

Table 2.1

PREVALENCE OF DEMENTIA IN DIFFERENT AGE GROUPS

AGE	PREVALENCE
65+	5%–8%
75+	15%–20%
85+	25%–50%

Data Source: American Psychiatric Association Practice Guidelines for the Treatment of Psychiatric Disorders: Compendium 2006, by American Psychiatric Association, 2006, Arlington, VA: American Psychiatric Publishing.

People with dementia lose their abilities at different rates, depending on what lies at the root of the disorder. Some conditions that cause dementia can be reversed—such as high fever, dehydration, vitamin deficiency and poor nutrition, bad reactions to medicines, problems with the thyroid gland, or a minor head injury. The degree of a dementia's reversibility often depends on how quickly the underlying cause is treated.

Irreversible dementia, on the other hand, is incurable. Alzheimer's disease (AD) is the most common form of irreversible dementia, but there are more than 100 other conditions that lead to dementia as well. This chapter identifies the most common types of dementia and discusses diagnosis and treatment options.

The Many Faces of Neurodegenerative Dementias

It isn't unusual for most people to use the terms "dementia" and "Alzheimer's disease" interchangeably. According to Martin Rossor (2003), AD has dominated our thinking about neurodegenerative disorders. But AD is just one type of dementia. Dementia involves the widespread impairment of cognitive function. It is expressed when an individual demonstrates—in different combinations—impairment in memory of events; memory and understanding of facts, language, thinking, and reasoning; and perception of the world. To differentiate among the types of dementia, one must understand what part of the brain has been affected. A quick review of the brain's anatomy will refresh the idea that cognitive function in the brain is modular, with particular areas of the cerebral cortex (i.e., the outside layer of the brain) specializing in particular functions. Currently, the only way to observe these changes—without a postmortem examination—is to examine an individual's loss of cognitive and motor abilities. Figure 2.1 shows the different parts of the human brain and is followed by Table 2.2, highlighting the key parts of the brain and their functions.

Mild Cognitive Impairment

While a gradual decline in cognition is a characteristic of normal aging, there is increasing evidence that some forms of cognitive impairment are recognizable as an early manifestation of dementia. Mild cognitive impairment (MCI) has long been recognized as a transition stage between normal cognition and dementia. MCI can affect many areas of cognition, such as memory, language, attention, reasoning, judgment, reading, and

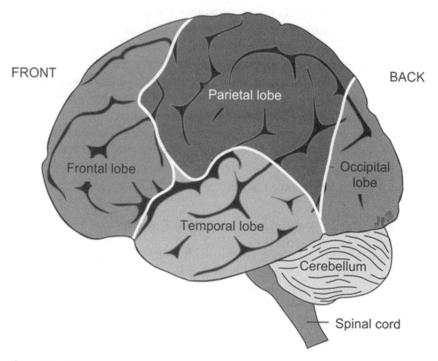

Figure 2.1 Different parts of the human brain.

writing, but those afflicted by it do not show other symptoms of dementia, such as impaired judgment or reasoning.

A number of criteria have been proposed to differentiate MCI from changes that come along with normal aging. The Mayo criteria are the ones most commonly applied (Petersen, Stevens, Ganguli, Tangalos, Cummings, et al., 2001) and include:

- Memory complaint, preferably corroborated by an informant
- Objective memory impairment (for age and education)
- Preserved general cognitive function
- Intact activities of daily living
- Not demented

There are two categories of MCI: amnestic and nonamnestic. Memory is the dominant problem in amnestic MCI and has been linked to Alzheimer's disease. Approximately 10%–15% of amnestic MCI converts to AD (Petersen, Stevens, et al., 2001). In nonamnestic MCI, memory

Table 2.2

COMMON PARTS OF THE BRAIN AND EACH OF THEIR FUNCTIONS

PART OF BRAIN	LOCATION	FUNCTION
Cerebellum	Located at the back.	Coordinates movement such as balance and muscle coordination.
Frontal lobe	Front part of the brain.	Involved in planning, organizing, problem solving, selective attention, personality, and a variety of higher cognitive functions, including behavior and emotions.
Temporal lobe	There are two temporal lobes, one on each side of the brain, located at about the level of the ears.	Responsible for differentiation of one smell from another and one sound from another. Also help in sorting new information and are believed to be responsible for short-term memory. Right lobe mainly involved in visual memory, while left lobe mainly involved in verbal memory.
Occipital lobe	Region in the back of the brain.	Mainly responsible for visual reception. Also contains association areas that help in the visual recognition of shapes and colors.
Parietal lobes	One of the two parietal lobes of the brain located behind the frontal lobe at the top of the brain.	Contain the primary sensory cortex, which controls sensation such as touch, pressure. Behind the primary sensory cortex is a large association area that controls fine sensation, such as judgment of texture, weight, size, shape. Right lobe important for sense of direction. Left lobe important for understanding spoken and/or written language.
Brain stem (pons and medulla oblongata)	The lower extension of the brain where it connects to the spinal cord.	Necessary for survival; controls functions such as breathing, digestion, heart rate, blood pressure, and arousal, that is, being awake and alert.

problems are not as predominant but include general impairments of cognition, such as impairments in language, visuospatial awareness, and attention. Also, the underlying causes of these impairments seem to be vascular, psychiatric, or neurologic. These patients convert to AD less often (2%) than those with amnestic MCI (University of California Davis, 2007). Nonamnestic MCI may progress to other types of syndromes, such as frontotemporal dementia, primary progressive aphasia, or dementia with Lewy bodies. But some people with MCI don't go on to develop any type of dementia. Some remain stable, while others even revert to normal.

For either subtype of MCI, there may be more than one underlying cause. The various causes generally are grouped into one of the following categories:

- *Neurodegenerative*—a disorder that gradually destroys brain cells (e.g., Alzheimer's disease, dementia with Lewy bodies, frontotemporal dementia)
- *Vascular*—a disorder that affects the blood vessels of the brain and the supply of oxygen and nutrients vital to brain cells, causing cell damage and death (vascular cognitive impairment)
- *Psychiatric*—certain psychiatric conditions that affect memory, concentration, and mood (e.g., depression)
- *Trauma*—physical injury to the brain that also may lead to cognitive difficulties; the potential cause is usually obvious (e.g., a history of severe head trauma)

When MCI progresses, memory problems become more noticeable. Family and friends may begin to notice signs, such as repeating the same question over and over again; retelling the same stories or providing the same information repeatedly; lacking initiative in beginning or completing activities; having trouble managing number-related tasks (e.g., bill paying); lacking focus during conversations and activities; and being unable to follow multistep directions.

It is difficult to make a diagnosis of MCI. First, not everyone exhibits all of the signs and symptoms of MCI. Second, other health issues may contribute to changes in memory. As a result, there is no established approach to diagnose MCI. A diagnosis of MCI is based on the results of a full diagnostic evaluation that includes neurological examinations, neuropsychological and psychiatric evaluations (to rule out depression and other emotional-health concerns), a physical examination including laboratory tests, and a review of the patient's past medical history and current medications. The evaluation is complemented by clinical observations of the patient's symptoms and their onset (i.e., sudden or gradual presentation, rate of progression) over time. Another valuable tool used to diagnose MCI is a memory test, which includes testing language skills, recall, attention span, and visual-spatial abilities. Depending on the results of this evaluation, further testing may be necessary, including bloodwork and brain imaging. This evaluation is similar to that given to individuals with more severe memory problems and is directed toward better defining the problem and looking for medical conditions that might have an effect on the brain.

Figure 2.2 provides a flow chart that could guide the classification process in a diagnostic setting. As the figure demonstrates, diagnosis can occur in stages:

Stage 1: The patient—or another individual with knowledge about the patient—expresses some concern about the patient's cognitive functioning.

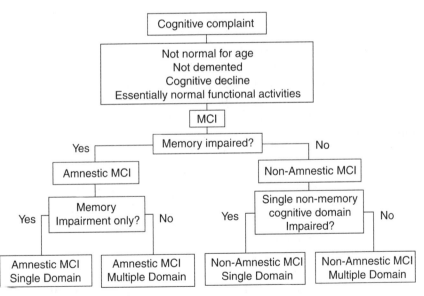

Figure 2.2 Decision process for making diagnosis of subtypes of mild cognitive impairment.
Source: "Mild Cognitive Impairment as a Diagnostic Entity," by R. C. Petersen, 2004, *Journal of Internal Medicine, 256,* pp. 183–194. Reprinted with permission from Blackwell Publishing.

Stage 2: The clinician determines whether the person is normal or demented, then assesses if a decline in function has occurred through a careful history obtained from the patient and preferably a collateral source.

Stage 3: If there is evidence of a decline in cognition, the clinician must determine if this change in cognition constitutes a significant impairment in functional activities such that the person might be considered as having a very mild dementia. But, if the functional impairment is not significant, the clinician may entertain the diagnosis of MCI, and the next task is to identify the clinical subtype.

Stage 4: The clinician should assess memory more carefully, perhaps with a word list learning procedure or paragraph recall. There are no generally accepted instruments for this determination, though neuropsychological testing may be useful.

Most patients diagnosed with MCI remain stable. It is currently estimated that people with MCI have a risk of developing dementia three to five times greater than that faced by others their age (DeCarli, 2003). Aging is a primary predictor of progression of MCI to AD. MCI is relatively unlikely to represent a predementia condition in patients less than 50 years old. But, with every year of age increase, MCI is slightly more likely to convert to AD. MCI does not always lead to dementia and can take many years to do so. In most cases, a person diagnosed with MCI will not undergo any medical treatment but will be regularly monitored for changes in memory. Counseling may assist people with MCI to find ways to adjust to the changes they are experiencing and to learn about ways to compensate for their memory difficulties.

There is no current treatment for MCI that has been sufficiently substantiated to have obtained FDA approval. Although there is no specific cure, several approaches using medication and nonmedication techniques can be useful for treating MCI. A number of psychoactive medications are used to achieve these goals. The only FDA-approved medications for dementia or cognitive impairment are the cholinesterase inhibitors, memantine, and the combination of ergoloid mesylates (approved for nonspecific cognitive decline). In addition, other drugs, including vitamin E, ginkgo biloba, and selegiline, are occasionally used for this purpose in selected patients, although they are not generally recommended, because their efficacy and safety are uncertain (APA Practice Guidelines, 2007). Researchers have discovered that donepezil (Aricept) may delay the onset of AD in people diagnosed with Amnestic MCI. Medications such as nonsteroidal anti-inflammatory drugs (NSAIDs) may reduce inflammation in the brain and might help slow the progression of AD (Veld, 2001). It is also critical for patients with MCI and their families to be educated and informed about MCI and the risk of AD.

Dementia

Dementia is an acquired, progressive decline in cognitive function due to damage or disease in the brain beyond what might be expected from normal aging. A typical early sign is impairment in recent memory, with the progression of memory disorder. Other aspects of cognitive deficits such as disorientation, anomia, aphasia, and acalculia may develop. Dementia is a nonspecific term that encompasses many disease processes, just as fever is attributable to many etiologies.

Symptoms of dementia can be classified as either reversible or irreversible depending upon the etiology of the disease, although dementia, by definition, is irreversible and will eventually result in death. Probably fewer than 10% of all dementias are reversible (Adelman & Daly, 2005).

Different degenerative diseases that cause the dementia syndrome tend to affect different areas of the cerebral cortex. Whether or not dementia can be treated (i.e., is reversible) depends on whether the deficits are localized in the brain or widespread.

Patients with a discrete abnormality, such as a loss of language or dysphasia, would—by implication—have focal, or localized, damage to the cerebral cortex. If the dysphasia occurred suddenly, it would most likely be at the onset of a stroke. In dementia, the onset of dysphagia is gradual and is more commonly a manifestation of late-stage dementia. A patient with widespread deficits would likely have a disease like AD, which diffusely affects the cerebral cortex, meaning that the damage is irreversible. The first purpose of a thorough medical evaluation is to distinguish between reversible and irreversible forms of brain failure.

Because of the complexity of the brain, neurodegenerative diseases manifest themselves in behaviors and impairments that overlap each other. Patients with dementia usually have multiple medical comorbidities. The costs of managing medical comorbidities in patients with dementia are usually higher than those for individuals without dementia (when age, gender, and specific disease conditions are controlled). Much of this is attributed to higher utilization of inpatient, home health, and short-stay skilled nursing facility services. Hill and associates (2002)

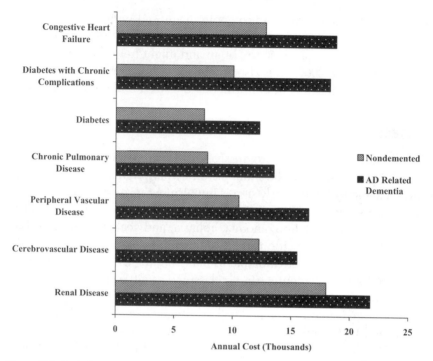

Figure 2.3 Costs for patients with both Alzheimer's disease and comorbid diseases versus patients with no dementia.
Source: "Alzheimer's Disease and Related Dementias Increase Costs of Comorbidities in Managed Medicare," by J. W. Hill et al., 2002, *Neurology, 58,* pp. 62–70. Reprinted with permission from Lippincott, Williams & Wilkins.

reported substantially higher costs for patients with both AD and comorbid diseases than for patients with no dementia (Figure 2.3).

TYPES OF DEMENTIA

The more scientists understand the similarities and differences among neurodegenerative diseases, the more patients, families, and caregivers will benefit. Let's take a look at the most common types of dementia, their diagnosis, and their treatment.

The major dementia syndromes include:

- Alzheimer's disease (AD)
- Multi-infarct dementia (MID)
- Dementia with Lewy bodies (DLB)

- Parkinson's disease dementia (PDD)
- Frontotemporal dementia (FTD)

Alzheimer's Disease

Alzheimer's disease is the most common dementia, accounting for the majority of the cases in the elderly. Alzheimer's disease accounts for 50%–75% of all cases of dementia in persons age 65 and older (Holland, 1999). It results in memory loss, personality changes, global cognitive dysfunction, and functional impairments. Loss of short-term memory is most prominent during the early stages of the disease. In the late stages, patients are totally dependent upon others for basic activities of daily living, such as feeding and toileting.

It is likely that AD was around hundreds of years ago, but its symptoms were mistaken for those of other illnesses. It was generally accepted that as people aged, they would inevitably lose their mental abilities. If an individual did demonstrate features that we now associate with AD, it was assumed that insanity, senility, or a hardening of the arteries was at the root of the problem. Early scientists did not have extensive knowledge of brain disorders since examinations of the brain could be conducted only after death.

It wasn't until 1907 that the German physician Alois Alzheimer offered a scientific explanation, which suggested that mental decline in the elderly was not a natural process, nor was it senile dementia. Arnold Pick, a physician in Prague, recruited Alzheimer to examine the brain of two patients, each of whom had suffered from prominent behavioral and language impairments. Alzheimer's key instrument was the microscope, with which he was able to identify and differentiate biological causes of dementia. Alzheimer confirmed the presence of abnormal inclusions—now known as Pick bodies—which were deposits of the tau protein. The discovery of abnormal protein deposits as related to brain disorders was a pivotal moment in medical history. The more scientists study abnormal protein functioning in the brain, the closer we get to pinpoint the exact cause of AD.

To understand AD from a biological perspective, scientists focus on the proteins associated with amyloid plaques and neurofibrillary tangles. The following sections present a description of the biological processes believed to cause Alzheimer's. The exact cause of AD is unknown. In fact, there is probably not one single cause, but a number of factors that come together in certain people to cause the disease. Chapter 3 presents causes of AD in detail.

Amyloid Hypothesis

According to the amyloid hypothesis, accumulation of beta-amyloid protein in areas of the brain related to memory is the primary influence driving AD pathogenesis (Figure 2.4). This results in production, aggregation, and deposition of the toxic amyloid beta peptide, which leads to disruption of cell-to-cell communication and eventually the death of neurons in the brain. The amyloid hypothesis remains the predominant scientific explanation for the cause of AD and is the culmination of more than a decade of scientific research from around the world.

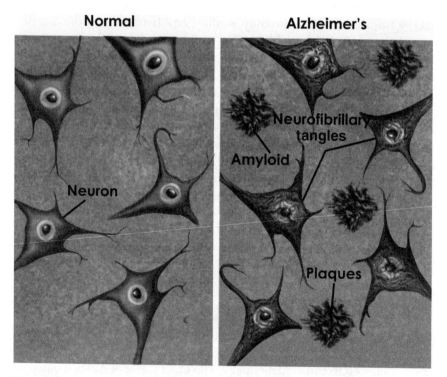

Figure 2.4 Deposition of the toxic amyloid beta peptide in Alzheimer's patients.

Tau Hypothesis

In addition to amyloid plaques, the second most pathological hallmark of AD is the tau protein. Tau is a cytoskeletal protein that binds and stabilizes microtubules (MTs), thereby maintaining the network of MTs that are essential for axonal transport in neurons. In AD, tau deforms and loses its ability to support the cell, eventually aggregating into neurofibrillary tangles (Figure 2.5). The Tau hypothesis suggests that these events culminate in neuronal dysfunction and degeneration, leading to the onset of AD.

Experts have documented the progression of symptoms associated with AD and developed several methods of identifying stages of AD. Staging systems provide useful frames of reference for understanding how the disease may unfold and for making future plans.

One lens that scientists use to define the stages of Alzheimer's identifies three general stages of the disease. What follows is a breakdown of

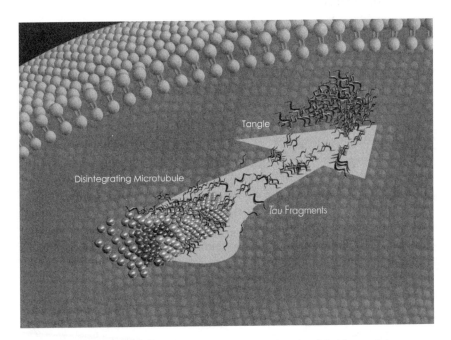

Figure 2.5 Intraneuronal accumulation of abnormally phosphorylated tau protein (neurofibrillary change).
Source: "2005–2006 Progress Report on Alzheimer's Disease," by National Institute on Aging, 2007d, NIH Publication Number 06-6047.

the early, middle, and late stages as defined by Reisberg, Ferris, deLeon, and Crook (1982):

1. Early Stage

A person in this stage is usually aware of the diagnosis and can participate in decisions affecting future care. Symptoms can include mild forgetfulness and communication difficulties, such as finding the right word and following a conversation. An individual may have difficulty learning new things and concentrating or may have a limited attention span. Some people stay involved in activities, while others become passive or withdrawn. The individual may also be frustrated by changing abilities and may become depressed or anxious. It is important to monitor the emotional well-being of the person. The individual may withdraw from usual activities and may become restless. Furthermore, the individual may also exhibit mild coordination problems.

2. Middle Stage

This stage brings a further decline in the person's mental and physical abilities. Memory continues to deteriorate as the person forgets his or her personal history and no longer recognizes family and friends. Increased confusion and disorientation to time and place result in requiring assistance in many daily tasks, such as dressing, bathing, and using the toilet. The person shows signs of mood shift and anger, as well as hostility. In response to the loss of abilities, a person may react in a number of ways. For example, he or she may become less involved in activities or repeat the same action or word over and over again. Some people become restless and pace or wander in this stage. Furthermore, the individual may have disrupted sleep patterns and may also experience language difficulties and visual spatial problems. It can be helpful to understand more about the disease and develop strategies to deal with these situations. The local Alzheimer's Society can provide education, resources, and support. Registering the person with the Safely Home, the Alzheimer Wandering Registry program, will provide peace of mind should the person become lost.

3. Late Stage

In this last stage, the person becomes unable to remember, communicate, or look after herself. There are significant behavioral changes, such as crying and groaning. The nonverbal methods of communications are lost. The individual sleeps longer and more often. Care is required 24 hours a day. Eventually, the person becomes bedridden, loses the ability to speak, has difficulty eating or swallowing, and loses control of bodily functions. Weight lose is a very common problem. This stage eventually ends with the person's death, often from secondary complications such as pneumonia.

Alzheimer's disease is a progressive disease, increasing in severity over time. The disease affects all races and ethnic groups. It seems to affect more women than men. Alzheimer's disease is considered a major public health problem. The cost of caring for people with AD is estimated at more than $100 billion per year in the United States. The average yearly cost per affected person is $20,000–$40,000, depending on the severity of the disease (eMedicineHealth, 2005a). This cost does not take into account the loss of quality of life for the affected person or the physical and emotional toll on family caregivers. Furthermore, AD is the fourth most common cause of death among older adults, particularly among women (Alzheimer's Association, 2008). People with AD live an average of 8 years after diagnosis but may survive anywhere from 3 to 20 years (Administration on Aging, 2007). The primary cause of death is intercurrent illness, such as pneumonia.

Diagnosis of AD is usually a clinical diagnosis, which is considered to be reasonably accurate. Laboratory tests cannot be solely relied upon to confirm the presence of the disorder and are mainly used to compliment a clinical diagnosis. Chapter 5 presents diagnosis of AD in detail. Typically, diagnosis of AD includes recording the patient's medical history, using an interview or questionnaire to identify past medical problems, difficulties in daily activities, and prescription drug use, among other things. The physician may wish to speak to a close family member who can supplement information. A physical examination follows and includes evaluations of hearing and sight, as well as blood pressure and pulse readings. Standard laboratory tests include blood and urine tests to measure blood count, thyroid and liver function, and levels of glucose and other blood-based indicators of illness, which can eliminate other possible conditions. A depression screening may also be conducted. Further testing includes neuropsychological testing using a variety of tools to assess memory, problem-solving ability, attention, vision-motor coordination, and abstract thinking (e.g., the ability to perform simple calculations in one's head). Finally, a "structural" brain scan such as a CAT scan (CT) or magnetic resonance imaging (MRI) may be recommended to rule out brain tumors or blood clots in the brain as the reason for symptoms. Many scientists are trying to determine if other brain-imaging techniques might be able to identify telltale signs of early Alzheimer's reliably enough to be used as diagnostic tools.

According to the National Institute on Aging (Alzheimer's Disease Education and Referral Center, 2007), no treatment has been proven to stop AD. Cases show, however, that taking the drugs donepezil, rivastigmine, or galantamine may help prevent some symptoms from becoming worse for a limited time in patients in the early and middle stages of the disease. The FDA recently approved the use of donepezil to treat moderate to severe AD. Memantine has been approved to treat moderate to severe AD, although it is limited in its effects. Some medicines may help control behavioral symptoms of AD such as sleeplessness, agitation, wandering, anxiety, and depression. Treating these symptoms often makes patients more comfortable and makes their care easier for caregivers. Chapter 7 presents details of medical and nonmedical management of AD.

Multi-Infarct Dementia

While it was once believed that a loss of blood supply to the brain was the main cause of dementia, it is now proven that blood flow reduction is a result, rather than a cause, of dementia. What can lead to dementia is death of brain tissue, which can occur either by a series of large or small strokes or by Binswanger's disease, a disease of the small arteries that carry blood from the heart to central parts of the brain. This type of dementia is referred to as multi-infarct dementia (MID), or vascular dementia. Multi-infarct dementia is the second most common form of dementia after AD. Approximately 10%–20% of people in the United States over age 65 who are experiencing dementia have MID (National Institute on Aging, Alzheimer's Disease Education and Referral Center, 2007). It usually affects people between the ages of 60 and 75 and is more likely to occur in men than women. In the United States, individuals of African descent have a higher incidence of MID than Whites.

Multi-infarct dementia is caused by an impaired blood supply to the brain. It develops gradually following a number of mini-strokes or transient ischemic attacks, which the person may not realize he or she is having. Multi-infarct dementia affects the cerebral cortex, which is the outer part of the brain. Subcortical vascular dementia (Binswanger's disease) involves vascular damage to the inner parts of the brain, particularly to the sheath of nerve cell fibers, which insulates the fibers in the brain. There is also a vascular dementia that involves both cortical and subcortical damage to the brain. There are rarer causes of vascular dementia that may affect some people with auto-immune inflammatory diseases that affect the arteries, such as systemic lupus erythematosus and temporal arteritis.

Risk factors for the development of multi-infarct dementia include a history of stroke, hypertension, smoking, and atherosclerosis. Atherosclerosis is the cause of many serious vascular problems, including heart attacks, cerebrovascular diseases, and peripheral vascular diseases, and may be associated with conditions such as diabetes mellitus, obesity, high cholesterol levels, and kidney disorders that require dialysis.

Symptoms of vascular dementia are similar to those of other dementias. The symptoms vary depending on the location and severity of the damage. Memory impairment is often an early symptom of the disorder, followed by judgment impairment. This often progresses in stepwise stages (i.e., periods of abrupt decline alternating with plateau periods of minimal decline) to delirium, hallucinations, and, finally, to impaired thinking. Personality and mood changes accompany the deteriorating mental condition, as well. Apathy and lack of motivation are common. Catastrophic reactions, where a person becomes withdrawn or extremely agitated, are also common. Confusion that occurs or is worsened at night is another common symptom.

Multi-infarct dementia is diagnosed on the basis of history, symptoms, signs, and tests and by ruling out other causes of dementia, including dementia due to metabolic causes. History may include a history of stroke or hypertension. History of the dementia often shows a stepwise progression of the condition. Other characteristics that suggest multi-infarct dementia rather than Alzheimer's disease include abrupt onset, somatic complaints, emotional changes, and focal neurologic signs and symptoms.

While no treatment can reverse brain damage that has already been caused by a stroke, treatment to prevent further strokes is very important. Such preventive measures involve the management of vascular risk factors, such as hypertension, diabetes, high cholesterol levels, and heart disease. Disorders that contribute to confusion—heart failure, decreased oxygen intake (hypoxia), thyroid disorders, anemia, nutritional disorders, infections, and psychiatric conditions (depression)—should be treated appropriately. Correction of coexisting medical and psychiatric disorders often greatly improves mental functioning. Medications, which include antipsychotics, beta-blockers, and serotonin-affecting drugs, may be required to control aggressive or agitated behaviors or behaviors that are dangerous to the person or to others. These are usually given in very low doses, with adjustment as required.

Dementia With Lewy Bodies

Dementia with Lewy bodies (DLB) is increasingly recognized clinically as one of the most common type of degenerative dementia, representing 15%–25% of all cases (McKeith et al., 2000). Dementia with Lewy bodies is characterized by two traits, which resemble PD and AD. The first trait is the presence of Lewy bodies, small, round inclusions found inside nerve cells that have long been associated with Parkinson's disease. Unlike Parkinson's disease, a brain disorder that is not classified as a dementia, DLB features Lewy bodies that have accumulated in the brain stem and cortical areas of the cerebral hemispheres. The second trait of DLB is the presence of amyloid plaques (i.e., the collection of abnormal beta-amyloid proteins), making it strikingly similar to AD. Dementia with Lewy bodies also shows neurofibrillary tangles, but they are far fewer in occurrence than with AD.

First described in the 1960s, DLB has a varied clinical presentation that shares features with those of other degenerative dementias. It was often overlooked pathologically because of the difficulty in identifying cortical Lewy bodies. When immunohistochemical stains were developed and exposed constituents of Lewy bodies, the prevalence of this disorder finally began to be recognized.

Challenges remain in defining DLB as an entity distinct from other degenerative dementias. Clinically, symptoms of DLB resemble those of both Parkinson's and Alzheimer's. Just as with Alzheimer's, people with DLB exhibit short-term memory deficits, visuospatial difficulties, and language disturbances. People with DLB also present with manifestations of Parkinson's disease—resting tremor, motor slowing, rigidity, reduced facial expression, stooped posture, and shuffling gait. But DLB has unique features of its own. In addition to dementia, DLB presents with the early appearance of visual hallucinations, difficulty with balance, reduced body movement, cognitive fluctuations, dysautonomia, sleep disorders, and neuroleptic sensitivity.

According to the National Institute of Neurological Disorders and Stroke (2007), the central feature of DLB is progressive cognitive decline, combined with three additional defining features: (1) pronounced "fluctuations" in alertness and attention (i.e., frequent drowsiness, lethargy, lengthy periods of time spent staring into space) or disorganized speech; (2) recurrent visual hallucinations, and (3) Parkinsonian motor symptoms (e.g., rigidity and the loss of spontaneous movement).

The Consortium on DLB (McKeith et al., 2005) also published guidelines highlighting three types of criteria for diagnosing DLB. They are as follows:

1   First, it is mandatory that a significant degree of cognitive impairment in two or more areas are present (i.e., it is a dementia).
2   Second, two or more of the following core features must be present:
    a   Marked and persistent fluctuations in attention or level of alertness
    b   Well-formed visual hallucinations
    c   Extrapyramidal motor signs (as may be seen in PD)
3   Third, supportive features may also suggest the diagnosis, including repeated falls, unexplained syncope (i.e., brief periods of loss of consciousness), other psychotic features like delusions, sleep disturbances (e.g., sleeping excessively, abnormal movements during sleep), and sensitivity to neuroleptics—a class of medication used to treat psychotic symptoms.

Distinguishing DLB from AD or PD is important because individuals with DLB are usually very sensitive to the extrapyramidal motor side effects associated with many neuroleptic drugs. Dementia with Lewy bodies patients should have minimal to no exposure to neuroleptic drugs, since their psychotic symptoms can be severe. Newer antipsychotic drugs, such as risperidone (Risperdal) and olanzapine (Zyprexa), may be better tolerated by individuals with DLB. Antipsychotics can cause a dramatic decline in function, sometimes with poor recovery after stopping these medications. Therefore, it is important to diagnose this condition and avoid using such agents, especially since visual hallucinations appear early in Lewy body dementia and antipsychotic medications are routinely used to treat such symptoms.

Dementia with Lewy bodies patients may, more so than AD and PD patients, particularly benefit from cholinesterase-inhibitor therapy. Acetylcholinesterase inhibitors may decrease confusion and cognitive fluctuations in DLB. These drugs generally do not worsen motor symptoms. These drugs also may be used for treatment of agitation and hallucinations associated with DLB (eMedicineHealth, 2005b). Psychotic symptoms, particularly visual hallucinations, may benefit from the use of cholinesterase-inhibitor agents, such as tacrine (Cognex) and donepezil (Aricept). If extrapyramidal motor signs are prominent in an individual with DLB, moderate use of anti-Parkinson's drugs to enhance dopamine function can be helpful but may exacerbate psychotic symptoms. Several reports have documented frequently good, and occasionally dramatic, responses of DLB patients to tacrine or donepezil treatment. This might possibly be attributed to the fact that DLB typically involves a greater loss of the brain chemical acetylcholine than does AD but is associated with fewer neurofibrillary tangles.

Through ongoing clinical, pathological, and therapeutic research investigations, it is hoped that an increased understanding of DLB and its relationships to both AD and PD will lead to more specific and effective interventions for all three disorders.

Parkinson's Disease Dementia

Parkinson's disease (PD) is a neurodegenerative disorder causing not only motor dysfunction but also cognitive, psychiatric, autonomic, and sensory disturbances. It is known as Parkinson's disease dementia (PDD). Dementia affects about 40% of patients with PD (Barone, Amboni, Vitale, & Bonavita, 2004); the incidence of dementia in these patients is up to six times that found in healthy people. Longitudinal studies suggest that up to 75% of patients with PD may eventually develop dementia (Williams-Gray, Foltynie, Lewis, & Barker, 2006). The clinical characteristics and course of PDD, its pathological features, and the most appropriate treatment are areas of current investigation.

Many patients with PDD experience psychosis. Psychotic symptoms in PDD patients are associated with major behavioral, cognitive, and functional problems (Leroi & Burns, 2007). Behavioral problems include apathy, personality changes, speech disturbances, and visual hallucinations. The most common manifestation of psychosis in PDD is visual hallucinations, but delusions, paranoid beliefs, agitation, and florid psychosis can also occur. Hallucinations and delusions in patients with PPD may have severe clinical consequences for those patients and their caregivers. When severe, PPD often surpasses the motor features of PD as a major cause of disability and mortality. Depression is also associated with PPD or early stage of PD onset.

The anatomic and pathologic basis of PDD is not fully understood. Magnetic resonance imaging and neuropathologic studies demonstrate more prominent global brain atrophy in PD patients with dementia than in those without dementia. It is also reported that cognitive deficits are the result of the interruption of frontal-subcortical loops that facilitate cognition and that parallel the motor loop (Merino & Luchsinger, 2004). Fibers from various areas of the cortex (e.g., posterior parietal, premotor) converge on the striatum (particularly the head of the caudate) and project to the prefrontal cortex via nigral, pallidal, and thalamic structures. Different areas of the caudate also project to different areas of the prefrontal cortex. Damage to any of the structures of the circuit can elicit the frontal-like cognitive deficits that characterize cognitive dysfunction in PD.

Psychosis has traditionally been considered as a dopaminergic drug-induced phenomenon, but factors intrinsic to the disease process itself also cause hallucinations and delusions. These factors may include Lewy body deposition in the limbic system, cholinergic deficits, and impairments of primary visual processing (Williams-Gray, Foltynie, Lewis, & Barker, 2006). As mentioned earlier, patients with PDD often experience neuropsychiatric symptoms that differ from those associated with other types of dementia. Despite this fact, PDD and DLB are distinct disorders, and whether or not they represent different presentations of the same disease is an area of debate and investigation.

An understanding of the pathophysiology underlying the symptoms associated with PPD is essential to the development of targeted therapeutic strategies. Postmortem studies suggest an association between Lewy body deposition and PPD, and indeed Parkinson's disease and DLB may form part of the same disease spectrum. Whether Lewy bodies actually play a causative role in cognitive dysfunction, however, is unknown. Deficits in neurotransmitter systems provide more obvious therapeutic targets, and dysfunction of dopaminergic, cholinergic, noradrenergic, and serotonergic systems have all been implicated; these may each underlie different features of PPD, perhaps explaining the heterogeneity of the syndrome.

There is currently no recommended treatment for PPD. Antipsychotic agents can worsen extrapyramidal symptoms, making them unsuitable for patients with this condition. Therapeutic intervention for cognitive and behavioral symptoms in PPD currently focuses on two main groups of drugs: cholinesterase inhibitors and atypical antipsychotics. A recent large, randomized-controlled trial suggests that cholinesterase inhibitors can produce a modest improvement in cognitive function, as well as psychotic symptoms, generally without an adverse effect on motor function (Hake, 2001). Certain atypical antipsychotics allow hallucinations, delusions, and behavioral problems to be brought under control with minimal deleterious effects on motor function and cognition, but their safety in elderly patients has recently been called into question. Deep brain stimulation does not appear to be a useful treatment for cognitive and psychiatric dysfunction in patients with PPD. Modafinil improves alertness in Parkinson's disease and warrants further investigation to establish its effects on cognitive performance.

Frontotemporal Dementia

Frontotemporal dementia (FTD) is a rare form of dementia that causes a slow, worsening decline of mental abilities. FTD occurs between the ages of 35 and 75 and only rarely after age 75 (Kumar-Singh & Broeckhoven, 2007). The age of onset for FTD is typically younger than that of AD, where the incidence increases dramatically after age 75. Both sexes are equally affected, and, in most cases, the onset is slow and insidious.

Frontotemporal dementia involves loss of nerve cells in the frontal lobes and the temporal anterior lobes of the brain. As with all dementias, FTD is caused by many underlying diseases, which include Pick's disease, corticobasal degeneration, and other unusual and rare diseases. For example, if Pick bodies develop in the brain, Pick's disease will cause clinical presentations of FTD in a patient. A major scientific breakthrough occurred in 1998 with the discovery that a mutation in the tau gene causes a form of FTD called frontotemporal dementia with Parkinsonism linked to chromosome 17 (FTDP-17).

The symptoms of FTD fall into two clinical patterns, depending on whether the damage has affected the right or left side of the front of the brain. The two clinical presentations, key to identifying FTD, are progressive aphasia and disorder of social behavior.

1   Progressive aphasia—a disorder of speech and language, caused by damage to the left side of the brain, that affects oral and written comprehension and production while spatial skills and memory remains intact. This can include Progressive Fluent Aphasia or Progressive Nonfluent Aphasia.

a   Progressive Fluent Aphasia (aka Semantic Dementia) occurs when patients have difficulty in understanding single words (i.e., names of objects) and express confusion when they are heard. This is evident in both oral and written communication (i.e., patients will try to describe a target word by talking around the target word). These patients have fluent speech and construct well-formed, grammatically correct sentences, but single word-comprehension is lost.

b   With Progressive Nonfluent Aphasia, single-word comprehension and expression remain intact, but the patient cannot retrieve grammatical forms, so words that allow one to form proper sentences are "lost." In essence, the patient has difficulty determining who did what to whom in a sentence. As a result, speech is disjointed and requires a lot of effort.

2   Disorder of personality and social behaviors caused by right-sided brain disease; symptoms include:

a   Uninhibited and socially inappropriate behaviors that seem insensitive to social norms and are far from the person's usual behavior (e.g., stealing, drinking out of the punch bowl at a party, blurting out rude comments, a general lack of empathy)

b   Hypersexuality, which leads to inappropriate sexual behavior (e.g., promiscuity, sexual demands on spouses, or even obsessive sexual fetishes involving celebrities)

c   Inappropriate rage responses (e.g., sudden outbursts of angry behavior that are triggered by minimal or even imagined causes)

d   Hyperoral behavior, an oral fixation that causes people to put food and other objects in their mouths. This obsessive behavior can lead to weight gain.

e   Other compulsive or repetitive behaviors (e.g., pacing, collecting things, or washing hands repeatedly)

f   Loss of concern about personal hygiene and personal appearance, loss of drive, social withdrawal, apathy

g   Memory loss, but not to the same degree present in those with AD, and it is usually not one of the first signs

Frontotemporal dementia is often misdiagnosed as a psychiatric problem or as Alzheimer's, since they share the same symptoms. The health care provider bases an initial diagnosis on history and symptoms, signs, tests, and the elimination of other causes of dementia, including dementia due to metabolic causes. Some disorders resemble FTD but can be cured, which makes a proper diagnosis extremely important. Although there is no definitive diagnostic test for FTD that can be done in a living patient, several options exist that can rule out conditions that appear to be FTD. Metabolic derangements, B-12 deficiency, and hypothyroidism must be included in the differential diagnosis. Multi-infarct dementia and pseudo-dementia (depression mimicking dementia), as well as chronic sedative usage, need to be ruled out, as well. Serum studies can detect B-12 deficiency, a low-functioning thyroid, or disorders affecting metabolism. Magnetic resonance imaging can detect the accumulation of small strokes, closed head injury, subdural hematoma, a brain tumor, or other forms of cancer, all of which mimic FTD.

Scientists and other experts on FTD are trying to promote a greater understanding of FTDs and other dementias in the hope of improving diagnosis. The earlier the medical community can properly diagnose the disease, the more likely the treatment strategies will halt its effects. Table 2.3 compares and contrasts FTD and AD, which are often confused.

An international group of clinical and basic scientists in a conference (McKhahnn et al., 2001) recommended the following clinical criteria for FTD diagnosis:

1 The development of behavioral or cognitive deficits is demonstrated by:
   a Early onset and progressive change in personality, characterized by difficulty in controlling or changing behavior, often resulting in inappropriate responses or activities (disorders of affect and social comportment)
   b Early onset and progressive changes in language, characterized by problems with expression of language or severe naming difficulty, and problems with word meaning (progressive aphasia).
2 The above deficits cause significant impairments in social or occupational functioning and represent a significant decline from a previous level of functioning.
3 The course is characterized by a gradual onset and continuing decline in function.
4 The deficits above are not due to other nervous system conditions (e.g., stroke), systemic conditions (e.g., thyroid disease), or substance-induced conditions.

Table 2.3

SIMILARITIES AND DIFFERENCES BETWEEN FRONTOTEMPORAL DEMENTIA AND ALZHEIMER'S DISEASE

FEATURES	FRONTOTEMPORAL DEMENTIA	ALZHEIMER'S DISEASE
Age at which disease generally occurs	■ Usually after age 40 and before age 65.	■ Usually after age 65.
Brain areas affected	■ Frontal and temporal lobes.	■ Starts in the medial termporal area, usually in the hippocampus. ■ Spreads to other areas of the brain.
Pathologic features	■ Loss of nerve cells. ■ No amyloid plaques. ■ Tau tangles seen in certain FTDs.	■ Loss of nerve cells. ■ Amyloid plaques. ■ Tau tangles.
Clinical features	■ Begins with personality and behavior changes; some patients may be hyperactive, while others seem apathetic. ■ Loss of empathy toward others. ■ Lack of insight into proper social conduct. ■ Memory is preserved early on. ■ Language difficulty. ■ Compulsive eating and oral fixations. ■ Repetitive actions. ■ Later in the disease, loss of motor skills, speech, and muscle movement.	■ Begins with memory loss. ■ Patients lose ability to learn new information. ■ Patients become unable to orient themselves to time and place. ■ Later in the disease, personality and behavior problems develop. ■ Possible hallucinations and delusions in later stages.

Source: "Frontotemporal Dementia: Growing Interest in a Rare Dementia," by Alzheimer's Disease Education and Referral Center, July 2002, *Connections, 9,* p. 4.

5   The deficits do not occur exclusively during a delirium.
6   The disturbance is not better accounted for by a psychiatric diagnosis (e.g., depression).

Trained and experienced health care professionals can also pinpoint FTD by collecting information from the following.

- A careful medical history and examination of behavioral changes that rely heavily on information from the family members and others close to the patient. This is necessary because patients lack the ability to recognize changes that have occurred or don't perceive their behaviors as problematic.
- A neuropsychological examination, which helps assess language, memory, executive functioning, and visual-spatial skills.
- Neuroimaging studies, such as a Positron Emission Tomography (PET) scan or a Single Proton Emission Computed Tomography (SPECT) scan, which determine where and how extensively brain regions have atrophied.

Treatment studies for FTD are in premature stages, but approaches derived from principles of medical therapeutics can be used to alleviate behavioral symptoms.

Practical strategies based on rational approaches and safety precautions can reduce the impact of behavioral symptoms. This could include making sure that the individual with FTD doesn't drive and avoids other situations where judgment is important.

Psychiatric medications, such as selective serotonin reuptake inhibitors or small doses of newer antipsychotic medications, can alleviate some of the more difficult behavior symptoms of FTD (National Institute on Aging, Alzheimer's Disease Education and Referral Center, 2007). Medications used for other conditions, like AD, PDD, and depression, can help slow down the progression of FTD. Antioxidants such as vitamin E and nonsteroidal anti-inflammatory agents can also alter the natural history of FTD. As can be expected, not all medications for treating dementia will have positive effects on individuals with FTD. Some medications that successfully treat other dementias, like cholinergic drugs and antipsychotic drugs that contain dopamine blockers, are ineffective or could be harmful to a person with FTD.

3

Causes of and Risk Factors for Alzheimer's Disease

While scientists know Alzheimer's disease involves progressive brain cell failure, they have not yet identified any single reason why cells fail.

Alzheimer's Association

WHY DO PEOPLE DEVELOP ALZHEIMER'S?

Alzheimer's disease (AD) is now the fourth leading cause of death in adults. Despite its growth among the elderly population, researchers still do not fully understand what causes AD. One thing is certain: It is a genetically complex neurodegenerative disorder and the leading cause of dementia in the elderly. And, a recent study confirmed that people who develop AD or dementia exhibit brain structure changes years before they show any signs of memory loss (Smith et al., 2007).

In the first chapter, we discussed the biological processes that cause symptoms of AD to present in an individual. We know that amyloid plaques and neurofibrillary tangles (which are presented in detail again in this chapter) contribute to the breakdown of the brain's nerve cells, leading to a gradual loss of cognitive and physical functions. But what sets off this physiological breakdown? Increased research efforts have determined a few factors that are proven to trigger these neurological changes, but no conclusive set of evidence exists that pinpoints one single factor as the main cause of AD. New research has shed light on a host of other factors that may cause AD, though additional findings need to be collected to confirm any consistent correlation. Consequently, the scientific community has agreed that—just like heart disease, cancer, and stroke—AD is not caused by one single factor but is the result of complex and related factors.

Before discussing causes and risk factors of AD, let's look at the three types of AD.

TYPES OF ALZHEIMER'S DISEASE

Early-Onset Alzheimer's Disease

This is a rare form of AD in which people are diagnosed with the disease before age 65. The age at onset in some families is as young as 35, and some cases have been cited where the disease began in the mid-20s. Fewer than 10% of all AD patients have this type of AD (Mayo Clinic. com, 2007f). People with Down's syndrome, often in their mid- to late 40s or early 50s, are at risk of being affected by this type. Younger people who develop AD have more of the brain abnormalities that are associated with AD. A condition called myoclonus—a form of muscle twitching and spasm—is also more commonly seen in early-onset Alzheimer's than in late-onset Alzheimer's (WebMD, 2007d). Early-onset Alzheimer's appears to be linked with a genetic defect on chromosome 14—a defect to which late-onset Alzheimer's is not linked (Mullan et al., 1995).

Late-Onset Alzheimer's Disease

This is the most common form of AD, accounting for about 90% of cases and usually occurring after age 65. Late-onset AD strikes almost half of all people over the age of 85 (WebMD, 2007d). Late-onset AD is not inherited in the same way as some cases of early-onset AD. Many factors combine to alter a person's risk of developing late-onset AD, so that some develop it in later life and others do not. Genetic and environmental factors are both involved. As mentioned earlier, most of these factors are not fully understood, but it is known that having a close family member with the condition increases risk, though only by a small amount. Studies suggest that a gene or genes on chromosome 10 may be risk factors for late-onset AD (Ertekin-Taner et al., 2000). Other factors such as other illnesses, diet, levels of activity and random chance, are probably more significant in the development of AD in later life. Late-onset dementia is also called sporadic Alzheimer's disease (Alzheimer Society, 2007).

Familial Alzheimer's Disease

Familial Alzheimer's disease (FAD) is a very rare type of Alzheimer's disease, accounting for fewer than 1% of all AD cases. Familial Alzheimer's disease usually strikes at a younger age, striking people in their 40s and 50s. In some extremely rare cases, people in their 30s have been known to develop it (WebMd, 2007d). As the name suggests, this type of Alzheimer's is known to be entirely inherited, that is, it runs in families. In these families, members of at least two generations can be documented to have AD (Cleveland Clinic Health System, 2004). This type is genetically inherited through a fault on chromosome 1, 14, or 21 (Edwardson & Morris, 1998).

CAUSES OF ALZHEIMER'S DISEASE

The causes of Alzheimer's are poorly understood. According to the National Institute on Aging (2006), AD disrupts each of the three processes that keep neurons healthy: communication, metabolism, and repair. As a result, nerve cells in the brain stop working, lose connections with other nerve cells, and eventually die. The destruction and death of nerve cells causes the memory failure, personality changes, problems in carrying out daily activities, and other features of the disease. These losses in memory and communication function are correlated with the brain content of two characteristic neuropathological lesions—beta-amyloid (Abeta) plaques and neurofibrillary tangles—which result in the death of brain cells and the breakdown of the connections between them. Abeta plaques (amyloid hypothesis) and neurofibrillary tangles are the primary hallmarks of AD. According to the amyloid hypothesis, accumulation of Abeta in the brain is the primary influence driving AD pathogenesis (Hardy & Selkoe, 2002). The rest of the disease process, including formation of neurofibrillary tangles containing tau protein, is proposed to result from an imbalance between Abeta production and Abeta clearance.

Beta-Amyloid (Abeta) Plaques

The production of Abeta is a normal cellular process. Abeta is a small fragment of a larger protein called amyloid precursor protein (APP). Amyloid precursor protein is a protein that appears to be important in helping neurons grow and survive. Amyloid precursor protein may help damaged neurons repair themselves and may help parts of neurons grow after brain injury (National Institute on Aging, 2006).

Amyloid precursor protein is associated with the cell membrane, the thin barrier that encloses the cell (Figure 3.1). After it is made, APP sticks through the neuron's membrane, partly inside and partly outside the cell. Enzymes act on the APP and cut it into fragments of protein, one of which is called beta-amyloid (Figure 3.2). Healthy brain cells clear away excess amounts of Abeta. In AD, the Abeta fragments begin clumping together outside the cell, and then join other molecules and non-nerve cells to form insoluble plaques (Figure 3.3). The plaques, combining with other molecules, neurons, and non-nerve cells, eventually cause neurodegenerative changes.

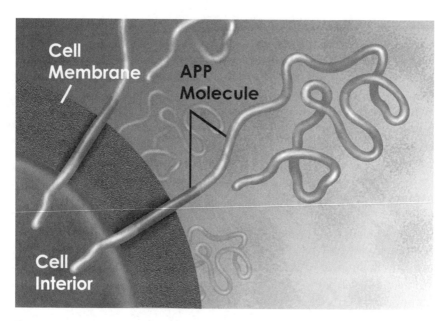

Figure 3.1 Amyloid precursor protein (APP) helps neurons grow and survive.
Source: "Alzheimer's Disease: Unraveling the Mystery," by National Institute on Health, December 2003, NIH Publication Number 02-3782.

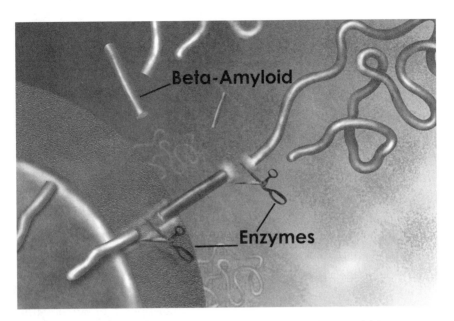

Figure 3.2 Enzymes cut APP into fragments of protein, called beta-amyloid.
Source: "Alzheimer's Disease: Unraveling the Mystery," by National Institute on Health, December 2003, NIH Publication Number 02-3782.

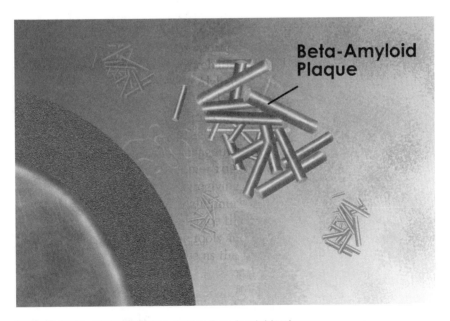

Figure 3.3 Clumping of beta-amyloid to form insoluble plaques.
Source: "Alzheimer's Disease: Unraveling the Mystery," by National Institute on Health, December 2003, NIH Publication Number 02-3782.

In AD, plaques develop in the hippocampus that helps to encode memories and in other areas of the cerebral cortex that are used in thinking and making decisions (Mattson, 1998). Although it has not been proven, researchers speculate that plaques build up much earlier than noticeable changes to brain functions can be seen.

Neurofibrillary Tangles

Healthy neurons have an internal support structure partly made up of structures called microtubules. These microtubules act like tracks, guiding nutrients and molecules from the body of the cell down to the ends of the axon and back. A special kind of protein, tau protein, keeps the microtubules stable and helps maintain the neuron's structure. Tau proteins are essential for normal brain function. In AD, tau protein is changed chemically, which makes it tangle up with other threads of tau, creating "neurofibrillary tangles" (Figure 3.4). When this happens, the microtubules disintegrate, collapsing the neuron's transport system. This may

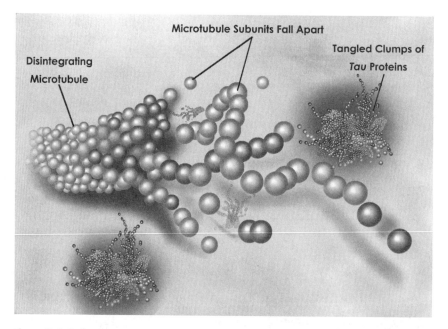

Figure 3.4 Formation of neurofibrillary tangles.
Source: "Alzheimer's Disease: Unraveling the Mystery," by National Institute on Health, December 2003, NIH Publication Number 02-3782.

result first in malfunctions in communication between neurons and later in the death of the cells. A small number of neurofibrillary tangles are a universal consequence of aging.

Some groups of neurons are preferentially affected by tangles in AD. For example, neurofibrillary tangles frequently occur in areas of the hippocampus that are involved in processing experiences prior to storage as permanent memories (Munoz & Feldman, 2000). This correlates with the clinical deficits observed in the early stages of AD in learning and in the creation of new memories, as well as with the relative preservation of established memories.

In elderly persons with AD, increasing evidence suggests a link between this neurodegenerative disease and vascular risk factors and atherosclerosis. The nature of this link remains speculative. Some studies suggest that the disease arises as a secondary event related to atherosclerosis of extracranial or intracranial vessels (Casserly & Topol, 2004). It is also suggested that atherosclerosis and AD are independent but convergent disease processes. This hypothesis is lent support by observations of shared epidemiology, pathophysiological elements, and response to treatment in both disorders. Studies related to the relationship between the degree of coronary and cerebral atherosclerosis and the extent of beta-amyloid accumulation strongly suggest that atherosclerosis-induced brain hypoperfusion contributes to the clinical and pathological manifestations of AD.

Oxidation and the Inflammatory Response

Since one theory behind the cause of Alzheimer's disease is the overproduction of Abeta, researchers are attempting to discover why excess beta-amyloid is toxic to nerve cells. Some researchers focus on two processes in the body that may be involved with Alzheimer's disease: *oxidation* and the *inflammatory process* (A.D.A.M. Healthcare Center, 2004a).

Oxidation is a cellular process known to play a role in many serious diseases, including coronary artery disease and cancers, and experts believe it may also contribute to Alzheimer's. One theory of beta-amyloid and its role in AD goes as follows.

As beta-amyloid breaks down, it releases unstable chemicals called oxygen-free radicals, which bind to other molecules through *oxidation*. Oxidation is the result of many common chemical processes in the body, but when oxidants are overproduced, they can cause severe damage in cells and tissue, including genetic material (DNA) in cells. One result of oxidation is the marshaling of immune factors to repair any injury. Overproduction of some of these immune factors produces a so-called *inflammatory response,* in which excess immune factors can actually damage the body's own cells. Inflammatory factors of specific interest in Alzheimer's research are the enzyme cyclooxygenase (COX) and its products called prostaglandins. Excess amounts of these inflammatory factors may increase levels of *glutamate,* an amino acid that excites nerves and, when overproduced, is a powerful nerve-cell killer. The inflammatory process has also recently been associated with the release of soluble toxins called amyloid-beta-derived diffusible ligands, which some investigators believe may prove to be key players in the destructive process of beta-amyloid.

Genetic Factors

It is now understood that genetic factors play a crucial role in determining whether one will develop AD. There are certain genes that have been identified as ones that increase the risk of developing AD, but there is no guarantee that the disease will develop. Other genes have been identified that practically guarantee the onset of Alzheimer's, but such genes are very rare, with only a few hundred individuals in the world carrying them. A major target of current AD research is to compare the concentration of factors responsible for beta-amyloid build-up in different people; genetic factors are believed to play a role in many cases.

Genes for Alzheimer's Disease

The genetics of AD is quite complex. It is known that AD tends to run in families. Currently, mutations in four genes, situated on chromosomes 1, 14, 19, and 21, are believed to play a role in AD (Peskind, 1996). Three of these (on chromosomes 21, 14, and 1) lead to the development of early-onset AD, as described earlier, which is much less common than late-onset AD. One gene, the Apolipoprotein E (ApoE) gene on chromosome 19, has been associated primarily with late-onset AD, although recent work suggests that its peak effect occurs earlier than originally thought. It has aroused intense interest because the great majority of the 4 million Americans diagnosed with AD developed the late-onset type of AD, after age 65.

Genetics 101

A refresher in genetics is crucial to understanding the genetic implications associated with AD. Every cell in the human body contains a set of 46 chromosomes, or 23 pairs. Each chromosome is made up of genes, which are actually tightly packed, condensed DNA strands that contain all of our genetic information. Just as our chromosomes come in pairs, so do our genes. Each gene—or specific subunit of DNA—codes for a protein or chemical that serves some specific function in the body.

Sometimes, during cellular reproduction, mistakes occur that change the genetic code of a chromosome. These errors can be silent (a polymorphism) or more prevalent (a mutation). A better way to understand the difference is to think of one common analogy that compares the gene to a long word made up of the letters DNA.

Polymorphism. In a "silent" error, the meaning of a word is not lost, despite a misspelling. Here's an example:

Chromosome 1: THEATRE

Chromosome 1": THEATER

In a polymorphism, the gene codes for the correct protein, despite the error.

Mutation. This type of error has more serious consequences. It occurs when a gene is misspelled in a way that results in the loss of the word's meaning. See this example:

Chromosome 1: GOOD

Chromosome 1": GXOD

In a mutation, the gene would code for a different protein, or the code would not be able to make a protein at all. Either way, the body would ultimately be lacking in a protein for which a normal chromosome would be able to code. Many diseases are the result of mutations.

Inheritance

If a mutation or polymorphism occurs, this error will be replicated as cells reproduce, meaning they can be passed on to future generations.

Whether or not these errors manifest themselves in an individual depends on the genetic makeup of the partners involved in reproduction. Conditions can be inherited in families in different ways.

Autosomal dominant conditions manifest in individuals when errors occur on the chromosomes numbered 1 through 22. Recall that every human cell contains 23 pairs of chromosomes; the 23rd chromosome pair is made up of the sex chromosomes and determines whether the body will develop as a woman (X pairs with X) or as a man (X pairs with Y). With autosomal dominant conditions, only one abnormal gene of the pair is necessary for an individual to be affected. And, since the chromosomes involved are not the sex chromosomes, both males and females in a family can receive the condition. Autosomal dominant conditions are passed from an affected parent to offspring with a 50% chance. Often, multiple people in one generation will be affected with autosomal dominant conditions.

Autosomal recessive conditions are passed on when both parents are carriers for a condition, meaning that they have one abnormal copy of the gene but do not express any clinical symptoms of a disease and are not at increased risk of developing the disease. If two parents are carriers of a condition, then the offspring that inherits both copies of the disease gene will be affected. Offspring have a 25% chance of inheriting a condition with an autosomal recessive condition. Autosomal recessive conditions appear frequently in individuals who have the same racial background, who marry within the same family, or who are from the same generation within a family (brothers and sisters).

Conditions that occur on the 23rd pair of chromosomes are known as X-linked and are passed to new generations maternally. Still other conditions are recognized as multifactorial, meaning that both genetic and environmental factors create the condition. It has been established that those with a first-degree blood relative with AD is 1.5 times more likely to develop AD than those who don't have a family history of AD (Lautenschlager et al., 1996). Despite this probability, it is no "guarantee" that the individual will develop Alzheimer's. In fact, many neurodegenerative conditions like Alzheimer's have been defined as multifactorial, since it seems that environmental conditions (e.g., head trauma, infection) can increase the risk of developing a brain disorder in addition to any possible genetic mutations. Multifactorial conditions do not always follow a specific pattern of inheritance, but better understanding of the genetic side of diseases will no doubt direct researchers and scientists to develop appropriate treatment options. Let's take a look at a few genes that scientists have already discovered have some relation to AD.

The Role of Chromosomes 21, 14, and 1

Early-onset AD or FAD strikes early and fairly often in certain families. Combing through the DNA of these families, researchers have found abnormalities in chromosomes 21, 14, and 1. The scientists found that some families have a mutation in selected genes on these chromosomes. On chromosome 21, the mutation causes an abnormal amyloid precursor protein (APP) to be produced. On chromosome 14, the mutation causes an abnormal protein called presenilin 1 (PS1) to be produced. On chromosome 1, the mutation causes yet another abnormal protein to be produced. This protein, called presenilin 2(PS2), is very similar to PS1. If just one of these genes inherited from a parent contains a mutation, the person will almost inevitably develop early-onset AD. This means that in these families, if one parent has early-onset AD, their children have about a 50–50 chance of developing the disease.

The chromosome 21 gene also intrigues Alzheimer's researchers because of its role in Down syndrome. People with Down syndrome have an extra copy of chromosome 21 and, as they grow older, usually develop abnormalities in the brain like those found in Alzheimer's disease.

Although early-onset AD is very rare and mutations in these three genes do not play a role in the more common late-onset AD, scientists have a few leads for researching causes of late-onset AD. First, scientists can conclude that genetics is indeed a factor in AD. Second, a few key players in the AD disease process have now been identified. Perhaps the most interesting finding is that mutations in APP can cause AD, highlighting the key role of beta-amyloid in the disease. Many scientists believe that mutations in each of these genes cause an increased amount of the damaging beta-amyloid to be made in the brain.

The Role of Apolipoprotein E

In addition to gene mutations on specific chromosomes, researchers have found that one form of the apolipoprotein E (ApoE) gene appears more often among patients with the more common, late-onset form of AD than among the general population. The ApoE gene makes a protein involved in carrying cholesterol in the bloodstream. Most evidence suggests that the ApoE gene does not directly cause AD but instead leads to the occurrence of the disease at an earlier age (though not as early as with early-onset AD). There are four different forms of the ApoE gene. Inheriting one of these forms—called E4—on chromosome 19 increases a person's risk of developing AD threefold. Inheriting two E4 copies of the gene increases risk 12 to 15 times. People with two copies of E4 also tend to develop AD earlier in life than the general population. The E4 version of ApoE is present in about 15% of all White people and is even more common in people of African descent. However, not all of these people develop AD, and not all people who have AD also have the E4 version of ApoE. This means that other environmental or genetic factors must also be present in order for a person to develop Alzheimer's.

RISK FACTORS FOR ALZHEIMER'S DISEASE

We now discuss all of the risk factors associated with AD, both definite and possible. Table 3.1 offers a complete list of definite and possible risk factors for AD. Among all risk factors, genetic risk as a cause of AD is an area of intense investigation, as we've just discussed.

Definite Risk Factors

According to Daniel Kuhn (1999), a *risk factor* or *susceptibility factor* is any circumstance or element that puts one at risk for developing a disease. Research has shown that the inhalation of tobacco smoke increases the risk of developing certain lung and heart diseases; high blood pressure and obesity increase the risk of developing heart disease; and exposure to asbestos increases one's risk of developing cancer. Alzheimer's

Table 3.1

RISK FACTORS OF ALZHEIMER'S DISEASE

DEFINITE RISK FACTORS	POSSIBLE RISK FACTORS
Age	Gender
Family history	Small strokes or cerebrovascular disease
Genetics and hereditary	Parkinson's disease
Down syndrome	Race and ethnicity
Head injury or brain trauma	Environmental toxins
Low educational/occupational status	Diet
Environmental toxins	Lack of exercise
Cerebrovascular disease	Stress
Parkinson's disease	Depression before onset of AD
Diabetes	

disease is no exception. The main difference is that research on AD is just beginning to scratch the surface. Increased investigations allowed the scientific community to recommend preventive measures for heart disease, and the medical community believes that the same trend will follow with continued AD research.

Age

Numerous studies have confirmed that as people get older, their chances of developing Alzheimer's increase. In fact, age is the greatest risk factor for AD (Tyas, Manfreda, Strain, & Montgomery, 2001). One in 10 individuals over the age of 65 and almost half of those over 85 are affected (Evans et al., 1989). "Age is critically important," confirmed Dr. John C. Morris (2006), a member of the board of directors of the Alzheimer's Association and Director and Principal Investigator of the Alzheimer's Disease Research Center at Washington University in St. Louis. "As the Boomers get older, people are interested in looking at risk factors that may be operating in midlife which could be modified and prevented, such as diabetes, high blood pressure, and high cholesterol."

As a person ages, the brain shrinks in size and neurons in certain areas atrophy or become faulty (Figure 3.5). These age-related changes are most likely responsible for some of the declines in cognitive abilities. However, the exact mechanisms for how this takes place are not entirely clear and are the subject of current research. It is still unclear why some elderly people develop AD, while others do not. This fact itself indicates that other factors are at play that contribute to the disease.

Recent research has identified a potential mechanism related to aging that may contribute to the development of AD. This potential mechanism is messenger RNA; mutations in messenger RNA have been reported in elderly humans and older rodents. The deletion of two consecutive bases in a protein results in an altered reading frame and, thus, a protein with an amino acid sequence unrelated to that specified in the original gene. The predicted abnormal forms of two proteins relevant to the pathogenesis of AD, ß-amyloid precursor protein and ubiquitin-B, and their corresponding altered messenger RNA have been found in the brains of patients with AD (van Leeuwen et al., 1998).

Head Injury and Brain Trauma

Recent studies have provided "very strong evidence that there is a connection between head trauma and at least some of the pathology of

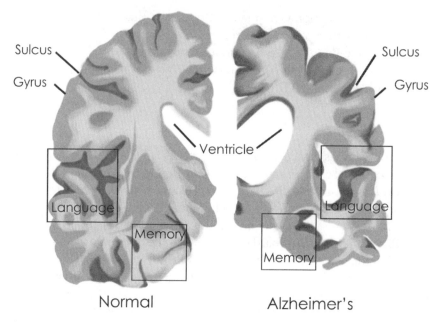

Figure 3.5 Shrinking brain along with neurons with age.
Source: "Mechanism of Possible Biological Effect of Activated Water on Patients Suffering From Alzheimer's Disease," by I. V. Smirnov, 2003, *Explore, 12.* Copyright © 2003 by Dr. Igor V. Smirnov, PhD, MS, USA.

Alzheimer's disease," Dr. Trojanowski said (Doskoch, 2000). It is possible that deposits that form in the brain as a result of a head injury may trigger the onset of AD. Punch Drunk Syndrome is a form of dementia commonly seen in professional boxers, since these individuals often suffer repeated blows to the head. The syndrome—as interpreted in the Adam Sandler film *Punch Drunk Love*—impairs memory, language, and other brain functions. Repeated impact to the head is not the only risk factor: Studies indicate that a severe blow to the head that results in a loss of consciousness (e.g., from a car accident or a fall) increases one's chances of developing Alzheimer's later on in life. At the World Alzheimer Congress 2000, Steven T. DeKosky, MD, and colleagues at the University of Pittsburgh Medical Center reported findings from neocortical samples taken from brain injury patients 1 and 3 days after injury. The samples, which were obtained by surgical resection and compared with postmortem samples from neurologically normal controls, revealed increases in amyloid precursor protein (APP), apolipoproteins E and D, and ß-amyloid (Aß). Many of the Aß deposits "had morphologic characteristics of classic amyloid plaques in AD," Dr. DeKosky and colleagues reported (Doskoch, 2000).

A Mayo Clinic (Nemetz et al., 1999) study published in the *American Journal of Epidemiology* found evidence that AD begins much earlier in people who previously suffered a head injury. Researchers looked for evidence of the onset of AD in medical records of more than 1,280 residents of Olmsted County, Minnesota, who had suffered traumatic brain injuries between 1935 and 1984 and who were at least 40 years old at last follow-up. They compared their results with those for a group of 689 community members diagnosed with AD but with no history of head trauma. They found that the median observed time from injury to onset of Alzheimer's was 10 years in the traumatic brain injury (TBI) group. This was significantly less than the expected time of 18 years to onset in the non-head-injury group. Although the overall incidence of Alzheimer's among TBI cases was similar to that expected, on the basis of rates for the Olmsted County population, the number of TBI cases with onset of Alzheimer's before age 75 was more than twice that expected. They say the results point toward a TBI interacting with other factors to hasten the onset of AD in susceptible individuals.

Several studies have found that Aß deposition occurs in a third of fatal head injury cases, even in children who survived only a few hours. The Aß is generally distributed throughout the brain; its presence does not correlate with the existence of cerebral contusions, increased intracranial pressure, or intracranial hematomas. Neurofibrillary tangles may also occur. The nature of pathology depends in part on injury severity—tangles do not seem to occur after mild trauma—but "I don't think there's much insight into how severe the injury has to be" to trigger AD-like pathology, Dr. Trojanowski said (Doskoch, 2000).

Down Syndrome

Down syndrome is a form of mental retardation that manifests in individuals who inherit an extra copy of chromosome 21 (i.e., have three copies instead of two). This extra chromosome can come from either parent. Autopsies reveal that almost all people with Down syndrome who live into their 40s exhibit changes in the brain—mainly plaques and tangles—that are consistent with AD. The occurrence of AD in people with Down syndrome increases dramatically from the age of 40 onward, but not all people with Down syndrome express Alzheimer's classic symptoms. This discrepancy is still not fully understood.

Researchers from the Institute of Psychiatry at King's College London have identified a molecule that could be targeted to treat the cognitive impairment in people with Down syndrome. They found that people with Down syndrome have higher levels of myo-inositol in their brains than people without the condition, and that increased levels of this molecule are associated with reduced intellectual ability (King's College London, 2005). The researchers also suspect that high levels of myo-inositol could play a role in predisposing people with Down syndrome to early-onset AD. The molecule is known to promote the formation of amyloid plaques, now considered to be a hallmark of Alzheimer's.

Low Education and Occupational Status

It has been proven that individuals with low educational and occupational status are at a higher risk of developing Alzheimer's, and those who received a higher education and have reached higher occupational status run a lower risk of developing the disease. This phenomenon may stem from the fact that highly educated people and those who have tapped into their intellect occupationally have developed more complex connections in their brains from childhood onward than those who did not. This has been explained as a consequence of a greater "brain reserve capacity" in people with high educational and occupational status. Smaller brains and head size may lead to fewer connections within the brain and have also been suggested in causation of AD (Letenneur et al., 1999).

Whether education and occupational level are true risk factors, independent of other environmental factors, is still under consideration. On one hand, people who are well educated might perform better on tests that measure intellectual ability than those with less education. Results from one brain-imaging study reported that dementia patients with high levels of education had greater perfusion deficits in functional scanning than dementia patients at similar levels of severity but with fewer years of schooling (Chiu, Lee, Hsiao, & Pai, 2004). Decreased synaptic connections are believed to correlate with lower educational level, suggesting that lack of early education may predispose people to AD by interacting with other risk factors.

On the other hand, well-educated individuals might express fewer symptoms of dementia, possibly because they have developed more complex connections in their brains in childhood, meaning that they have extra capacity to cope with the physical changes to the brain associated with dementia (Alzheimer's Society, 2007c). Prominent figures such as former president Ronald Reagan and the artist Norman Rockwell prove that people with keen intellects are not immune to developing AD. Education and occupation are often linked to socioeconomic status, and other lifestyle factors must be included in the equation when it comes to determining risk factors for AD (Hall, Gao, Unverzagt, & Hendrie, 2000).

Family History

It is believed that persons who have a history of AD in their family are two to three times more likely to develop the disease further on in life as presented in familial Alzheimer's disease (FAD) (Memorystudy.org, 2007). The greater the number of family members who have suffered from the disease, the greater the risk. However, most cases of Alzheimer's are a result of both genetics and other contributing factors, and the hereditary form only accounts for about 5% of all cases. Fewer than 1% of AD cases are inherited, mostly those with onset before age 65. However, evidence suggests that by age 90, about one-half of the first-degree relatives of AD patients develop dementia (Mohs, Breitner, Silverman, & Davis, 1987).

Possible Risk Factors

In his book, *Alzheimer's Early Stages,* Daniel Kuhn (1999) defines possible risk factors as "those suspected of being somehow linked to Alzheimer's disease but not yet proven to have a consistent association with the disease" (p. 50). Kuhn also adds that—like most of the other risk factors associated with Alzheimer's—additional research is needed to clarify their role, since thorough studies about these possible factors have not been carried out. The next sections discuss a few new directions of research that have possible associations with AD.

Gender

The majority of people with AD are women. It is believed that about twice as many women as men have AD. This might be partly correlated with the fact that women tend to live longer than men and that women may have gender-specific risk factors that affect them but not men. Despite women's greater longevity, studies have shown that women have a higher chance of developing AD than men. The reason for this disparity is still unclear. Some hypothesize that depleted estrogen levels may be related to developing AD (Paganini-Hill & Henderson, 1994), although recent studies have demonstrated the opposite (Hebert, Scherr, McCann, Beckett, & Evans, 2001).

Studies have found that women with AD tend to have lower scores on the Mini-Mental State Examination than men (Buckwalter, Sobel, Dunn, Diz, & Henderson, 1993). Women may also have greater deficits in language skills than men (Hebert et al., 2000), and psychiatric and behavioral problems may also be more frequent in women with AD than in men with AD (Cohen et al., 1993). Not only do twice as many women as men have AD, but women who do develop AD tend to have more severe disease and tend to survive longer after the onset of AD than men.

Ethnicity

Another inborn trait that puts one at risk for AD is race and ethnic origin. The rate of cognitive decline in people with AD appears to be slower among African Americans than among non-African Americans (Barnes et al., 2005). Another study reports that the first-degree relatives of African Americans with AD have a higher cumulative risk of dementia than do those of Whites with AD. Thus, they face a greater familiar risk for dementia (Green, Cupples, Go, Benue, & Edeki, 2002). Yet another study revealed that African Americans and Hispanics were at a much greater risk of developing AD than were members of other racial groups. This study determined that African Americans were four times as likely as European Americans to develop Alzheimer's by age 90, and the results were shown to be unrelated to educational levels (Tang et al., 2001). The presence of an APOE-(epsilon)4 allele is a determinant of AD risk in Whites, but African Americans and Hispanics have an increased frequency regardless of their APOE genotype. These results suggest that other genes or risk factors may contribute to the increased risk of AD in African Americans and Hispanics (Kukull & Martin, 1998).

Smoking

Most people are aware of the scientific evidence that nicotine in cigarettes contributes to heart and lung diseases. In the case of AD, controversy surrounds the issue because evidence supports both sides—some studies show that nicotine has preventive effects, while others show that smokers are at high risk for developing Alzheimer's. Studies have indicated that nicotine may actually protect one from developing AD. With the onset of AD, acetylcholine neurotransmitter is depleted, yet nicotine acts in much the same way as acetylcholine and is particularly helpful in enhancing memory. More research is necessary to determine the true value of nicotine in the context of AD.

Conversely, studies have suggested that cigarette smoking is a clear contributor to memory loss in the elderly. In light of the fact that vascular disease can lead to dementia and that nicotine causes vascular disease, it remains to be seen whether cigarette smoking will ever be established as a preventive measure for AD.

Alcohol

A high consumption of alcohol can lead to a vitamin B-1 deficiency, particularly among alcoholics who replace nutritious foods with alcohol. People who drink excessive amounts of alcohol over a long period of time significantly increase their risk of developing a form of AD. This form is better known as Korsakoff's syndrome and often causes memory impairments in affected individuals (DeAngelo & Halliday, 2005). However, there is no proved correlation between memory loss and alcohol and the development of AD. Some research has even suggested that moderate amounts of red wine, which contains anti-oxidants, might help to reduce the risk of dementia and AD (Alzheimer's Society, 2007b).

Nutrition

Diet can affect a person's risk of developing many types of illness, including AD. A healthy and balanced diet, which enables a person to maintain a normal body weight, will reduce the likelihood of developing high blood pressure or heart disease, both of which put a person at greater risk of developing AD. It is also believed that too much saturated fat can cause a narrowing of the arteries, making a heart attack or stroke more likely. Heart attacks, strokes, and vascular disease increase a person's risk of developing vascular dementia, thus AD.

People who have AD often have low levels of folic acid in their blood, but it is not clear whether this is a result of the disease or if they are simply malnourished as a result of their illness. Mattson suggests that consuming adequate amounts of folic acid—either in the diet or by supplementation—could be beneficial to the aging brain and help protect it against Alzheimer's and other neurodegenerative diseases (Duan et al., 2002).

Exercise

Through research, scientists are learning that some of the risk factors for heart disease and stroke, such as high blood pressure and high cholesterol, may increase the risk of AD. Lack of exercise may be another indicator. Researchers have reported that healthy people who reported exercising regularly had a 30%–40% lower risk of dementia (Larson et al., 2006). They concluded that older people who exercise three or more times a week are less likely to develop Alzheimer's and other types of dementia, according to a study.

Stress

Cases have existed where individuals appeared to develop AD immediately following a major life change, such as the death of a spouse, divorce, or retirement. Scientists have therefore begun investigating psychological stress as a risk factor of AD, though controversy surrounds the relationship. Researchers at the University of California–Irvine say that stress hormones can rapidly accelerate the formation of the brain lesions that cause Alzheimer's disease. On the basis of these findings, the researchers suggest that managing stress and reducing certain medications used by the elderly could significantly slow down the progression of the disease (Billings, Green, McGaugh, & LaFerla, 2007). A previous study of nearly 800 Catholic nuns, priests, and brothers found that those plagued by negative emotions, such as depression and anxiety, had about twice the risk of Alzheimer's of those who took a more laid-back approach to life.

Depression

A study from the researchers at the Mount Sinai School of Medicine, in New York, shows that there is a link between people who have a lifetime history of major depressive disorder and Alzheimer's (Rapp et al., 2006). Their research found that such people are more likely to be diagnosed with AD. Other studies have shown that people with depression had more plaques and tangles in the hippocampus (plaques and tangles are a key feature of AD). People with Alzheimer's disease with a history of depression and who were depressed at the time of diagnosis showed more pronounced neuropathological changes in the hippocampus. The research also found that people with a lifetime history of major depressive disorder were more likely to have a rapid decline toward Alzheimer's.

It has not been determined whether depression is a true risk factor or whether it marks the onset of AD, and further investigation needs to be conducted before any conclusive statements are made that relate the two.

Other Diseases

Cerebrovascular Disease and High Blood Pressure. When blood supply to the brain is impeded, damage may occur in the brain, which can lead to a form of dementia known as vascular dementia. A study of American Catholic nuns demonstrated that individuals who suffer from transient ischemic attack (TIA) are more likely to express symptoms of AD than those who do not. Some studies have reported an association between Alzheimer's disease and systolic hypertension. Scientists have also found that high levels of lipids in midlife can double the risk of dementia in later life; these factors reduce blood supply to the brain and are under consideration as possible risk factors for developing Alzheimer's (Kivipelto, Helkala, Laakso, Hänninen, & Hallikainen, 2001). Consequently, lowering high blood pressure and high cholesterol levels appears to reduce the risk of AD in elderly patients (A.D.A.M. Healthcare Center, 2004a). Although, hypertension is strongly linked to memory and mental difficulties, stronger evidence is needed to prove any causal relationship between hypertension and AD.

Parkinson's Disease. Parkinson's disease is a disorder that impairs the movement of hands, arms, and legs in an individual. There is an interchangeable pattern of association between AD and Parkinson's: Of individuals with Parkinson's, 20%–30% develop symptoms of Alzheimer's, often in the late stages of Parkinson's, and most people in the late stages of AD exhibit symptoms of Parkinson's disease.

Diabetes. Results of a study published in the *Archives of Neurology* suggest that those with diabetes have a 65% higher risk of developing AD (Arvanitakis, Wilson, Bienias, Evans, & Bennett, 2004). It was generally assumed that this happens because the blood vessel and heart disorders associated with diabetes are also risk factors for AD. But now there's strong evidence that people with high insulin levels—prior to even developing diabetes—are already on the road to developing AD (DeNoon, 2005). High insulin levels are known to cause blood vessels to become inflamed. Inflamed tissues send off chemical warning signals, which, in turn, set off an avalanche of tissue-damaging effects. Insulin doesn't just cause inflammation in the lower body; it also causes inflammation in the brain. One dangerous effect of this insulin-caused brain inflammation is increased levels of beta-amyloid in the brain—the twisted protein that forms the sticky plaques associated with AD.

Environmental Factors

Obesity. Obesity joins a growing list of lifestyle risk factors for Alzheimer's—high cholesterol, high blood pressure, and diabetes. It has been shown that being extremely overweight or obese increases the likelihood of developing AD. Researchers found a strong correlation between body mass index and high levels of beta-amyloid; with every unit increase in body mass index at age 70, the chance of developing Alzheimer's increased by 36% (Gustafson, Rothenberg, Blennow, Steen, & Skoog, 2003).

Estrogen. Several studies of hormone replacement therapy have shown that postmenopausal women who take estrogen may have a lower risk of developing AD (Zandi et al., 2002), and a few small trials claim to have found improvement in female patients with AD who are taking estrogen. Other research has shown that women with AD who are treated with estrogen show no sign of improvement. Currently, research is inconclusive as to the exact role, if any, that hormone replacement therapy may play in relation to AD. Since hormone replacement therapy may be recommended for reasons other than AD, women should be aware of the risks and benefits of estrogen use.

Anti-Inflammatory Drugs. As discussed earlier, inflammation in the brain may contribute to AD. The brains of AD patients show evidence of mild active inflammation, including microglial and complement activation, and the presence of inflammatory cytokines. Epidemiological retrospective studies have been conducted to determine the risk of developing AD among patients receiving anti-inflammatory drugs or having conditions, such as arthritis, in which these drugs are routinely used. Studies have shown that nonsteroidal anti-inflammatory drugs (NSAIDs) may slow the progression of Alzheimer's, though clinical trials have not demonstrated a benefit from these drugs.

   Other studies have set out to explore whether drugs can slow down the progression of Alzheimer's in those who already are diagnosed with the disease or whether certain NSAIDs could prevent Alzheimer's in healthy older people at risk of the disease. Research into the use of anti-inflammatory drugs to prevent or suspend Alzheimer's is still in very preliminary stages.

Toxicity. One long-standing theory is that overexposure to certain trace metals or chemicals may cause Alzheimer's (Markesbury, 1996). It is also known that ingestion of toxic metals can lead to brain damage. Trace levels of many metals have been found in the brains of people with AD. Aluminum is one particular element that is known to affect the nervous system. One theory proposed that the common occurrence of being exposed to aluminum could cause AD. At first, medical scientists thought this theory was absurd. Aluminum, they believed, accumulated merely as a result of a destructive process caused by some other factor. In recent years, however, the aluminum hypothesis has been gaining respect. In studies where the brains of experimental animals were injected with aluminum, an acute encephalopathy accompanied by neuronal inclusions was produced that resembled neurofibrillary tangles. Studies have also discovered a direct association between the level of aluminum in municipal drinking water and the risk of AD (Armstrong, Anderson, Cowburn, Cox, & Blair, 1992).

Some individuals in occupations that expose them to certain chemicals have been shown to be at increased risk of developing AD. A study conducted by Canadian researchers demonstrated that individuals who worked with glues, pesticides, and fertilizers were at an increased risk of AD (Canadian Study of Health and Aging Working Group, 1994). Another smaller study suggested that exposure to electromagnetic fields may also have the same effect (Sobel, Dunn, Davanipour, Qian, & Chui, 1996), and a U.S. study showed similar results in people who were exposed to the organic solvents benzene and toluene (Kukull, Larson, Bowen, McCormick, & Teri, 1995).

This chapter has reinforced the common belief in the medical community that AD and other neurodegenerative conditions are considered multifactorial conditions. AD is not considered to be a true genetic disorder (with the exception of early-onset AD). Genetics is classified as a definite risk factor for AD, but even though an individual may have a genetic composition that puts him at increased risk of developing AD, it does not mean that he will definitely develop the disease. Similarly, a person who doesn't inherit the gene still might develop AD. As you've just learned, factors involving the environment also increase one's risk of developing the disease.

4 Symptoms of Alzheimer's Disease

Some change in memory is normal as we grow older, but the symptoms of Alzheimer's disease are more than simple lapses in memory.

Alzheimer's Association

Alzheimer's disease (AD) attacks the brain long before it takes a form that is recognizable to an outsider. The early signs of AD often go unnoticed by loved ones, mistaken for old age, forgetfulness, and even depression. When the disease does manifest itself, it takes the form of abnormal cognitive functions and behavioral patterns, with changes in memory, movement, judgment, abstract reasoning, and behavior. Since a recognizable pattern is often difficult to pinpoint, family members are often unaware that AD is brewing underneath. In some cases, a dramatic change in lifestyle may expose the disease's development, or the person with AD may complain about her symptoms. Often, it takes years for symptoms to surface that are severe enough to turn to a medical professional for help.

People who develop dementia or Alzheimer's disease experience brain structure changes years before any signs of memory loss begin (Smith et al., 2007). AD takes from 7 to 10 years to develop completely. In some cases, brain functions diminish one by one, but usually they deteriorate simultaneously. In others, some functions remain intact and the person never progresses to experience the disease's severe stages. It is also important to note that even if some of AD symptoms are present, it doesn't mean that a person definitely has AD. It *could* just be a normal part of aging. To a normal person, it is hard to tell the difference at first. For this reason, defining stages to the disease is extremely important.

Another factor that contributes to the difficulty of diagnosing Alzheimer's is the patient's resistance to the changes in lifestyle. It is common for people with AD to subconsciously compensate for the loss of their cognitive functioning. They may retreat from activities that are too demanding—such as working, socializing, playing cards—to disguise the fact that they are simply unable to perform certain tasks that they once easily managed. They may avoid new situations, since they demand recent memory, and pass certain responsibilities to their spouse, such as paying bills and grocery shopping. It is natural to feel embarrassed and even confused about the impairments one is experiencing, but, usually, these efforts are not deliberate attempts to cover up symptoms. It is, most likely, a subconscious reaction to the changes in memory and thinking.

The life span of AD can potentially be quite long, so it is usually categorized into three levels to frame its progression. Early stages are called mild AD; middle stages are called moderate AD; and final stages are called severe AD. As mentioned before, symptoms vary from person to person, but the general description of the stages provided in this chapter are the most commonly observed, "classic" symptoms in each stage.

In AD's early stages, symptoms are very subtle, and it is during this stage that family members, and even the person with AD, tend to overlook the symptoms. Short-term memory begins to dissolve, and normal activities become slightly more difficult to complete than usual. Attention span reduces, and the person with AD may get lost or disoriented and experience slight personality changes, like mood swings. People with Alzheimer's tend to be less motivated to complete activities or tasks. They may become stubborn and be resistant when presented with new challenges.

As AD takes over the brain, even more symptoms continue to emerge or old symptoms worsen. Speech problems, inability to identify familiar objects, forgetting how to use ordinary objects like a pencil, and forgetting to turn off the stove or lock the front door are classic symptoms that characterize the disease's middle stages. People with the disease will more frequently forget words or names during conversations. As this forgetfulness begins to make itself obvious, a person with AD will retreat from social situations, avoiding conversations and keeping quiet to avoid making mistakes. This shame can lead to other medical problems, like depression and antisocial behavior, which deserve equal attention from a medical professional.

Odd behavior is another noticeable symptom that can help pinpoint the presence of AD. A person might misplace objects, leaving books in the freezer or plates in the washing machine. A person with AD will also repeatedly ask the same questions, to the point of irritation. People with AD can also be easily provoked, becoming uncharacteristically angry.

As mentioned earlier, AD typically develops slowly and causes a gradual decline in cognitive abilities, and it may take a person from 7 to 10 years to progress to a stage of severe dementia (Mayo Clinic, 2006a). Modern medicine has enabled people with AD to live an average of 8 years and as many as 20 years or more from the onset of symptoms as estimated by relatives (U.S. Congress Office of Technology Assessment, 1987). Again, these numbers vary, since progression and severity differ from person to person. One fact remains: Most people with AD die not of the disease itself but of other complications, like pneumonia, urinary tract infections, or concussions (Alzheimersinfo101.org, 2007). And, earlier symptoms of the disease respond well to various treatments. All of these facts point to one thing—early diagnosis is vital to a person with AD. Defining the stages of AD is one of the best ways to notice symptoms and to recruit a medical professional to make an early diagnosis.

It is important to understand that the information is stored in three different parts of your memory: the short-term memory, the recent memory, and the remote memory. Information stored in the short-term memory may include the name of a person you met a few minutes ago. Information stored in the recent memory may include what you ate for breakfast today. Information stored in the remote memory includes things that happened years ago, such as memories of childhood (Information from your family doctor, 2003).

The medical community has crafted several staging systems, which identify early to late stages of AD. These systems are used as measures that can aid in pinpointing or ruling out Alzheimer's and in keeping treatment and lifestyle options aligned with the progressive stages of the disease. This chapter begins with a brief summary of the most common symptoms of AD. You'll then learn how these symptoms are separated in different manners depending on the staging system applied.

THE 10 WARNING SIGNS OF ALZHEIMER'S DISEASE

The Alzheimer's Association has identified a checklist of 10 common symptoms—warning signs—for identifying AD. It is important to point out that many of these symptoms overlap (Alzheimer's Association, 2005c). For instance, loss of memory makes it difficult to recall objects, which makes conversations difficult, which might lead an individual with Alzheimer's to withdraw from social settings. The checklist is important because the presence of these symptoms doesn't always mean the individual has Alzheimer's. If an individual is withdrawing, she may be depressed, which can be treated with the help of a psychiatrist or a psychologist. But, if an individual is demonstrating several of these behaviors, it is absolutely necessary to recruit a team of experts to assess whether the person has AD. Only then the treatment process can begin.

To grasp the subtleties in AD's manifestations, it helps to think of two major areas of change—a decline in cognitive functions and changes in behavior. These changes are different from normal, age-related memory and behavioral changes. Making the distinction is no easy task, which is why knowledge of all the possible warning signs is so important.

Symptoms of Cognitive Decline

1. Memory Loss That Affects Day-to-Day Function

The first and most evident symptom of AD is a difficulty in remembering recent episodes—those events that took place within the past hour, day, or week. New learning is impaired, but remote memory, which enables the recall of events from the distant past, often remains intact. For example, a person with AD may be able to recall the house she grew up in as a child, but she may become disoriented in her present home and not know where she is for a moment. This subtle difference—being able to recall early memories, while forgetting more recent events—is one reason that the disease is mistaken for absentmindedness. On the surface, an individual with AD appears to be thinking and behaving normally, despite the neurological changes that are taking place internally.

Forgetfulness may take many different forms, starting out as mild and erratic. People with Alzheimer's may forget appointments or conversations or repeat the same questions. They may forget to turn off the stove or forget where outlets are in the house. At first, these incidences seem random and unrelated, so family members don't associate the unusual events with AD. One theme is clear—as AD begins to take its toll in the form of memory loss, family members often downplay the symptoms, dismissing them as a natural part of aging. Often, after a third party comes into the picture and points out the "obvious," the family members are able to recognize that these disconnected incidents are part of a medical problem. Later on, when the individual can't remember personal information, such as where he was born or what he did for a living or the name of a close relative, it's undeniable that some form of dementia may be present.

2. Difficulty Performing Familiar Tasks

People with AD first experience sporadic impairments in everyday functions, which can vary from misplacing keys to forgetting where the bank is. Simple tasks, such as eating, getting dressed, bathing, and grooming, are eventually lost with AD, but, in the beginning, one is usually able to keep these repetitive functions intact.

3. Problems With Language

People with AD demonstrate a loss of verbal communication—not necessarily with mechanics of speech (though this aspect of speech is impaired in later stages), but rather with the rules of speech. For example, they may forget simple words or forget the name of an object, like a pen, and substitute words that don't make sense. Or, since their ability to process information is delayed, they might have to take long pauses in a conversation. They may not be able to articulate their thoughts as well, and the depth or richness of their vocabulary may be lost.

4. Disorientation and Confusion of Time and Place

Considering the subtle nature of Alzheimer's early symptoms, it sometimes takes a significant change in the routine of an affected person for the disease to reveal itself. For example, a person with AD may get lost while on vacation, or the death of a loved one might force an individual with AD to manage independently, until it becomes apparent that she can no longer handle the details of everyday life.

It may not take a drastic change to notice that a person's confusion is straying from behavior associated with normal aging. A person may forget where he is, or he may not recognize places or people that should be familiar. He might forget the day or even the year.

5. Poor or Decreased Judgment

Since logic and reasoning are necessary to make sound judgments and these skills are lost with AD, a person with AD may make choices that are not appropriate, and, in some cases, even dangerous. A case has been reported of a woman who gave her life savings away to a neighbor and of another woman who turned up her thermostat to a scorching 85 degrees, which almost killed her. Milder instances of poor judgment include leaving the house without shoes or wearing pajamas in inappropriate public settings.

6. Decline in Abstract Thinking and Reasoning

As Alzheimer's takes its toll on an individual, tasks that require practical problem solving may become impossible to complete. Balancing a checkbook, which requires an understanding of numbers and math, may be difficult if the individual forgets how to compute even simple arithmetic equations. Tasks that involve a series of steps, such as driving a car, cooking a meal, or following directions, may be difficult to handle.

7. Misplacing Things

In line with other losses in judgment or reason, a person with AD may put things in inappropriate places. Misplacing things is a common occurrence, and everyday items (i.e., reading glasses, hearing aid, keys) may end up in strange places, like the refrigerator.

Behavioral Symptoms

Not all people in the early stages of AD express noncognitive, or behavioral, symptoms. Every case is different, and some people might demonstrate these behaviors only later on. Regardless, it is important to note that behavioral symptoms are just as relevant in detecting AD as cognitive symptoms.

8. Changes in Mood and Behavior

Behavioral changes may surface, such as unusual anger, irritability, restlessness, even silence. It has been seen that people with Alzheimer's become short-tempered and less inhibited in speech, cursing more or becoming more outspoken and opinionated. These outbursts are symptoms of the disease and should not be taken personally. Antisocial behavior may be mitigated if the trigger to the outbursts can be identified and minimized in the future—perhaps a certain threatening situation could be avoided, for example.

9. Changes in Personality

Some people may act out of character—an aggressive person may become passive; a nurturing wife may become self-absorbed and insensitive. Delusional thinking may also emerge. For example, a person with Alzheimer's may be convinced that her spouse is having an affair, despite all evidence to the contrary.

10. Lack of Motivation or Initiative

A person with AD may stop acting like his "old self." He may become confused, suspicious, or withdrawn. The most recognizable change is a lack of initiative and motivation. People with Alzheimer's may become apathetic toward activities that they once enjoyed. They might need prompting to become involved in normal activities, such as housework or social obligations. These changes are often misinterpreted as depression. Although depression and AD are interrelated, early-stage depression may be due solely to AD.

OTHER COMMON WARNING SIGNS OF ALZHEIMER'S DISEASE

The following are seven early warning signs of AD (WebMD, 2005).

1 Asking the same question over and over again
2 Repeating the same story, word for word, again and again
3 Forgetting how to cook, or how to make repairs, or how to play cards—activities that were previously done with ease and regularity
4 Losing one's ability to pay bills or balance one's checkbook
5 Getting lost in familiar surroundings or misplacing household objects
6 Neglecting to bathe, or wearing the same clothes over and over again, while insisting that one has taken a bath or that one's clothes are still clean

7   Relying on someone else, such as a spouse, to make decisions or answer questions one previously would have handled themselves

If someone has several or even most of these symptoms, it does not mean that the person definitely has the disease. It does mean that person should be thoroughly examined by a medical specialist who has been trained in evaluating memory disorders, such as a neurologist or a psychiatrist, or by a comprehensive memory disorder clinic with an entire team of experts with knowledge of memory problems.

FIRST SIGNS OF ALZHEIMER'S DISEASE

The early stage of AD is an area of much intrigue and research, since an early diagnosis can help the family and the individual participate equally in coping with the disease and anticipating the changes in lifestyle. The early signs of AD is consistent impairment of recent memory and, often, difficulty with spatial relations and poor judgment. Frequently the individual has difficulty with reasoning and language. The person may experience disorientation and poor concentration. Many of the symptoms overlap with the 10 warning signs discussed—as would be expected—but there are a few other behavioral symptoms, such as delusions, changes in sexuality, and diminished or lost sense of smell, that are worth noting. These symptoms may appear at the same time as memory loss or develop over time.

Difficulty With Spatial Relations

Agnosia is a term used to describe impairment of visual and spatial skills (i.e., the ability to discern between shapes and sizes and relate them to three-dimensional space). When people with Alzheimer's develop agnosia, their brains distort visual images, making it difficult to judge distances and recognize familiar shapes or objects. This phenomenon of a lack of depth perception may play itself out when a person with AD climbs the stairs. The person may stumble as a result of miscalculating where the steps are.

Changes in Sexuality

In most cases, diminished sex drive is more prevalent than a heightened sex drive. Men may have difficulty keeping an erection, and women may have difficulty with vaginal lubrication.

Diminished Coordination

Hand-eye coordination and rapid hand movements are affected in those with AD. This motor impairment can affect one's ability to drive, walk, or write. But most other physical functions are typically intact in the early stages of AD.

Diminished Sense of Smell

Though this is not a strong indicator of Alzheimer's, it has been suggested that people with AD tend to lose their sense of smell.

Abnormal Sleep Patterns

Another common change relates to a patient's sleep patterns. A person with AD may sleep during the day and be wide awake at night or may sleep for extended periods of time and have a low energy level in general.

THE FOUR A'S OF ALZHEIMER'S DISEASE

As mentioned repeatedly, cognitive disabilities are common in AD. A quick and easy way to identify these disabilities in AD is to apply the Four As—amnesia, aphasia, apraxia, and agnosia (Alzheimer's Foundation of America, 2007). Does the individual in question display any of the following?

Amnesia—Amnesia is the loss of memory. As pointed out, recent memory is lost first with dementia and remote memory remains intact until midway through the disease. Recent memory includes memory for facts or events that occurred within the past several hours, and remote memory refers to events that occurred months or years ago. For example, people with AD may forget names of people they met recently.

Aphasia—Aphasia is the inability to understand spoken or written words or the inability to communicate. Most aphasic patients develop communication deficits during the middle stages of AD. Receptive aphasia (i.e., the inability to understand spoken word) limits the patient's ability to understand instructions. For example, people with AD may not find the right words to communicate correctly (e.g., the word for "fork").

Apraxia—Apraxia is the inability to carry out a sequence of activities related to motor tasks, and this will limit a person's ability to participate in specific types of activities of daily living. Persons with AD begin to lose ability to perform complicated motor tasks early in the disease. The disabilities vary from individual to individual. For example, some people cannot put food on a fork and into their mouth but can still play a musical instrument. Others cannot dress themselves but can still shave. Persons with AD frequently lose fine motor skills and visual spatial ability, limiting their capacity for fine motor tasks. People in the early stage of Alzheimer's usually retain good skills; however, middle-stage people have multiple deficits, and late-stage persons frequently lack basic motor skills. (e.g., talking, walking, and self-feeding).

Agnosia—Agnosia is the inability to recognize preprogrammed sensory inputs. People with AD may forget faces, the appearance of specific objects (visual agnosia), or the "feel" of specific objects, as seen in tactile agnosia. People may have difficulty recognizing objects or familiar people (e.g., not able to recognize a son or daughter), while retaining an abundance of information about the objects or person. Persons with AD may be unable to touch objects and recognize them from the "feel." Sensory stimulation tasks may present a challenge to some Alzheimer's persons, while others may retain this ability. People also forget specific smells. Patients may not recognize specific objects as sharp or dangerous, although they can tell you that scissors can cut.

If a person is displaying any of these behaviors, further investigation should be conducted. Staging systems are an effective tool that can highlight symptoms of AD and identify how far along the disease has progressed.

STAGING SYSTEMS: THE PROGRESSION OF ALZHEIMER'S DISEASE

The remainder of this chapter outlines a few tools used in the medical community to delineate the many stages of AD. Each staging system focuses on different aspects of the disease, though there is overlap among all the tools. Some systems are primarily concerned with the loss of different skills or functions. Others focus on the cognitive impairments and use their increasing severity as markers for each stage. Regardless, by studying all the available systems, one will be able to see when the common symptoms began to present and how they become amplified as AD takes over the brain. Used in combination, these tools can assist a caretaker or loved one—even the individual afflicted—to take notice of signs of possible dementia and seek out appropriate care. Table 4.1 presents three stages of AD.

Table 4.1

COMMON STAGES OF ALZHEIMER'S DISEASE

STAGE/DURATION	DESCRIPTION
Stage I Forgetfulness stage Typically lasts from no time at all to about 5 years.	■ Apparent only to client or possibly family ■ No longer handles financial matters well ■ Covers up ■ Denial ■ Changes in social behavior
Stage II Confusional stage Can last anywhere from 2 to 12 years.	■ Definite impairment ■ Severe forgetfulness ■ Impaired orientation ■ Impaired concentration ■ Rambling speech ■ Past memories fairly intact ■ Moodiness ■ Lessened awareness ■ More problems with learning new material ■ Flattened affect ■ Takes less part in activities ■ Activity level will do nothing to defend against the deterioration
Stage III Demential stage Lasts approximately from 1 to 3 years.	■ Severely disoriented ■ Severely confused ■ Hallucinations, paranoid ideation ■ Agitation ■ Wandering; needs total supervision ■ Severely impaired judgment ■ Incontinence ■ Swallowing difficulties ■ Motor problems ■ Visual spatial problems, severe in nature ■ Infectious diseases

Adapted from "The Global Deterioration Scale for Assessment of Primary Degenerative Dementia," by B. Reisberg, S. H. Ferris, M. J. deLeon, and T. Crook, 1982, *American Journal of Psychiatry, 139,* p. 1137.

Table 4.2

FOUR STAGES OF ALZHEIMER'S DISEASE

INITIAL SYMPTOMS	MILD SYMPTOMS	INTERMEDIATE SYMPTOMS	SEVERE SYMPTOMS
Begins to show mild forgetfulness and has trouble with short-term memory of recent events, activities, names of familiar people or places.	Confusion and memory loss begin, as do disorientation of time and place and trouble performing routine tasks. Noticeable changes in personality, judgment, focus, and attention.	Difficulty performing the normal activities of daily living (e.g., feeding and bathing). Increased agitation and anxiety occur, along with erratic sleeping patterns, wandering and pacing, increased difficulty recognizing faces and recalling names.	Loss of speech, bladder control; requires full time care.

Table 4.2 breaks down the symptoms into four stages, and its simplicity demonstrates the progressive nature of the disease. Note the difference between mild and intermediate symptoms. Each stage is interdependent with the other, meaning that the symptoms from the earlier stages remain and the new symptoms are incorporated into the individual's behavior. Also, remember that every person is different, so all people with Alzheimer's will not display each and every symptom.

Table 4.3 presents detailed summary of the symptoms of AD from the early to the late stages and is a reference tool created by the Alzheimer's Association–South Central Wisconsin Chapter.

Figure 4.1 gives a visual representation of the classic symptoms of AD. These common symptoms can appear alone or overlap. One thing is clear: as the disease progresses, it becomes harder and harder for a person with AD to take care of himself or herself independently. The figure is also a solid representation of the high degree of variation with which AD manifests itself from person to person. Not all people will experience all these symptoms, but the figure shows the range of symptoms that is possible from the early to the late stages.

Table 4.3

ALZHEIMER'S DISEASE, EARLY TO LATE STAGES

EARLY STAGE	MIDDLE STAGE	LATE STAGE
The early stage of Alzheimer's disease typically lasts from almost no time at all to about 5 years. People in this stage generally show the following characteristics and/or symptoms:	The middle stage of Alzheimer's disease can last anywhere from 2 to 12 years. Symptoms described in the early stage become more obvious and evident. People in this stage generally show the following characteristics and/or symptoms:	The late stage of Alzheimer's disease lasts approximately from 1 to 3 years. People in this stage typically show the following characteristics and/or symptoms:

EARLY STAGE

Problems remembering most recent information; short-term memory loss
- Is unable to recall what was learned a few minutes, hours, or days ago
- Has no sense of recognition, as if the information was never given in the first place
- Has intact long-term memory; memories from years past are the clearest
- Repeats stories, statements, and requests

Difficulty performing familiar tasks
- Not turning on the oven or forgetting ingredients in an old familiar recipe
- Changes in follow-through or ability to pay bills, balance checkbook
- Changes in ability to follow through with usual grocery shopping routines

MIDDLE STAGE

Continues to remember less and less; forgets more quickly than in early stages
- Can't remember visits right after you leave
- Eventually forgets own name, names of spouse, children, and others
- Increasingly repeats statements, requests, actions

Increased difficulty or inability to perform familiar tasks
- May only be able to perform one step of a task at a time when instructed
- Needs help with everyday things such as bathing and dressing
- Has decreased attention span

Lack of or poor judgment
- Unable to judge safe conditions
- May act in unsafe ways (no coat in winter, leaves stove on)
- May act in inappropriate ways (undress in public, act out sexually)

LATE STAGE

Little or no short-term memory remains
- May have unpredictable moments when a memory surfaces or the person responds to something from the past
- Is only in the present now

Inability to perform tasks
- Unable to bathe, dress, eat, and go to the bathroom without assistance
- May be able to perform a small, very simple step of a task with assistance

(continued)

77

Table 4.3

ALZHEIMER'S DISEASE, EARLY TO LATE STAGES (continued)

EARLY STAGE	MIDDLE STAGE	LATE STAGE
Altered or decreased judgment ■ Changes in ability to set usual limits on purchases (buying everything offered for sale on TV, or writing checks to any salesperson who comes to the door or solicits over the phone or through the mail) ■ Putting items in unusual places (firewood in clothes dryer, portable phone in the refrigerator) ■ Dressing inappropriately for weather	*Language changes* ■ Unable to find the right word or remember names of simple objects ■ May be unable to understand what is being said ■ Is able to communicate non-verbally—body language, emotions ■ May be able to react to non-verbal communication of others but may misinterpret	*Complete lack of judgment* *Unable to use words to communicate* ■ Communication becomes mostly nonverbal ■ May groan, scream, or make grunting noises
Language Changes ■ Forgetting names of common objects ■ Difficulty coming up with the right words to use—talks around things	*Changes in mood, behavior and personality* ■ May be suspicious, irritable, teary or silly ■ Anxiety and frustration become more evident; may begin to have difficulty with emotional and impulse control and his effect on others ■ May imagine he hears or sees things that are really not there ■ May have increased restlessness, wandering, and/or noticeable decrease in functioning later in the day	*May want to put everything into mouth, or touch, or grab for everything* *Cannot recognize family or self in mirror* *The ability to perceive the environment through the senses continues to decline through the senses* ■ May have trouble chewing and/or swallowing ■ May lose ability to walk ■ Likely to be incontinent of urine and stool
Changes in mood, behavior, personality ■ Engages in behaviors that are out of character, such as crying, swearing, angry outbursts, rudeness, or withdrawal from usual activities ■ Having a numb or flat emotional response to an event that would usually get a more connected response, such as a death in the family or a car accident ■ Wearing dirty clothes when usually immaculate in appearance	*Confused about time and place* ■ Doesn't know where she is ■ Loses all sense of time ■ May confuse day and night *Loses ability to abstract thinking* ■ Loses personality and/or sense of self; loses ability to understand	

Disorientation to time and place

- Not knowing consistently where he or she is
- Getting lost in familiar places
- Not knowing the time of day, day of week, month, or year

Problem with abstract thinking

- Changes in ability to make patterns from data or to interpret meaning of something he is seeing
- Loss of initiative; unable to conceptualize how to start a task but can finish it once told/shown
- Unable to make patterns from data and reliably interpret the meaning of what she is seeing or hearing
- Unable to hold onto two thoughts or ideas at the same time

Changes in the ability to perceive the environment through the senses

- Visual changes in depth perception makes print and pattern confusing; pattern in a rug may appear as holes in floor, shadows may become frightening holes or seem strange and threatening, and it might seem as if the car she is riding in is continually going to crash into things
- Smell and tastes are altered. Foods may taste different and/or appetite may be diminished because of taste and smell changes
- Sense of touch is altered with regards to ability to interpret temperature; may no longer feel how hot a radiator, stove, or frying pan is
- Hearing is altered. Sound discrimination becomes more difficult; everything may sound garbled. The ability to mask out background sounds in order to focus becomes increasingly difficult

Changes occur physically

- May lose control of bladder and/or bowel function
- May be less steady when walking or develop an altered gait
- May begin losing weight

Source: "Planning Guide for Dementia Care at Home: A Reference Tool for Care Managers," Developed by the Alzheimer's Association—South Central Wisconsin Chapter, the Wisconsin Alzheimer's Institute, and the Wisconsin Bureau of Aging and Long Term Care Resources, Division of Disability and Elder Services, Department of Health and Family Services (3/2004 Revision) Document Number PDE-3195, Part 2.

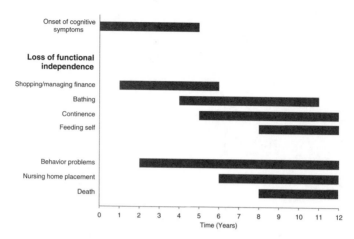

Figure 4.1 Typical occurrence of manifestations of Alzheimer's disease.
Source: "Advances in the Treatment of Alzheimer's Disease," by P. D. Sloane, 1998, *American Family Physician, 58,* p. 1579. Copyright © 1998 American Academy of Family Physicians. All rights reserved. Adapted with permission.

WHAT NEXT?

In an ideal world, once it is clear that an individual has AD, the family and caregivers can seek out assistance and prepare for a comfortable future, despite the uncomfortable circumstances. Unfortunately, many detrimental societal and psychological factors come into play once a diagnosis has been made. Lisa Snyder, LCSW, at the University of California, has identified six common themes among people diagnosed with Alzheimer's disease—denial, ambivalence, resistance to change, fear, memory loss, and low self-esteem (Bryce, 2000). Just like the symptoms of AD, these factors can be identified and addressed so that proper actions can eventually be implemented. Let's take a look at each of these themes in detail.

Denial

Denial is a normal, psychological defense that everyone uses to cope with an uncomfortable issue or situation. People diagnosed with AD may feel like dissociating themselves from the diagnosis because of the stigma attached to the disease. Even the close community outside an individual—their family, friends, coworkers—may not want to accept the diagnosis, since they will also be affected in some way. It is also possible that a person with Alzheimer's may forget that he has the disease. In either case, people with AD and their families need emotional support to help them through accepting and eventually pursuing proper treatment.

Ambivalence in Disclosing the Diagnosis

With so many gray areas surrounding AD, there are many myths about the disease. Is it contagious? Will one be ostracized by the community? These negative attitudes can proliferate without proper education about Alzheimer's. It all starts in the doctor's office. If the doctor does not disclose the diagnosis in a healthy, productive manner, the chain of ambivalence will continue and proliferate.

Wanting Things to Stay the Same

Alzheimer's disease is progressive—it's always changing. This lack of control over one's life is alarming and difficult to accept. This resistance to change is a common phenomenon among people diagnosed with AD.

Fear of the Future

As an individual with Alzheimer's loses the ability to function normally, a fear that one is losing a part of oneself arises. "What's going to happen to me?" is a question that many with the disease ask.

Day-to-Day Experiences of Memory Loss

Memory loss that changes from one day to the next is an unusual challenge to cope with, according to people with AD. "I take a step before doing something and ask, 'Am I the same person? Can I do this?'"

Changes in Self-Esteem and Self-Concept

Alzheimer's disease places people in a life where change is constant, making it hard for them to define themselves. A mother's maternal skills may gradually diminish, an editor may lose his ability to recall words.

People with Alzheimer's disease should remember that they are still people who will continue to be remembered for their role and qualities they had in the past and the ones they will hold in the future. Since long-term memory often stays intact, even in AD's late stages, one can engage in activities that recall one's previous interests and talents, which can enhance peace of mind and autonomy.

5

Diagnosis and Assessment of Alzheimer's Disease

It's time to change the way doctors diagnose Alzheimer's disease, says an international panel of experts.

WebMD

This chapter explores the impact of obtaining an accurate diagnosis and identifying diagnostic tools for AD that have proven to be reliable. Diagnosis of Alzheimer's is difficult, because there are no definite tests for the disease. The diagnosis is made clinically through a systemic assessment that eliminates other possible causes. A diagnosis of AD is "probable," meaning that other causes of the symptoms have been ruled out and the most likely cause is AD (Mayo Clinic, 2007).

At present, there are only two ways to confirm the presence of AD in an individual. One option is a postmortem, which can establish beyond doubt whether AD was present. Another option is a brain biopsy, a surgical procedure in which brain tissue is removed and examined for tiny lesions characteristic of AD. Though this method is reliable, undergoing a brain biopsy is a dangerous procedure, and it is rarely recommended as a diagnostic tool. There is currently no single test that accurately diagnoses AD, so physicians use a variety of assessments and laboratory measurements to make a diagnosis.

EARLY DIAGNOSIS

The diagnosis of AD is its own burden, often leading people with AD and their families to avoid testing or evaluation (Tangalos, 2003). A recent study shows that a diagnosis of AD is typically delayed by nearly 3 years from the start of symptoms (WebMD, 2005). People with AD and their families should know that there are a number of benefits to an early diagnosis.

Early diagnosis may help people avoid taking unnecessary medications and therapies and may help them and their family members to make better and timely decisions. Early diagnosis also allows families to address legal, financial, and personal matters, while enabling people with AD to take a part in the process (Tangalos, 2003). Early diagnosis also increases the opportunity to make maximum use of treatments and services available to people with AD; early intervention may enhance drug therapy outcomes. There is growing evidence that an early diagnosis and targeted management can preserve function and independence and promote quality of life for people with AD and their caregivers.

Alzheimer's disease is not only a problem of memory; it is also an impairment of problem solving. An understanding of the manifestations of the various stages is necessary to effectively take care of a patient throughout the continuum of disease progression. With early diagnosis, a plan of care—including measures to enhance patient safety—may be implemented.

ACCURATE DIAGNOSIS OF ALZHEIMER'S DISEASE

Studies have shown that the clinical diagnosis of AD is often inaccurate when compared with neuropathologic findings (Silverman & Thompson, 2006). Accuracy continues to improve, but physicians cannot be 100% sure of an AD diagnosis. Physicians, through testing and "process of elimination," can diagnose probable Alzheimer's with almost 90% accuracy (Simon, 2000).

Other diseases that can cause similar symptoms can be ruled out in the process and treated. A report from the World Alzheimer Congress 2000 stated that in a group of people showing minor memory problems, AD was the cause in less than half of the cases; in fact, about 20% had problems that could be reversed with treatment (Simon, 2000). The report also stated that depression, thyroid disease, high blood pressure, and alcohol dependence are among many other illnesses whose symptoms mimic those of AD. An accurate diagnosis of dementia is essential since many of these disorders are treatable. In the early stages of Alzheimer's, memory loss may go unrecognized or be attributed to normal aging. Once other potential problems are ruled out, it is likely that the diagnosis of AD is accurate. The sooner the family is confident of the Alzheimer's diagnosis, the sooner the treatment can begin to help alleviate the symptoms and possibly slow the progression of the disease.

MAKING THE DIAGNOSIS

There is currently no single test that can detect AD, thus making the diagnosis of AD complex and time-consuming. To reach an accurate diagnosis, sometimes a person has to see a number of health care professionals. In 1984, the National Institute of Neurological and Communicative Disorders and Stroke and the Alzheimer's Disease and Related Diseases Association (NINCDS-ARDA) established diagnostic criteria designed for research purposes and clinical definition (McKhann et al., 1984). Again, in 2001, the American Academy of Neurology (AAN) recommended a classification for the diagnosis of AD (Knopman et al., 2001). This classification is divided into definite, probable, and possible AD. According to AAN, in addition to histopathological confirmation, definite AD requires the clinical finding of dementia as determined by the Mini-Mental Status Exam (MMSE) or other standardized neuropsychological testing; the exam must demonstrate deficits in two or more areas of cognition with progressive memory loss in the absence of delirium.

We'll now discuss the main diagnostic tools, which for simplicity can be divided into three categories—history and physical exam, neuropsychological assessment, and neurodiagnostic tests. Table 5.1 summarizes the Alzheimer's diagnostic process.

History and Physical Exam

The diagnosis of AD begins with a complete medical history and thorough physical exam.

Patient History

History includes a thorough review of the individual's family history and a detailed evaluation of changes in mental abilities, personality, mood, and

Table 5.1

DIAGNOSIS AND ASSESSMENT OF ALZHEIMER'S DISEASE

HISTORY AND PHYSICAL EXAM	NEUROPSYCHOLOGICAL ASSESSMENT	NEURODIAGNOSTIC TESTS

Patient history
Physical
    examination
	Mini-Mental State
	    Examination
	Mini-Cog Test
	Clock Drawing Test
	Brief Cognitive Rating Scale
	Neuropsychiatric Inventory
	    Questionnaire
	Severe Impairment Battery
	Alzheimer's Disease
	    Cooperative Study Activities
	    of Daily Living
	Activities of Daily Living
	Instrumental Activities
	    of Daily Living
	Functional Staging Score Test
	Numeric Pain Rating Scale
	Faces Pain Rating Scale
	Discomfort Scale for Dementia
	    of the Alzheimer's Type
	Checklist of Non-Verbal
	    Indicators
	Pain Assessment Checklist for
	    Seniors with Limited Ability
	    to Communicate
	Pain Assessment for the
	    Dementing Elderly
	Pain Assessment in
	    Advanced Dementia
		Laboratory tests
		Computer tomography
		Magnetic resonance imaging
		Positron emission tomography
		Single photon emission
		    computed tomography
		Magnetic resonance
		    spectroscopy imaging
		Electroencephalography
		Electrocardiogram

behavior, including when and how the individual's symptoms developed (Harvard Health Publications, 2007). The individual, family members, caregivers, and friends may be asked questions regarding the person's symptoms at present and in the past. There will be questions about past illnesses and about family medical and psychiatric history. The physician will obtain a history of medical conditions affecting other family members, especially whether they may have had AD or a related disorder.

A history from the individual helps the physician assess a person's past and current health situation. Full disclosure of a person's past and current medical conditions and procedures, surgeries, and traumas, and a complete list of medications, vitamins, herbs, and supplements is necessary to determine a diagnosis. Information about diet, lifestyle, and family history of disease is also important.

Frequently, an inciting event that disrupts coping skills—such as a hospitalization or the death of a spouse—draws the attention of family members to a person's memory problems. Generally, AD is characterized by a gradually progressive decline that occurs over years, and it is important to ascertain the period during which the memory symptoms developed. The family may describe an acute onset of memory impairment that follows the inciting event, but careful questioning frequently elucidates memory problems that predate that time and indicate a gradually progressive course (Carlsson, Gleason, & Asthana, 2005). The progressive loss of memory in recent events is highlighted, with examples of missed appointments, bills paid late, and stories repeated on the phone. A decreased initiative and planning ability is often quite striking, with reduced participation in conversation.

In addition to memory decline, the diagnosis of AD requires a change in one other intellectual domain, such as using language, recognizing objects and people, using tools, planning, and adjusting to circumstances, that interferes with activities of daily living (ADLs) and represents a decline from a previous level of functioning (Gauthier, 2000). An estimate of a person's baseline level of functioning may be based on educational background as well as on occupational history, including detailed information on the highest-level tasks associated with his vocation (Carlsson, Gleason, & Asthana, 2005). For persons who have not worked outside the home, questions about hobbies, household management, and volunteer activities may provide important information about the patient's previous level of functioning.

Information is obtained about physical complaints or symptoms, such as loss of coordination, sudden vision problems, or weakness (Harvard Health Publications, 2007). Changes in instrumental activities of daily living (IADLs) such as using the telephone, grocery shopping, managing finances, doing laundry, and driving can help identify areas in which there is functional decline (Carlsson, Gleason, & Asthana, 2005). A history of cardiovascular disease or associated risk factors, coronary artery bypass surgery, head injury, seizures, depression, Parkinson's disease, or alcohol abuse may help clarify the underlying cause of memory loss. Also obtained is comprehensive information about incidents that risked the patient's safety—having car accidents, getting lost, wandering, managing medication, starting kitchen fires, being an unwitting victim of financial scams, and hunting or other use of firearms. Information is gathered on depression, tremors, rigidity, falls, dysphagia, urinary incontinence, symptoms of stroke or transient ischemic attack, waxing and waning level of consciousness, and visual hallucinations (Carlsson, Gleason, & Asthana, 2005). This may seem like a lot of information, but the person's history is part of the foundation for the physician's diagnostic workup. It enables the physician to construct a list of possible diagnoses that will guide the medical evaluation that follows (Harvard Health Publications, 2007).

Physical Exam

The physical examination is part of the diagnosis process and enables the physician to assess the overall physical condition of the patient. If the patient has a medical complaint, the physical exam provides the physician with more information about the problem, which helps determine an appropriate plan of treatment.

A complete physical exam includes assessment of conditions that could cause dementia. The physician will also assess risk factors for dementia, such as family history, education and occupation status, alcohol use, head injury, and heart disease. A physical exam may include evaluation of disorders as diverse as heart failure, liver disease, kidney failure, thyroid disorders, and respiratory diseases, which can cause dementia-like changes (Carlsson, Gleason, & Asthana, 2005).

A complete neurological exam including muscle tone and strength, coordination, speech, reflexes, senses, eye movement, and the pupils' reaction to light will be conducted to access the health of specific areas of the brain (Alzheimer's Association, 2007b). These types of abnormalities are not usually features of early AD. For example, unequal reflexes or weakness on one side of the body suggests localized brain damage such as stroke or tumor, while tremors or other involuntary movements may indicate a degenerative disorder such as Parkinson's disease (Carlsson, Gleason, & Asthana, 2005).

Neuropsychological Assessment

Neuropsychological testing studies the relationship between the brain and behavior. It provides critical adjunctive information for the diagnosis of conditions such as dementia. It enables a clinician to analyze a patient's cognitive status, as well as emotional, psychological, motor, and sensory functions (Alzheimer Research Forum, 2007).

Neuropsychological assessment is used when the patient is having serious problems with memory, concentration, ability to remember words and names or to understand language, and a variety of other symptoms (WebMD, 2007c). Neuropsychological assessment can also help a physician and a family better understand the effect of a disorder on the person with AD's everyday functioning. Such quantitation provides a number of benefits:

- Neuropsychological testing is a relatively sensitive and specific diagnostic tool for AD and can help distinguish AD from other neurological illnesses.
- Testing provides a way to track and document the progression of the disease.
- Tests allow for the systematic description of the various symptoms that are being experienced by the patient so that each can be addressed for optimal care.

There are a number of neuropsychological tests available to clinicians for the diagnosis of AD. The next section covers the most commonly used assessment in a clinical setting to assess cognition, function, and pain in dementia.

Mini-Mental State Examination

The Mini-Mental State Examination (MMSE) is a brief test that measures the cognitive status in adults and measures a person's problem-solving skills, attention span, counting skills, and memory. It consists of a simplified, scored form with 11 questions (Table 5.2). The test asks the patient a series of questions to collect basic information concerning their surroundings. This portion of the MMSE will give the physician insight into whether there has been damage to different areas of the brain. It requires only 5–10 minutes to administer, making it practical for screening at-risk populations (Tangalos et al., 1996). The MMSE may not be useful at the extreme ends of the 30-point scale to determine who is or is not impaired. It also may not be useful at the higher levels, particularly in younger patients.

Mini-Cog Test

The Mini-Cog Test, developed by Dr. Soo Borson and colleagues and endorsed by the American Geriatrics Society, is used in screening older adult patients for dementia. It is a very simple and quick test carried out

Table 5.2

THE MINI-MENTAL STATE EXAMINATION (MMSE)

CATEGORY	POINTS	QUESTIONS
1. Orientation	10	■ Year, season, date, day of week, and month ■ State, county, town, or city ■ Hospital or clinic, floor

2. Registration	3	■ Name three objects: Apple, table, penny
		  ■ Each one spoken distinctly and with brief pause
		  ■ Patient repeats all three (one point for each)
		■ Repeat process until all three objects learned
		■ Record number of trials needed to learn all three objects

3. Attention and calculation	5	■ Spell WORLD backwards: DLROW
		  ■ Points given up to first misplaced letter
		  ■ Example: DLORW scored as two points only

4. Recall	3	Recite the three objects memorized in 2, Registration

5. Language	9	Patient names two objects when they are displayed
		  ■ Example: Pencil and watch (two points each)
		Repeats a sentence: "No ifs, ands, or buts"
		Follows three-stage command:
		  ■ Take a paper in your right hand
		  ■ Fold it in half
		  ■ Put it on the floor
		Reads and obeys the following:
		  ■ Close your eyes
		  ■ Write a sentence
		Copies the design (picture of two overlapped pentagons)

Source: "Mini-Mental State: A Practical Method for Grading the Cognitive State of Patients for the Clinician," by M. F. Folstein, S. Folstein, and P. R. McHugh, 1975, *Journal of Psychiatric Research, 12,* pp. 196–197. Copyright © 1975 Elsevier.

in the primary care setting and takes about 3 minutes to administer (American Association for Geriatric Psychiatry, 2003). The test consists of a three-item recall—also included in the MMSE—in which the person is asked to repeat three unrelated words and then asked to recall the three words. Those who are unable to recall any of the three words are categorized as probably demented. If they can recall all three words, then they are categorized as probably not demented. The Mini-Cog test results only contribute to a diagnosis of dementia. The test cannot be used in isolation as a diagnostic test for AD.

Clock Drawing Test

The Clock Drawing Test (CDT) is a simple test that can be used as part of a neurological test or as a screening tool for Alzheimer's and other types of dementia (Wolf-Klein, Silverstone, Levy, & Brod, 1989). The person undergoing testing is asked to draw a clock and to put the numbers in their appropriate locations. The patient is then instructed to draw specific hours on the clock (i.e., 3:00 or 11:15). There are a number of scoring systems for this test. The AD Cooperative Scoring System is based on a score of five points. Patients are scored as follows:

1 point for the clock circle

1 point for all the numbers being in the correct order

1 point for the numbers being in the proper special order

1 point for the two hands of the clock

1 point for the correct time

A normal score is 4 or 5 points.

The test can provide huge amounts of information about general cognitive and adaptive functioning such as memory and how people are able to process information and vision (About.com, 2007). A normal CDT (i.e., the clock is normally constructed) almost always predicts that a person's cognitive abilities are within normal limits and that the person is probably not demented. If the person draws a clock that is in any way abnormal, she is considered probably demented. The CDT does offer specific clues about the area of change or damage. Research varies on the ability of the CDT to differentiate between, for example, vascular dementia and AD.

Brief Cognitive Rating Scale

The Brief Cognitive Rating Scale (BCRS) is an assessment tool to be used with the Global Deterioration Scale (GDS) for assessment of

Table 5.3

THE BRIEF COGNITIVE RATING SCALE (BCRS)

Axis I: Concentration	Rating
No objective or subjective evidence of deficit in concentration.	1
Subjective decrement in concentration ability.	2
Minor objective signs of poor concentration (e.g., subtraction of serial 7s from 100).	3
Definite concentration deficit for persons of their backgrounds (e.g., marked deficit on serial 7s from 100; frequent deficit in subtraction of serial 4s from 40).	4
Marked concentration deficit (e.g., giving months backwards or serial 2s from 20).	5
Forgets the concentration task. Frequently begins to count forward when asked to count backwards from 10 by 1s.	6
Marked difficulty counting forward to 10 by 1s.	7

Axis II: Recent memory	Rating
No objective or subjective evidence of deficit in recent memory.	1
Subjective impairment only (e.g., forgetting names more than formerly).	2
Deficit in recall of specific events evident upon detailed questioning. No deficit in recall of major recent events.	3
Cannot recall major events of previous weekend or week. Scanty knowledge (not detailed) of current events, favorite TV shows, and so on.	4
Unsure of weather; may not know current president or current address.	5
Occasional knowledge of some events. Little or no idea of current address, weather, and so on.	6
No knowledge of any recent events.	7

Axis III: Past memory	Rating
No subjective or objective impairment in past memory.	1
Subjective impairment only. Can recall two or more primary school teachers.	2
Some gaps in past memory upon detailed questioning. Able to recall at least one childhood teacher and/or one childhood friend.	3
Clear-cut deficit. The spouse recalls more of the patient's past than the patient. Cannot recall childhood friends and/or teachers but knows the names of most schools attended. Confuses chronology in reciting personal history.	4
Major past events sometimes not recalled (e.g., names of schools attended).	5
Some residual memory of past (e.g., may recall country of birth or former occupation).	6
No memory of past.	7

Table 5.3

THE BRIEF COGNITIVE RATING SCALE (BCRS)

Axis IV: Orientation	Rating
No deficit in memory for time, place, identify of self or others.	1
Subjective impairment only. Knows time to nearest hour, location.	2
Any mistakes in time > 2 hours: day of week > 1 day; date > 3 days.	3
Mistakes in month > 10 days or year > 1 month.	4
Unsure of month and/or year and/or season; unsure of locale.	5
No idea of date. Identifies spouse but may not recall name. Knows own name.	6
Cannot identify spouse. May be unsure of personal identity.	7

Axis V: Functioning and self-care	Rating
No difficulty, either subjectively or objectively.	1
Complains of forgetting location of objects. Subjective work difficulties.	2
Decreased job functioning evident to coworkers. Difficulty traveling to new locations.	3
Decreased ability to perform complex tasks (e.g., planning dinner for guests, handling finances, marketing, etc.).	4
Requires assistance in choosing proper clothing.	5
Requires assistance in feeding, and/or toileting, and/or bathing, and/or ambulating.	6
Requires constant assistance in all activities of daily life.	7

Total score

Source: "The Brief Cognitive Rating Scale (BCRS): Findings in Primary Degenerative De-mentia (PDD)," by B. Reisberg et al., 1983, *Psychopharmacology Bulletin, 19,* pp. 48–49. Reprinted with permission from MedWorks Media Global, LLC.

primary degenerative dementia to help stage a person suffering from a primary degenerative dementia such as AD (Reisberg, Schneck, Ferris, Schwartz, & deLeon, 1983). This assessment tool tests five different areas known as axis, four cognitive and one functional (Table 5.3). For the first four axis (i.e., cognitive), a clinician will ask a variety of questions to determine the level of impairment. The results of the fifth axis (i.e., functioning) are determined primarily by observation. After a score is determined for each axis, the clinician totals the results and divides by 5. This answer will result in a stage corresponding on the GDS. The tester can also use the Functional Assessment Staging (FAST) scale for a more accurate assessment, which is described later in further detail.

Neuropsychiatric Inventory Questionnaire

The Neuropsychiatric Inventory Questionnaire (NPI-Q) is a rapidly administered instrument that provides a reliable assessment of behaviors commonly observed in patients with dementia (Cummings, Frank, Cherry, Kohatsu, & Kemp, 2002). The NPI-Q is a validated self-administered tool and is a brief, rapid, informant-based instrument that provides a reliable assessment of behaviors commonly observed in persons with AD (Table 5.4). The NPI-Q may be a useful tool because it assesses the severity of the symptom in the persons with dementia and the distress the symptom causes the caregiver.

Severe Impairment Battery

The Severe Impairment Battery (SIB) was proposed in 1990 in order to evaluate the cognitive abilities of people for whom standard cognitive measures are no longer adapted (Hugonot-Diener et al., 2003). Its purpose was to analyze different cognitive domains on the basis of the residual capacities of people with cognitive impairment. SIB is used to evaluate the cognitive function of severely impaired patients (i.e., those with an MMSE score < 15). It consists of a 0–100-point scale, based on a patient's performance of simple tasks in six major subscales: attention, orientation, language, memory, visuospatial ability, and construction. Persons with progressive dementia invariably evolve to a stage where they can no longer be tested by standard neuropsychological tests.

Alzheimer's Disease Cooperative Study–Activities of Daily Living

Alzheimer's Disease Cooperative Study–Activities of Daily Living (ADCS-ADL) was developed to describe performance of ADL by individuals with AD to identify which ADL are useful for assessment of people in clinical trials (Galasko et al., 1997). It is a 42-item evaluation

Table 5.4

NEUROPSYCHIATRIC INVENTORY QUESTIONNAIRE (NPI-Q)

Please answer the following questions based on *changes* that have occurred since the patient first began to experience memory problems.
Circle "yes" only if the symptom(s) has been present in the *past month*. Otherwise, circle "no." If circling yes, use the legend below to rate Severity (how it affects the patient) and Caregiver distress (how it affects you).

Severity
1 = Mild (noticeable, but not
    a significant change)
2 = Moderate (significant, but not
    a dramatic change)
3 = Severe (very marked or
    prominent; a dramatic change)

Caregiver distress
0 = Not distressing at all
1 = Minimal (slightly distressing, not
    a problem to cope with)
2 = Mild (not very distressing,
    generally easy to cope with)
3 = Moderate (fairly distressing, not
    always easy to cope with)
4 = Severe (very distressing,
    difficult to cope with)
5 = Extreme or very severe (extremely
    distressing, unable to cope with)

	Answer	Severity	Caregiver distress
Delusions Does the patient believe that others are stealing from him or her, or planning to harm him or her in some way?	Yes No	1 2 3	0 1 2 3 4 5
Hallucinations Does the patient act as if he or she hears voices? Does he or she talk to people who are not there?	Yes No	1 2 3	0 1 2 3 4 5
Agitation or aggression Is the patient stubborn and resistive to help from others?	Yes No	1 2 3	0 1 2 3 4 5
Depression or dysphoria Does the patient act as if he or she is sad or in low spirits? Does he or she cry?	Yes No	1 2 3	0 1 2 3 4 5
Anxiety Does the patient become upset when separated from you? Does he or she have any other signs of nervousness, such as shortness of breath, sighing, being unable to relax, or feeling excessively tense?	Yes No	1 2 3	0 1 2 3 4 5

(continued)

Table 5.4

NEUROPSYCHIATRIC INVENTORY QUESTIONNAIRE (NPI-Q) *(continued)*

	Answer	Severity	Caregiver distress
Elation or euphoria Does the patient appear to feel too good or act excessively happy?	Yes No	1 2 3	0 1 2 3 4 5
Apathy or indifference Does the patient seem less interested in his or her usual activities and in the activities and plans of others?	Yes No	1 2 3	0 1 2 3 4 5
Disinhibition Does the patient seem to act impulsively? For example, does the patient talk to strangers as if he or she knows them, or does the patient say things that may hurt people's feelings?	Yes No	1 2 3	0 1 2 3 4 5
Irritability or lability Is the patient impatient and cranky? Does he or she have difficulty coping with delays or waiting for planned activities?	Yes No	1 2 3	0 1 2 3 4 5
Motor disturbance Does the patient engage in repetitive activities, such as pacing around the house, handling buttons, wrapping string, or doing other things repeatedly?	Yes No	1 2 3	0 1 2 3 4 5
Nighttime behaviors Does the patient awaken you during the night, rise too early in the morning, or take excessive naps during the day?	Yes No	1 2 3	0 1 2 3 4 5
Appetite and eating Has the patient lost or gained weight, or had a change in the food he or she likes?	Yes No	1 2 3	0 1 2 3 4 5

Source: "The Validation of the NPI-Q, A Brief Clinical Form of the Neuropsychiatric Inventory," by D. I. Kaufer et al., 2000, *Journal of Neuropsychiatry and Clinical Neuroscience, 12*(2), pp. 233-239. Reprinted with permission.

test that provides information about cognitive deficits and functional and behavioral manifestations of the disease. It consists of a series of questions to elicit a person's ability to perform one of the ADLs. The scores depict the range from total independence to total inability.

Activities of Daily Living

There are many ADL scales, but the Katz ADL is the most appropriate instrument to assess functional status as a measurement of the client's ability to perform ADL independently (Wallace & Shelkey, 2007). Clinicians typically use the tool to detect problems in performing activities of daily living and to plan care accordingly. The Katz ADL is most effectively used among older adults in a variety of care settings and compares baseline measurements (i.e., those taken when the client is well) to subsequent measures.

The Katz ADL scale is used widely to determine degrees of a patient's functional impairment and measures bathing, dressing, toileting, transferring, continence, and feeding (Table 5.5). The Index ranks adequacy of performance in six functions: bathing, dressing, toileting, transferring, continence, and feeding. Clients are scored yes/no for independence in each of the 6 functions. A score of 6 indicates full function, 4 indicates moderate impairment, and 2 or less indicates severe functional impairment. The ADL instrument can be repeated to determine changing needs for assistance.

Instrumental Activities of Daily Living

A separate IADL allows a health professional to establish the levels at which an elderly individual functions when caring for himself and performing the more sophisticated tasks of everyday life (Tangalos, 2003). The IADL scale includes 8 items: telephoning, shopping, preparing food, housekeeping, doing laundry, driving or using another mode of transport, managing finances, and taking responsibility for own medication. This instrument measures seven areas of more complex activities required for optimal independent functioning (Table 5.6). As with the ADL scale, the IADL instrument may be repeated periodically to determine the need for more support. An in-home assessment may identify environmental supports needed to maximize the patient's function, ensure the patient's safety, and minimize the primary caregiver's distress.

Table 5.5

THE KATZ ADL SCALE

ACTIVITIES Points (1 or 0)	INDEPENDENCE (1 point) *No* supervision, direction, or personal assistance	DEPENDENCE (0 points) *With* supervision, direction, personal assistance, or total care
Bathing Points:_____	Bathes self completely or needs help in bathing only a single part of the body such as the back, genital area, or disabled extremity.	Needs help with bathing more than one part of the body, getting in or out of the tub or shower. Requires total bathing.
Dressing Points:_____	Gets clothes from closets and drawers and puts on clothes and outer garments complete with fasteners. May have help tying shoes.	Needs help with dressing self or needs to be completely dressed.
Toileting Points:_____	Goes to toilet, gets on and off, arranges clothes, cleans genital area without help.	Needs help transferring to the toilet, cleaning self or uses bedpan or commode.
Transferring Points:_____	Moves in and out of bed or chair unassisted. Mechanical transferring aides are acceptable.	Needs help in moving from bed to chair or requires a complete transfer.
Continence Points:_____	Exercises complete self-control over urination and defecation.	Is partially or totally incontinent of bowel or bladder.
Feeding Points:_____	Gets food from plate into mouth without help. Preparation of food may be done by another person.	Needs partial or total help with feeding or requires parenteral feeding.

Source: "Progress in the Development of the Index of ADL," by S. Katz, T. D. Down, H. R. Cash, and R. C. Grotz, 1970, *Gerontologist, 10,* p. 21. Copyright © The Gerontological Society of America. Reproduced by permission of the publisher.

Table 5.6

ASSESSMENT OF INSTRUMENTAL ACTIVITIES OF DAILY LIVING (IADL)

A. Ability to use telephone
1. Operates telephone on own initiative; looks up and dials numbers, and so on.   1
2. Dials a few well-known numbers   1
3. Answers telephone but does not dial   1
4. Does not use telephone at all   0

A. Ability to use telephone	1

B. Shopping
1. Takes care of all shopping needs independently   1
2. Shops independently for small purchases   0
3. Needs to be accompanied on any shopping trip   0
4. Completely unable to shop   0

C. Food Preparation
1. Plans, prepares, and serves adequate meals independently   1
2. Prepares adequate meals if supplied with ingredients   0
3. Heats, serves, and prepares meals or prepares meals but does not maintain adequate diet   0
4. Needs to have meals prepared and served   0

D. Housekeeping
1. Maintains house alone or with occasional assistance (e.g., "heavy work domestic help")   1
2. Performs light daily tasks such as dishwashing, bed making   1
3. Performs light daily tasks but cannot maintain acceptable level of cleanliness   1
4. Needs help with all home maintenance tasks   1
5. Does not participate in any housekeeping tasks   0

E. Laundry
1. Does personal laundry completely   1
2. Launders small items; rinses stockings, etc.   1
3. All laundry must be done by others   0

F. Mode of Transportation
1. Travels independently on public transportation or drives own car   1
2. Arranges own travel via taxi but does not otherwise use public transportation   1
3. Travels on public transportation when accompanied by another   1
4. Travel limited to taxi or automobile with assistance of another   0
5. Does not travel at all   0

G. Responsibility for own medications
1. Is responsible for taking medication in correct dosages at correct time   1
2. Takes responsibility if medication is prepared in advance in separate dosage   0
3. Is not capable of dispensing own medication   0

H. Ability to handle finances
1. Manages financial matters independently (budgets, writes checks, pays rent, bills, goes to bank), collects and keeps track of income   1
2. Manages day-to-day purchases but needs help with banking, major purchases, etc.   1
3. Incapable of handling money   0

Source: "Assessment of Older People: Self-Maintaining and Instrumental Activities of Daily Living," by M. P. Lawton and E. M. Brody, 1969, *Gerontologist, 9,* p. 181. Copyright © The Gerontological Society of America. Reproduced by permission of the publisher.

Functional Assessment Staging Test

Functional Assessment Staging Test (FAST) was developed to assess a person's ability to perform daily and necessary life activities throughout the entire course of AD (Sclan & Reisberg, 1992). The test evaluates the changes in functional performance (Table 5.7). The FAST consists of a checklist of functions required for daily living that is divided into seven major stages, from normality (FAST stage 1) to severe dementia (FAST stage 7). Stages 6 and 7 are further divided into 11 substages (6a to 6e and 7a to 7f), each of which is based on specific functional deficits.

FAST evaluates the progression of functional decline in clients with uncomplicated dementia or AD. It also provides an indication of the level of care that is required for a person who has AD. The information learned from these tests helps determine whether a person has AD with an accuracy rate of about 90%.

Pain Assessment

An estimated 70% of older adults suffer from chronic pain (Mobily, Herr, Clark, & Wallace, 1994). However, assessing pain in elders with dementia, especially those with late-stage dementia, is challenging. Therefore, pain is frequently overlooked during probable Alzheimer's diagnosis assessment, but it not only affects functional status and the quality of life in people with AD but also leads to agitation and behavioral changes.

In the disease's early stages, complaints of discomfort or pain by persons with probable AD are considered as reliable as those of cognitively intact persons. As AD advances, pain often goes unreported because persons with AD can't communicate what they are feeling. This loss has a significant emotional impact on caregivers and also affects their ability to monitor the comfort and well-being of the individual with AD. Developing effective ways to help caregivers identify pain in individuals with impaired communication may improve quality of life for individuals with dementia and their caregivers.

Many pain scales are validated for use in adults. The two self-report pain assessment tools most commonly used in the clinical practice—the Numeric Pain Rating Scale and the Faces Pain Rating Scale—are considered useful in the early state of AD. Studies have been conducted comparing different pain scales in patients with dementia. Findings report that 86% of persons with an MMSE score of <15 could locate pain on themselves (Wynne, 2000). From this and other studies, it appears

Table 5.7

FUNCTIONAL ASSESSMENT STAGING TEST (FAST)				
FAST STAGE	**FUNCTIONAL ASSESSMENT**	**NO**	**YES**	**MONTHS**[a]
1	No difficulties, either subjectively or objectively.			
2	Complains of forgetting location of objects; subjective word finding difficulties only.			
3	Decreased job functioning evident to coworkers; difficulty in traveling to new locations.			
4	Decreased ability to perform complex tasks (e.g., planning dinner for guests; handling finances).			
5	Requires assistance in choosing proper clothing for the season or occasion.			
6a	Difficulty putting clothing on properly without assistance.			
6b	Unable to bathe properly; may develop fear of bathing. Will usually require assistance adjusting bath water temperature.			
6c	Inability to handle mechanics of toileting (i.e., forgets to flush; doesn't wipe properly).			
6d	Urinary incontinence, occasional or more frequent.			
6e	Fecal incontinence, occasional or more frequent.			
7a	Ability to speak limited to about half a dozen words in an average day.			
7b	Intelligible vocabulary limited to a single word in an average day.			
7c	Nonambulatory (unable to walk without assistance).			
7d	Unable to sit up independently.			
7e	Unable to smile.			
7f	Unable to hold head up.			

Note: Functional staging score = Highest FAST Stage checked.
[a] Number of months deficit has been noted.
Source: "Functional Assessment Staging (FAST)," by B. Reisberg, 1988, *Psychopharmacological Bulletin, 24,* p. 656. Reprinted with permission from MedWorks Media Global, LLC.

that using self to locate pain is the most reliable way to locate pain in those with significant cognitive impairment.

High completion failure rates have been noted in those with mild to moderate dementia (Agarwal, 2002). As the disease progresses to its middle and late stages, people with AD pose particular challenges because facial expressions and affect are often blunted from the disease process itself, and each individual may express pain in uniquely different ways. Patients may have difficulty reporting and identifying where they are experiencing pain. These people are dependent on health professionals to evaluate and treat discomfort through the observation of pain behaviors or facial expressions.

A pain assessment tool for advanced dementia allows a third party to observe a patient's discomfort, since the person cannot verbally express it. Although numerous scales exist, seven types of behavioral tools will be discussed here: Numeric Pain Rating Scale, Nonverbal Behavioral Pain Scale, Discomfort Scale for Dementia of the Alzheimer's Type, Checklist of Nonverbal Pain Indicators, Pain Assessment for the Dementing Elderly, Pain Assessment Checklist for Seniors with Limited Ability to Communicate and Pain Assessment in Advanced Dementia.

Numeric Pain Rating Scale (NPS). NPS is considered a useful pain assessment tool in Alzheimer's early stage. This scale is best used with individuals who can correctly express themselves. The most commonly used visual analog pain rating scale, it is a 100-mm line with 0 (no pain) at one end and 10 (worst pain possible) at the opposite end (Table 5.8). The person is asked to rate pain intensity by picking the number that most closely represents the level of pain that the person is experiencing.

Nonverbal Behavioral Pain Scale. Nonverbal Behavioral Pain Scale is also known as Faces Pain Rating Scale (FPS). FPS uses a series of faces that range from happy to sad with tears (Table 5.9). The person is asked to pick the face that best represents the pain that he is experiencing. It is best used with individuals who may be lacking in verbal skills but who

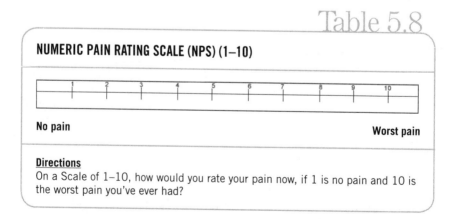

Table 5.8

NUMERIC PAIN RATING SCALE (NPS) (1–10)

| 1 | 2 | 3 | 4 | 5 | 6 | 7 | 8 | 9 | 10 |

No pain   **Worst pain**

<u>Directions</u>
On a Scale of 1–10, how would you rate your pain now, if 1 is no pain and 10 is the worst pain you've ever had?

Table 5.9

FACES PAIN RATING SCALE (FPS)

<u>Directions</u>
Ask person to point to the face that best reflects how he or she feels.

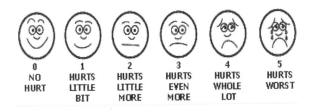

0	1	2	3	4	5
NO HURT	HURTS LITTLE BIT	HURTS LITTLE MORE	HURTS EVEN MORE	HURTS WHOLE LOT	HURTS WORST

can point to the face that best indicates how they feel. This scale is found to be an effective measure of pain in early dementia but has not been found as effective with those who have moderate to severe dementia. It is also believed by some that this scale is more a measure of depression than of pain for those with dementia.

Discomfort Scale for Dementia of the Alzheimer's Type (DS-DAT). Pain assessment is a particular challenge among individuals with advanced dementia, who lack the ability to formulate and express their experience of discomfort (Smith, 2005). The Discomfort Scale for Dementia of the Alzheimer's Type (DS-DAT) is an instrument that assesses discomfort in patients with severe dementia. This tool was developed on the assumption that discomfort can be observed, even though it may not be verbally expressed by the persons (Hurley, Volicer, Hanrahan, & Volicer, 1992). This scale is interesting because it requires no verbal response from the older person; it is simply a 5 minute observation assessment scale. Since persons with AD cannot voluntarily control their expressions or demeanor, observed markers are used as external markers of internal states. One assumption underlying the development of the DS-DAT is that indicators of discomfort in persons with AD are similar to those in infants and children.

The DS-DAT is a nine-item list requiring 5 minutes of observation to rate nonverbal behavior that is predictive of distress in persons at rest (Table 5.10). Items measuring frequency, intensity, and duration are correlated with a score that corresponds to a person's level of discomfort.

Table 5.10

THE DISCOMFORT SCALE FOR DEMENTIA OF THE ALZHEIMER'S TYPE (DS-DAT)

BEHAVIORAL INDICATOR	FREQUENCY (5 MIN)	DURATION (< 1 MIN) (≥ 1 MIN)	INTENSITY (HIGH) (LOW)
Noisy breathing Negative sounding noise on inspiration or expiration, breathing looks strenuous, labored, or wearing; respirations sound loud, harsh or gasping; difficulty breathing or trying hard at attempting to achieve a good gas exchange; episodic bursts of rapid breaths or hyperventilation.			
Negative vocalizations Noise or speech with a negative or disapproving quality; hushed low sounds such as a constant muttering with a guttural tone; monotone, subdued, or varying pitched sound with a definite unpleasant sound; faster rate than a conversation or drawn out as in a moan or groan; repeating the same words with a mournful tone; expressing hurt or pain.			
Lack of content facial expression Pleasant, calm-looking face; tranquil, at ease or serene; relaxed facial expression with a slack unclenched jaw; overall look is one of peace.			
Sad facial expression Troubled look on face, looking hurt, worried, lost, or lonesome; distressed appearance, sunken, "hound dog" look with lackluster eyes; tears, crying.			

Frightened facial expression

Scared, concerned looking face; looking bothered, fearful, or troubled; alarmed appearance with open eyes and pleading face.

Frown

Face looks strained; stern or scowling look, displeased expression with wrinkled brow and creases in the forehead; corners of the mouth turned down.

Lack of relaxed body language

Easy open-handed position; looking of being in a restful position and may be cuddled up or stretched out; muscles look of normal firmness and joints are without stress; look of idle, lazy, or "laid back"; appearance of "just killing the day"; casual.

Tense body language

Extremities show tension; wringing hands, clenched fist, or knees pulled up tightly; look of being in strained or inflexible position.

Fidgeting

Restless impatient movement; acts squirmy or jittery: appearance of trying to get away from hurt area; forceful touching, tugging, or rubbing of body parts.

Source: "Assessment of Discomfort in Advanced Alzheimer Patients," by A. C. Hurley, B. J. Volicer, P. A. Hanrahan, S. Houde, and V. Volicer, 1992, *Research in Nursing & Health, 15,* p. 373. Copyright © 1992. Reprinted with permission of John Wiley & Sons.

Before observation begins, the rater must wait 15 minutes after an intervention that may have caused pain or discomfort for the person, such as a position change or feeding. Since the invention of the DS-DAT, a modified version, which contains only six items, has become available. Three of the items that were reportedly hard to interpret—sad facial expression, frowning, and relaxed body language—are removed. Although this scale was found to be just as useful as the original version, it too is complicated and time consuming and requires expertise.

Checklist of Nonverbal Pain Indicators (CNPI). CNPI was designed to measure pain behaviors in postoperative cognitively impaired adults, both

Table 5.11

CHECKLIST OF NONVERBAL PAIN INDICATORS (CNPI)		
	WITH MOVEMENT	**AT REST**
Vocal complaints: nonverbal expression of pain demonstrated by moans, groans, grunts, cries, gasps, sighs.		
Facial grimaces and winces: furrowed brow, narrowed eyes, tightened lips, dropped jaw, clenched teeth, distorted expression.		
Bracing: clutching or holding onto siderails, bed, tray table, or affected area during movement.		
Restlessness: constant or intermittent shifting of position, rocking, intermittent or constant hand motions, inability to keep still.		
Rubbing: massaging affected area.		
Vocal complaints: verbal expression of pain using words such as "ouch" or "that hurts"; cursing during movement, or exclamations of protest such as "stop" or "that's enough."		
	Total score	

Source: "The Checklist of Nonverbal Pain Indicators (CNPI)," by K. S. Feldt, 2000, *Pain Management Nursing, 1,* p. 18. Copyright © 2000 Elsevier.

at rest and during activity (Feldt, 2000). It is a 6-item scale. Like the DS-DAT, items are scored for an interpretation of pain severity. The presence of a pain indicator is scored as 1, while the absence of the indicator is scored as 0. The subscores, as well as a total score, are summed both at rest and during activity (Table 5.11). There is no specific cutoff score to indicate pain severity; but the presence of any of the behavioral indicators may be indicative of pain and requires further assessment, intervention, and monitoring by the clinician.

Pain Assessment Checklist for Seniors With Limited Ability to Communicate (PACSLAC). PACSLAC is a clinically useful scale for assessing pain in patients with dementia (Fuchs-Lacelle & Hadjistavropoulos, 2004). It is the most valid and user-friendly behavioral scale for assessing pain in the elderly with limited communication skills. PACSLAC is a 60-item behavioral checklist covering four subscales designed to identify and assess pain among seniors with severe cognitive impairments (Table 5.12). It takes about 5 minutes to complete, and the initial psychometric evidence is very encouraging.

Pain Assessment for the Dementing Elderly (PADE). PADE is a tool for assessing pain in individuals with advanced dementia (Villanueva, Smith, Erickson, Lee, & Singer, 2003). It consists of three parts with a total of 24 items:

- Part 1: physical pain, which includes observable facial expression, breathing pattern and posture
- Part 2: global assessment involves proxy evaluation of pain intensity
- Part 3: functional, including ADL (dressing, feeding oneself, transfers from wheelchair to bed).

The items are rated using several different scoring methods. While some items are rated on a 4-point Likert scale, others are multiple-choice, with some items scored on a visual analog scale. While some items are scored retrospectively, others are not.

The different scoring methods make scoring interpretation absent and the scale complex, as it is confusing or difficult to interpret. The scale includes different scoring methods, so calculating cutoff scores for pain to determine sensitivity and specificity seems difficult. With practice, PADE requires 5–10 minutes of clinicians' time to complete. Given the scoring complexity, however, this is probably an underestimation.

Table 5.12

PAIN ASSESSMENT CHECKLIST FOR SENIORS WITH LIMITED ABILITY TO COMMUNICATE (PACSLAC)

Facial expressions	Present	Social/personality/mood	Present
Grimacing		Physical aggression	
Sad look		(e.g. pushing people and/or	
Tighter face		objects, scratching others,	
Dirty look		striking, kicking)	
Change in eyes (squinting,		Verbal aggression	
dull, bright, increased		Not wanting to be touched	
movement)		Not allowing people near	
Frowning		Angry/mad	
Pain expression		Throwing things	
Grim face		Increased confusion	
Clenching teeth		Anxious	
Wincing		Upset	
Opening mouth		Agitated	
Creasing forehead		Cranky/irritable	
Screwing up face		Frustrated	

Activity/body movement		Other	
Fidgeting		Pale face	
Pulling away		Flushed, red face	
Flinching		Teary eyed	
Restless		Sweating	
Pacing		Shaking/trembling	
Wandering		Cold and clammy	
Trying to leave		Changes in sleep	
Refusing to move		(please circle):	
Thrashing		Decreased sleep or	
Decreased activity		Increased sleep during day	
Refusing medications		Changes in appetite	
Moving slow		(please circle):	
Impulsive behavior		Decreased appetite or	
(e.g., repetitive		Increased appetite	
movements)		Screaming/yelling	
Uncooperative/resistant		Calling out (i.e., for help)	
to care		Crying	
Guarding sore area		A specific sound or	
Touching/holding sore area		vocalisation	
Limping		For pain "ow," "ouch"	
Clenched fist		Moaning and groaning	
Going into fetal position		Mumbling	
Stiff/rigid		Grunting	

Source: "Development and Preliminary Validation of the Pain Assessment Checklist for Seniors With Limited Ability to Communicate (PACSLAC)," by S. Fuchs-Lacelle and T. Hadjistavropoulos, 2004, *Pain Management Nursing, 5,* pp. 48–49. The PACSLAC is copyrighted by Shannon Fuchs-Lacelle and Thomas Hadjistavropoulos (Copyright © 2002) and is reprinted here with permission. No further reproduction, presentation, translation, or publication of the PACSLAC is authorized without the expressed, written consent of the copyright holders. Requests for such permissions may be directed to the attention of Dr. Thomas Hadjistavropoulos at thomas.hadjistavropoulos@uregina.ca

Pain Assessment in Advanced Dementia (PAINAD). PAINAD is a scale that is clinically very popular—an easy-to-use, valid, and reliable pain assessment tool for cognitively impaired nonverbal individuals (O'Malley et al., 2006). It consists of five items: breathing, negative vocalization, facial expression, body language, and consolability, with a scale of 0–2 for each item (Table 5.13). An objective description of each of the five items is outlined in the scale. Total scores range from 0 (no pain) to 10 (maximal pain). This scale is the only scale available for patients with advanced dementia who demonstrate significant changes in behavior secondary to pain.

Table 5.13

PAIN ASSESSMENT IN ADVANCED DEMENTIA (PAINAD)

ITEMS	0	1	2	SCORE
Breathing independent of vocalization	Normal	Occasional labored breathing. Short period of hyperventilation.	Noisy labored breathing. Long period of hyperventilation. Cheyne-Stokes respirations.	
Negative vocalization	None	Occasional moan or groan. Low level speech with a negative or disapproving quality.	Repeated troubled calling out. Loud moaning or groaning. Crying.	
Facial expression	Smiling or inexpressive	Sad. Frightened. Frowning.	Facial grimacing.	
Body language	Relaxed	Tense. Distressed pacing. Fidgeting.	Rigid. Fists clenched, Knees pulled up. Pulling or pushing away. Striking out.	
Consolability	No need to console	Distracted or reassured by voice or touch.	Unable to console, distract or reassure.	

Source: "Development and Psychometric Evaluation of the PAINAD (Pain Assessment in Advanced Dementia) Scale," by V. Warden, A. C. Hurley, and L. Volicer, 2003, *Journal of the American Medical Directors Association, 4,* p. 14. Reprinted with permission from Lippincott Williams & Wilkins.

Neurodiagnostic Tests

Neurodiagnostic tests include laboratory tests, imaging studies, and electrodiagnostic studies. Lab tests are performed to rule out infections or conditions such as vitamin deficiency, diabetes, anemia, chemical abnormalities, medication levels, and hormonal disorders, disorders of the thyroid, kidneys, or liver, or other factors that can cause dementia symptoms. Brain images cannot detect AD, but these studies are necessary to rule out other conditions such as stroke and brain tumors that can also cause dementia or dementia-like symptoms. Electrodiagnostic studies may include electroencephalogram and electrocardiogram that can either contribute to or rule out a diagnosis of AD.

Laboratory Tests

Blood tests are routine when a diagnosis of dementia is suspected.
   Blood tests measure the following.

1   *White blood cells,* which can indicate the presence of infection or an immunodeficient disease or process.
2   *Red blood cells,* which can show changes in the cells' size due to vitamin or mineral deficiencies. People with Alzheimer's disease often have normal blood counts, as the disease does not usually cause changes to the body systems except the brain. The test will help to exclude other diseases that may mimic the signs of dementia. Larger red cells may indicate B-12 or folic acid deficiencies. Smaller red cells can indicate iron deficiencies.
3   *Platelet count,* which can show problems with clotting.
4   *Blood chemistry,* which, for dementia, looks at calcium, cholesterol, various enzymes, glucose, potassium, and sodium levels. These blood chemicals will indicate abnormalities with the kidney, liver, circulatory function and other problems that might be affecting the functioning of other organs. Many body systems and chemicals in the blood can affect the brain. It is important to exclude and treat any conditions or diseases that may be causing symptoms of dementia.
5   *Thyroid* blood test for dementia, which can detect under- or overactivity of the thyroid that can cause cognitive and behavioral problems.
6   *Erythrocyte Sedimentation Rate (ESR)* test for dementia, which will check for any autoimmune disease.

7 *Venereal disease (VDRL)* test for dementia, which, although not as routinely undertaken as in the past, remains an optional test that may be done in areas where there are high rates of syphilis.

8 *Urinalysis,* which is evaluated to detect abnormalities, such as abnormal levels of sugar or protein. This test may be used to rule out other disorders that may be causing symptoms similar to those of AD.

9 *Lumbar Puncture,* which is not a routine diagnostic test for persons with dementia but should be done if metastatic cancer, meningitis, tertiary syphilis, hydrocephalus, encephalitis, demyelinating disease, immunosuppression, or inflammatory disease is suspected (Daly, 1999). It can also be performed to exclude people showing apparent dementia-type symptoms who are suffering from rare diseases of the central nervous system. The American Academy of Neurology does not recommend this test as it is not any better at diagnosing AD or dementia than clinical judgment. Research is being undertaken into the levels of tau and amyloid protein levels in the cerebrospinal fluid. It is hoped that levels may help in the future diagnosis of AD.

Imaging Studies

Computed Tomography (CT or CAT) and Magnetic Resonance Imaging (MRI) scans are usually not used to diagnose AD; rather, they are used to confirm or rule out such problems as tumor, hemorrhage, stroke, and hydrocephalus, which can masquerade as AD. These scans show atrophy of the brain that is characteristic of AD in its later stages.

A Positron Emission Tomography (PET) scan works by showing the difference in brain activity between a normal brain and one affected by AD. It reveals the region of the brain that affects AD, and recent studies indicate that PET can supply important diagnostic information and even confirm AD. Positron emission tomography scans can also help differentiate AD from other forms of dementia disorders, such as vascular dementia, Parkinson's disease, and Huntington's disease.

A Single Photon Emission Computed Tomography (SPECT) scan can be used to see how blood flows in certain regions of the brain and is useful in evaluating specific brain functions. This may reveal abnormalities that are characteristic of AD.

Magnetic Resonance Spectroscopy Imaging (MRSI) is used to study changes caused by brain tumors, strokes, seizure disorders, AD, depression, and other diseases affecting the brain. Computed tomography and MRI scans reveal the anatomic structure of the brain, while SPECT and PET scans provide images of brain activity based on blood flow, oxygen consumption, or glucose use. But none of these imaging techniques reveals the microscopic changes in brain tissue that characterize Alzheimer's disease and thus can't identify the disease with certainty.

Electrodiagnostic Studies

Electroencephalography (EEG) is often used to study various brain processes, such as perception, memory, language, and emotion, and is most helpful in identifying disorders that mimic AD. An EEG may be done to detect abnormal brainwave activity. Electroencephalography is usually normal in patients with mild AD and many other types of dementia, but EEG abnormalities do occur in delirium and in Creutzfeldt-Jakob disease, which are causes of dementia. Electrocardiogram (ECG or EKG) may be used to help rule out other cardiac conditions that may be causing symptoms similar to those of AD.

DIFFERENTIAL DIAGNOSIS

Many treatable conditions share the same symptoms as AD. Differentiating whether a person has AD or an illness that mimics AD is a delicate, complex process that is extremely important for an individual. If a physician or group of physicians can rule out other illnesses, treatment and planning for the person with AD can begin. If differential diagnosis reveals another cause of the symptoms, proper treatment can be administered and the patient can seek the appropriate care.

In the early stages of AD, a multitude of neurodegenerative diseases that are associated with the development of dementia including Pick's disease, Lewy body disease, and progressive supranuclear palsy, as well as other diseases such as vascular dementia and Creuztfeldt-Jakob disease. Most of these entities can be differentiated from AD by the clinical history and a careful examination (Tavee & Sweeney, 2003). Furthermore, symptoms and potentially treatable diseases that may mimic the dementia caused by AD include depression, thyroid disease, vitamin B-12 deficiency, normal-pressure hydrocephalus, and neurosyphilis, all of which should be effectively ruled out in the evaluation of AD (Tavee & Sweeney, 2003).

As we discussed in this chapter, physicians integrate several diagnostic tools to make an assessment of whether or not a patient has AD. These tools—history, physical examination, neuropsychologic testing, laboratory studies, and neuroimaging studies—can also reveal the presence of the conditions that mimic AD.

A physical examination can rule out AD, though this is tricky, since a patient can be suffering from a multitude of illnesses. A patient with gait apraxia, dementia, and urinary incontinence, for example, will be thought to have normal-pressure hydrocephalus, but vascular dementia sometimes occurs in addition to AD (Bejjani & Hammer, 2005). Diffuse Lewy body dementia surfaces with symptoms of hallucinations, mild Parkinson's symptoms, mental status changes, alterations in alertness and attention, and sensitivity to neuroleptic drugs—which can also occur with Alzheimer's disease. Parkinson's disease manifests in symptoms of tremor and rigidity, which come before any cognitive symptoms appear. Myoclonic jerks can suggest Creutzfeldt-Jacob disease, a rare dementia that progresses very rapidly (Daly, 1999). Myoclonus can also be found with dementia associated with anemia or liver failure.

Neurological examinations are not as effective in determining if an individual has Alzheimer's unless he or she is in very advanced stages of the disease; most patients in the early to middle stages of AD will have normal results on such exams. However, if a neurological exam uncovers focal neurologic signs, which indicate focal brain lesions, a patient might be suffering from multi-infarct dementia (including the rare disorders in multiple sclerosis and brain abscesses).

Neuroimaging tests are helpful in indicating some illnesses that mimic AD, but not all are equally effective—some tests identify certain conditions better than others. Computed tomography and MRIs are not effective with subcortical disorders, such as Parkinson's disease, progressive supranuclear palsy, Lewy body disease, strionigral degeneration, and disorders caused by neuroleptic medications. Subcortical vascular dementia—aka Binswanger disease—often occurs in patients with hypertension, diabetes mellitus, and hypercholesterolemia. These disorders typically cause memory deficits, while language remains intact, but motor functioning and executive functioning are impaired.

Neuroimaging studies can help in accurately diagnosing frontal lobe dementias, including Pick disease, frontotemporal lobe atrophy with Pick bodies, or motor neuron disease (Daly, 1999). In the early stages of frontal lobe dementias, behavioral changes begin to surface, including marked changes in judgment and mild defects in memory and visuospatial orientation. Disinhibition, compulsiveness, impatience, and sexual inappropriateness are also prominent symptoms.

Another area of differential diagnosis deals with the symptom of depression. People with Alzheimer's disease express symptoms of depression, such as a sad or blunted affect and feelings of worthlessness and hopelessness (Daly, 1999). People with AD tend to minimize their cognitive defects, while a normal depressed person will complain or be more unwilling to cooperate in cognitive tests. Another key difference noted between a normal depressed person and a depressed AD person is that a normal depressed person is less able to make and carry out plans and concentrate than is a person with AD. People with AD have marked visuospatial impairments and often express neurovegetative symptoms. Normal depressed persons have cognitive deficits associated with pain and physical complaints. There might also be a history of previous depression in the individual and/or her family.

Depression and Alzheimer's disease often overlap, and the diagnosis may be confirmed by a therapeutic trial of antidepressant medications (Daly, 1999). It also may be difficult to differentiate dementia from delirium. Persons with alcohol-related dementia typically confabulate and have preserved social skills, which is another shared symptom of depression. Dementia and depression are very difficult to distinguish, but it isn't uncommon for them to coexist.

Dementias take on two forms. They either present without prominent motor signs or they present with prominent motor signs (Geldmacher & Whitehouse, 1997). Dementias without prominent motor signs include Alzheimer's disease, frontotemporal dementia, and Creutzfeld-Jakob and other prion diseases. Dementias characterized at onset by prominent motor signs include dementias with Lewy bodies, idiopathic Parkinson's disease, progressive supranuclear palsy, cortico-basal ganglionic degeneration, hydrocephalus, Huntington's disease, and vascular dementia. Diagnostic tools used to conclude the presence of these dementias include a careful history, mental status screening, laboratory and imaging studies, and neuropsychologic testing. Genetic testing is also available, but its use is controversial and raises complex ethical questions.

6 Progression of Alzheimer's Disease

The rate of progression varies widely among individuals. Most people with Alzheimer's don't die of the disease itself, but of pneumonia, a urinary tract infection, or complications from a fall.

Mayo Clinic

Alzheimer's disease (AD) is a progressive illness, which means that symptoms worsen over time. How fast the disease progresses, and what pattern symptoms might follow, varies from individual to individual, but symptoms develop over the same general stages in all individuals. AD eventually affects nearly all brain functions, including memory, movement, language, behavior, judgment, and abstract reasoning.

Researchers and physicians use a number of scales to measure the progression of symptoms over time, which can define as many as seven distinct stages of the disease (Fisher Center for Alzheimer's Research Foundation, 2007). With AD, three broad phases are typically recognized: mild, moderate, and severe. The symptoms commonly seen in each stage are summarized in this chapter, but it is important to realize that there may be some overlap among the stages and that people may not experience every single one of these symptoms.

STAGES OF ALZHEIMER'S PROGRESSION

Staging systems provide useful frames of reference for understanding how the disease may unfold and for making future plans. But it is important to note that not everyone will experience the same symptoms or progress at the same rate (Alzheimer's Association, 2007). Furthermore, AD typically develops slowly and causes a gradual decline in cognitive abilities, usually over a span of 7 to 10 years (MayoClinic.com, 2006). After symptoms begin, people live, on average, 8 to 10 years (Merck Manual of Health & Aging, 2007). As mentioned earlier, progression is unpredictable. In most cases, cognitive symptoms appear at the beginning of the disease to 3 years after onset, many times before diagnosis (AlzheimersOnline, 2007). Functional and behavioral problems follow and can be evident any time within 1.5–6 years. Placement in a nursing home may be needed at any point from the 2.5-year mark on. Figure 6.1 gives a general overview of the progression of AD, and the gradual decline in the Mini-Mental State Examination (MMSE) score, from the time cognitive, functional, and behavioral symptoms first appear.

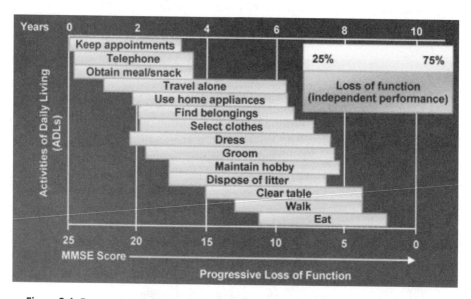

Figure 6.1 Progression of Alzheimer's disease.
Source: "An Integrated Approach to the Management of Alzheimer's Disease: Assessing Cognition, Function and Behaviour," by D. Galasko, 1998, *European Journal of Neurology, 5*, p. 512. Reprinted with permission.

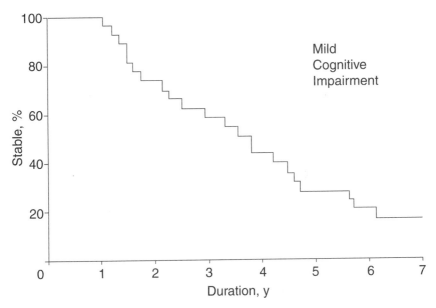

Figure 6.2 Progression of mild cognitive impairment.
Source: "Current Concepts in Mild Cognitive Impairment," by R. C. Petersen et al., 2001, *Archives of Neurology, 58,* p. 1986. Copyright © American Medical Association.

Figure 6.2 shows the survival curve of persons characterized as having a mild cognitive impairment for 6 years. Approximately 80% have converted to dementia during this time.

Figure 6.3 shows mild to moderate and moderate to severe stages of AD progression. People vary in the length of time spent in each stage and in which stage symptoms appear. Because the stages overlap, it is difficult to definitely place a person in a particular stage. However, the progression is always toward a worsening of symptoms. The stages identify groups of symptoms that reflect worsening brain decay and increasing dependence on caregivers. The end result of Alzheimer's is death, whether caused by the inability of the brain to keep the body going or by another disease or injury along the way.

Staging systems are considered to be helpful for understanding how the disease generally progresses. A number of staging systems have been developed to describe progression of AD. Let's take a look at a few staging systems commonly used today.

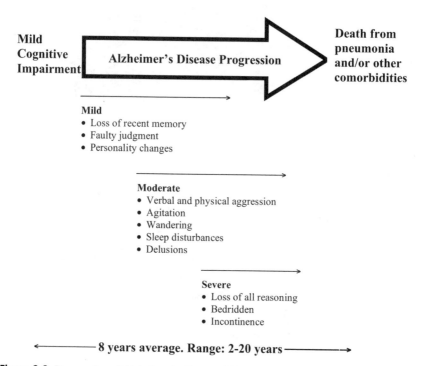

Figure 6.3 Progression of Alzheimer's disease from mild to severe stage. Limitations in activities of daily living (ADLs) and instrumental activities of daily living (IADLs) among people age 70 and above with AD.

The Three-Stage Model

It is difficult to place a person with AD in a specific stage because every individual with Alzheimer's progresses differently. However, symptoms usually follow a certain pattern in cognitive, behavioral, and physical deterioration. Therefore, these stages generally overlap (Gwyther, 1985).

Stage 1

Stage 1 lasts 2–4 years from the time a person starts developing the symptoms. Symptoms start with recent memory loss, which begins to affect a person's job performance. An individual has difficulty remembering familiar phone numbers and has trouble handling money or paying bills. At times the person may be disoriented about places, loses initiative, and takes longer with routine chores. He may arrive at wrong time or places. The individual loses spontaneity, the spark or zest for life. Mood and personality changes begin. The person has difficulty coping with the situation and becomes anxious about his symptoms and starts avoiding people. The individual has poor judgment, and decision making becomes a problem.

Stage 2

During Stage 2, memory loss and confusion continue to increase and the attention span shortens. The individual starts having problems recognizing close friends and/or family members and starts repeating statements and/or movements and becomes restless. She becomes restless, especially in late afternoon and at night. Also, she has a perceptual motor problem, with occasional muscle twitches or jerking. The individual has difficulty organizing thoughts and thinking logically and cannot find the right words; she makes up stories to fill in blanks. The person becomes suspicious, irritable, and fidgety and has loss of impulse control. The individual is afraid of bathing and has trouble dressing. The individual gains and then loses weight and may show signs of delusion. She requires full-time supervision.

Stage 3

Stage 3 is the terminal stage. The person cannot recognize family and the image of himself in the mirror. He has little capacity for self-care and loses weight even with a good diet. At this stage, the individual is not capable of communicating with words and cannot control bowel or bladder. The person may have seizures or experience difficulty with swallowing. The person eventually dies of infection or aspiration pneumonia or other similar conditions.

Functional Assessment Staging of Alzheimer's Disease (FAST)

The FAST staging system was developed by Dr. Barry Reisberg (1988) at the New York University Medical Center, Aging and Dementia Research Center. Functional assessment staging shows the progression of Alzheimer's in 16 stages/substages.

Stage 1

No cognitive decline (i.e., normal adult). No subjective complaints of memory deficit. No memory deficit evident on clinical interviews.

Stage 2

Very mild cognitive decline (i.e., forgetfulness, or normal older adult). No objective evidence of memory deficit on clinical interview. No objective deficits in employment or social situations. Appropriate concern regarding symptoms. Subjective complaints of memory deficit, most frequently in the following areas: (a) forgetting where one has placed familiar objects; and (b) forgetting names one formerly knew well.

Stage 3

Mild cognitive decline (i.e., early confusional or early AD). Earliest clear-cut deficits. Manifestations may take the form of the following: (a) patient may have gotten lost when traveling to an unfamiliar location; (b) coworkers become aware of patient's relatively low performance level; (c) word and name-finding deficit becomes evident to intimates; (d) patient may read a passage of a book and retain relatively little material; (e) patient may demonstrate decreased facility in remembering names upon introduction to new people; (f) patient may have lost or misplaced an object of value; and (g) concentration deficit may be evident on clinical testing. Objective evidence of memory deficit obtained only with an intensive interview. Denial begins to become manifest in patient. Mild to moderate anxiety accompanies symptoms.

Stage 4

Moderate cognitive decline (i.e., late confusional or mild AD). Clear-cut deficits on careful clinical interview. Inability to perform complex tasks. Deficits manifest in the following areas: (a) decreased knowledge of current and recent events; (b) deficit in memory of one's personal history; (c) concentration deficit elicited on serial subtractions; (d) decreased ability to travel, handle finances, and so on. Frequently no deficit in the following areas: (a) orientation to time and person; (b) recognition of familiar persons and faces; and (c) ability to travel to familiar locations. Denial is a dominant defense mechanism. Flattening of affect and withdrawal from challenging situations occur.

Stage 5

Moderately severe cognitive decline (i.e., early dementia or moderate AD). Patient can no longer survive without some assistance. Patient is unable during interview to recall a major relevant aspect of her current life (e.g., an address or telephone number of many years, the names of close family members, such as grandchildren, the name of the high school or college from which she graduated). Frequently some disorientation to time (i.e., date, day of the week, season) or to place. An educated person may have difficulty counting back from 40 by 4s or from 20 by 2s. Persons at this stage retain knowledge of many major facts regarding themselves and others. They invariably know their own names and generally know their spouse's and children's names. They require no assistance with toileting and eating but may have some difficulty choosing the proper clothing to wear.

Stage 6

Severe cognitive decline (i.e., middle dementia or moderately severe AD). May occasionally forget the name of the spouse upon whom he is entirely dependent for survival. Will be largely unaware of all recent events and experiences in his life. Retains some knowledge of his past life, but his recollection is very sketchy. Generally unaware of surroundings (i.e., the year, the season). May have difficulty counting from 10, both backward and sometimes forward. Will require some assistance with activities of daily living (e.g., may become incontinent, will require travel assistance but occasionally will display ability to find familiar locations). Diurnal rhythm frequently disturbed. Almost always recalls his own name. Frequently continues to be able to distinguish familiar from unfamiliar persons in his environment. Personality and emotional changes occur. These are quite variable and include (a) delusional behavior (e.g., patients may accuse their spouse of being an imposter, may talk to imaginary figures in the environment or to their own reflection in the mirror); (b) obsessive symptoms (e.g., person may continually repeat simple cleaning activities); (c) anxiety symptoms, agitation, and even previously nonexistent violent behavior may occur; and (d) cognitive abulla (i.e., loss of willpower because an individual cannot carry a thought long enough to determine a purposeful course of action) develops.

Person will also demonstrate the following:

- 6a—Requires assistance dressing
- 6b—Requires assistance bathing properly
- 6c—Requires assistance with mechanics of toileting
- 6d—Urinary incontinence
- 6e—Fecal incontinence

Stage 7

Very severe cognitive decline (i.e., late dementia or severe AD). All verbal abilities are lost. Frequently there is no speech at all—only grunting. Urinary incontinence requires assistance with toileting and feeding, loss of basic psychomotor skills (e.g., unable to walk, sit, or control head movement). The brain appears to no longer be able to tell the body what to do. Generalized and cortical neurologic signs and symptoms are frequently present.

- 7a—Speech ability limited to about a half-dozen intelligible words
- 7b—Intelligible vocabulary limited to a single word
- 7c—Ambulatory ability lost
- 7d—Ability to sit up lost
- 7e—Ability to smile lost
- 7f—Ability to hold up head lost

Global Deterioration Scale (GDS)

A seven-stage model describes the typical course of the disease (Reisberg, Ferris, De Leon, & Crook, 1982). A modified version of the seven-stage model of AD progression follows:

Stage 1

Is defined as a normal adult with no decline in function or memory.

Stage 2

Very mild decline; Stage 2 is defined as a normal older adult who has some personal awareness of functional decline. People complain of memory deficits and of forgetting the names of familiar people and places. This might be regarded as a feature of natural aging, rather than a disease process.

Stage 3

- ■ Mild decline; Stage 3 is defined as early AD.
- ■ Characteristics of the disease are noticeable deficits in demanding job situations. Anxiety can become a feature as the symptoms

and/or realization of the situation becomes apparent. Denial becomes a feature, and memory deficits become apparent only under intensive interview. Signs include one or more of the following: the person may get lost traveling to an unfamiliar location; colleagues notice low performance; names and word-finding deficits become evident to those close to the person; ability to recall information from a passage in a book becomes difficult; the ability to remember a name of a person newly introduced to the patient is affected; patient may misplace or lose a valuable object; and concentration may begin to become affected.

Stage 4

- Mild AD.
- Usually there is no deficit in recognizing familiar faces, in the ability to travel to places the patient knows, or orientation in time and person. The patient begins to require assistance in complicated tasks, such as planning a party or handling finances. He or she may exhibit problems remembering his or her life and events and have trouble concentrating and traveling.
- Denial and a flattening of mood becomes a feature. A tendency to back away from dealing with difficult or challenging situations becomes evident.

Stage 5

- Moderate, midstage severe decline AD.
- People with moderate Alzheimer's now cannot get by without assistance. They need help choosing proper attire. There is some disorientation in time; in interviews they may be unable to recall important information of their current lives, but they can still remember major information about themselves, their family, and others.

Stage 6

- Moderately severe decline AD.
- People with Alzheimer's by this stage of the disease start to forget significant amounts of information about themselves and their surroundings. They may forget names of their spouses, require assistance dressing, require assistance bathing properly, and then require assistance with the mechanics of toileting. Urinary incontinence and disturbed patterns of sleep become features.

- At this stage of Alzheimer's, personality and emotional changes become more apparent, and very apparent in some. This may manifest in delusional or obsessive behavior; there may be acute anxiety and even violent behavior. Because people cannot remember information long enough to act on their thoughts, they lose willpower (cognitive abulla).
- Fecal incontinence may also be a feature of the disease at this point.

Stage 7

- Very severe decline, late stage AD.
- In severe Alzheimer's, speech ability becomes limited to just six or seven words, and intelligible vocabulary is limited to a single word. Patients lose the ability to walk, sit up, and smile and eventually cannot hold up their head. The brain now appears unable to tell the body what to do.

The Five-Stage Scale of Alzheimer's Progression

Harvard Health Publications (2007) divides AD into five stages to describe progression of the disease.

Stage I

Memory problems appear. Initially, they may seem like slight absentmindedness and may go unnoticed by others. Some Alzheimer's patients are quite successful at hiding these symptoms, but this becomes increasingly difficult. They may lose or misplace valuable objects. They may not fully absorb what they read or hear, and their performance on the job or in social situations begins to suffer. They may become confused in new surroundings or lost in an unfamiliar part of town. Word-finding problems or aphasia may begin at this stage.

The first personality change is usually a loss of spontaneity. Alzheimer's patients may avoid situations that challenge their abilities and may become withdrawn, apathetic, moody, depressed, irritable, or anxious. They typically deny that their problems are serious, even to themselves, and may blame others for their failures. The family may assume that the person is under stress or suffering from an emotional problem.

Stage II

The patient's memory problems are now more obvious to others. Because it's difficult for people with Alzheimer's to retain new information, they may lose the thread of conversations. They sometimes have difficulty recalling current events, such as who the president is, and even bits of information from their own personal history, such as where they attended school. Their ability to perform mathematical calculations suffers, and they may no longer be able to manage their own finances. Depression often becomes prominent at this stage, further hampering the patient's ability to function.

Impaired reasoning and judgment make traveling more difficult. Although patients at this stage may be able to find their way around familiar areas, their ability to handle unexpected events is impaired, which makes driving risky. In addition, dishonest people can now more easily victimize them. Patients at this stage can have a striking lack of insight into their problems. They may refuse any assistance with finances but forget to pay bills; insist on driving but have a series of fender-benders; continue to cook but repeatedly scorch empty pots on the stove.

Stage III

Memory can fluctuate daily or even hourly. Alzheimer's patients sometimes forget major events in their lives, and yet continue to deny having memory problems. As they try to fill memory gaps, their conversation may become disjointed and filled with irrelevant content. Often they are unaware of the date or the time of year.

The continuing deterioration of memory makes people feel insecure, which they may express as paranoia and anger. They may accuse others of hiding things, stealing, or plotting against them. Their emotions are unstable, and their relations with others may be marred by rapid mood swings that have no apparent cause. They may have episodes of crying, angry outbursts, and agitation.

At this stage, the Alzheimer's patient is no longer able to survive without some assistance. Although able to manage many basic activities of daily living, such as using the toilet and eating, they only partially complete some tasks because they cannot remember all the steps involved. Their grooming and choice of clothes may be the most obvious sign of this difficulty. A simple decision, such as which sweater to wear, can be overwhelming to a person with dementia.

The decreased ability to think forces the person to withdraw from social activities that require active participation. Undemanding activities such as attending a concert may still be enjoyable, but going to a dinner party would be bewildering. The inability to handle potentially stressful situations causes anxiety, which can trigger catastrophic reactions such as shouting, cursing, or hitting others.

Stage IV

Dramatic changes occur as the Alzheimer's patient progresses to more advanced dementia. For the first time, the person may look ill. His language skills are considerably reduced, and memory impairment becomes so profound that everything can seem unfamiliar and threatening. Some knowledge of the past is usually retained, but it is fragmented.

Patients tend to be less withdrawn at this stage, but they often develop behavior problems. They have difficulty comprehending what others say or do, which can lead to a variety of emotional reactions, including delusions (accusing the spouse of infidelity or being an imposter, talking to imaginary people, believing the reflection in a mirror is a stranger), obsessive behavior (repeatedly cleaning an object, endlessly removing and replacing the contents of a drawer), agitation (pacing, hand-wringing, asking the same question repeatedly), and catastrophic reactions. Sleep disturbances are common. The patient may awaken at night with hallucinations; feeling frightened and disoriented, she may be unable to go back to sleep. Wandering at night can become a major problem.

Another problem for caregivers is the patient's fear of bathing, which is common in the middle stages of dementia. Problems with movement and coordination often emerge at this stage. The patient may walk with slow, shuffling steps and require assistance with bathing, dressing, and eating. Weight loss can occur from difficulties with chewing and swallowing. Incontinence often develops at this stage because patients do not remember where the toilet is, cannot manage their clothes, or do not recognize the body's signals.

Stage V

This stage has been called "the long good-bye." All language skills have been lost, and there seems to be very little left of the patient's "self." Behavior problems diminish, and motor skills decline until the person can no longer walk, sit up, chew and swallow food, or control bladder and bowel movements. Brain activity is disturbed, which may result in seizures. As the brain shuts down, the patient becomes unresponsive, lapses into a coma, and finally dies.

DEVELOPMENT OF COGNITIVE, BEHAVIORAL, AND PHYSICAL PROBLEMS

Cognitive Impairment

Alzheimer's disease is a chronic process with gradual deterioration of cognitive ability. Primary cognitive problems of AD include memory impairment, language disturbance, and impaired executive function, abstract thinking, and visuospatial deficits. As Alzheimer's progresses, a decline of logical thinking, judgment, problem-solving ability, executive functioning, and planning is expected (Yellowitz, 2005). The confusion and disorientation of mid-stage AD makes it increasingly difficult to maintain normal behaviors. The result may be inappropriate behavior in social situations or getting lost in one's own house. The person with AD can become a danger to self or others. There is no question that finding solutions to cognitive decline associated with Alzheimer's is a central area in geriatrics. The range, frequency, and severity of cognitive deficits and problem behaviors associated with AD put family caregivers under physically demanding and unremitting stressors.

Cognitive impairment makes the strongest contribution to both the development of long-term functional dependence and decline in function (Aguero-Torres et al., 1998). The presence of psychotic symptoms may further increase this dependence.

Behavior Problems

People with AD suffer from a variety of behavioral problems. In the advanced stage of the disease, people with AD become more and more helpless and dependent. Decline in logical thinking, judgment, and problem-solving ability are common among people with AD, particularly in the disease's later stages. As the symptoms of Alzheimer's progress, the person becomes more emotionally fragile (Helpguide.com, 2007a). At first, there may be a sense of grief and dread that accompanies the awareness of having a progressive terminal illness. Eventually though, the diagnosis of Alzheimer's is forgotten and the ability to be rational fades. Logical thinking can no longer be used to help alleviate fear and confusion. As problems with memory and judgment increase, the person with AD can become a danger to self or others. There is a gradual loss of cognitive abilities, which gives rise to odd behavioral problems that often drives caregivers to their limits (e.g., putting everything in their mouth, playing with their own excrement). Physical deterioration is also inevitable with AD progression.

Some behaviors have more of a psychological basis—driven by anxiety, paranoia, or hallucinations (Alzheimer's Association, 2007). Anxiety in people with AD may result from a fear of becoming a burden to friends or family members or from a fear of being left alone. It is often associated with suspiciousness. It should also be remembered that some of these behavioral problems in people with advance stage of AD, especially agitation, may be caused by delirium (Morley, 2007). Delirium is an extremely dangerous altered state of consciousness whose symptoms include confusion, distractability, disorientation, disordered thinking and memory, illusions and hallucinations, and hyperactivity. Other behavior problems include agitation, irritability, wandering, restlessness, sleep disturbances, aggressiveness, screaming, and inappropriate sexual behavior.

Depression is very common among people who have AD. It is estimated that clinically significant depression occurs in about 20%–40% of people with AD (Alzheimer's Association, 2003a). In many cases, they become depressed when they realize that their memory and ability to function are getting worse. Depressive symptoms in Alzheimer's may come and go, in contrast to memory and thinking problems that worsen steadily over time. People with AD suffering from depression may refuse to help with their own personal care. They may wander away from home more often. People with Alzheimer's and depression may be less likely to talk openly about wanting to kill themselves, and they are less likely to attempt suicide than depressed individuals without dementia. Men and women with Alzheimer's experience depression with about equal frequency.

Sleep disturbances associated with AD include increased frequency and duration of awakenings, decrease in both dreaming and nondreaming stages of sleep, and daytime napping (Alzheimer's Association, 2003b). Similar changes occur in the sleep of older people who do not have dementia, but these changes occur more frequently and tend to be more severe in people with AD. Alzheimer's patients may reverse their sleep-wake cycle, causing daytime drowsiness and nighttime restlessness—a condition called *sundowning*. It is very common for those with AD to become increasingly agitated as daylight fades away into night. These sleep disturbances often increase as AD progresses. Some people with Alzheimer's disease sleep too much while others have difficulty getting enough sleep. When people with Alzheimer's cannot sleep, they may wander during the night, be unable to lie still, or yell or call out, disrupting their caregivers. Studies have shown that sleep disturbances are associated with increased impairment of memory and ability to function in people with Alzheimer's. There is also evidence that sleep disturbances may be worse in more severely affected people with AD.

Wandering

Wandering is a common behavior in AD and is usually an attempt to communicate after language skills have been lost (Mayo Clinic.com, 2007d). Wandering made the disease critical to the field of search and rescue, because people with AD not only wander—they also easily become lost. AD can erase a person's memory of once-familiar surroundings and make adaptation to new surroundings extremely difficult. As a result, people with Alzheimer's sometimes wander away from their homes or care centers and turn up—frightened and disoriented—far from where they started. Wandering is also associated with too much stimulation, such as multiple conversations in the background; even the noise of pots and pans in the kitchen can trigger wandering. Because brain processes slow down as a result of Alzheimer's disease, the person may become overwhelmed by all the sounds and start pacing or trying to get away.

Normal adults rely upon three intact systems to know where they are in space (dbs Productions, 2007): (1) short- and long-term memory to identify landmarks; (2) a sense of time and speed to judge distance; and (3) an intact visual-spatial sense to know direction angles and expected arrival times between landmarks. All three of these systems are impaired in people with AD.

A person with Alzheimer's is disorientated and unable to judge potentially dangerous places and situations (Kennard, 2006c). For this reason, people with AD who tend to wander are said to be *critically wandering*. Critical wandering is considered dangerous to AD persons because they will not cry out for help or respond to shouts; they will not leave many physical clues; they may attempt to travel to a former residence or wander to a favorite location, which can be far away, and further increase their chances of getting lost or getting into a dangerous situation; and they may have a previous history of wandering.

People suffering from severe Alzheimer's have a higher incidence of critical wandering and are at more risk of danger. Wandering is among the most unsettling and even terrifying behaviors displayed by people with Alzheimer's. Wandering among individuals with AD may increase if the caregivers are young, less educated, overburdened, or depressed (Sink, Covinsky, Barnes, Newcomer, & Yaffe, 2006). Despite the best preventive efforts, especially in the home environment, critical wandering may still occur. Wandering also may be related to:

- Medication side effects
- Memory loss and disorientation
- Attempts to express emotions, such as fear, isolation, loneliness, or loss
- Curiosity
- Restlessness or boredom
- Stimuli that trigger memories or routines, such as the sight of coats and boots next to a door, a signal that it's time to go outdoors (Mayo Clinic, 2005)

Eating Disturbances

Eating impairment is well documented in the late stage of AD. Typical eating behaviors of an Alzheimer's patient include requiring constant reminders to open the mouth, verbally resisting food or spitting it out, pocketing food in the cheeks without swallowing, and clenching teeth. Abnormal eating behaviors can also be subtler, such as fluctuations in appetite, delusions about food, increased distractibility at meal time, and changes in food preferences (White, 2004). People with AD may develop a taste and smell dysfunction as the disease progresses. Severe eating problems put people with Alzheimer's at risk for weight loss, dehydration, and malnutrition.

As the disease progresses and more damage to the brain occurs, people with AD often have difficulty in swallowing. The brain is no longer capable of coordinating swallowing and breathing. Aspiration of food or fluids into the lungs may occur, which increases the likelihood of developing aspiration pneumonia, since inappropriate substances end up in the lungs, promoting bacterial growth.

Physical Impairment and Personal Care

In addition to becoming increasingly cognitively impaired, an individual with AD becomes progressively physically impaired. Patients gradually lose the ability to care for themselves and eventually become completely dependent on others (Medicine Online, 2007). Access to the bubble-like world to which they retreat becomes more difficult as language deteriorates. They lose their memory, and *repetitive movements* might emerge, including rocking, undressing, and walking up and down. People are also less able to establish and maintain eye contact and appear to see through people. They no longer recognize themselves in the mirror and don't appear to know their closest relatives. Patients will increasingly become less interested in personal hygiene. They will forget how to comb their hair, clean their teeth, and change clothes.

Often people become increasingly rigid toward the end of their life—their face becomes expressionless and rigid, the jaws clench, and the body stiffens. This can lead to difficulties with eating and falling. Daily activities for persons with AD tend to change as the disease progresses. AD tends to limit concentration and cause difficulties in following directions. These factors can turn simple activities into daily challenges. Daily functioning of the patient is often affected because AD is characterized by a steady loss of intellectual and social abilities.

Figure 6.4 presents limitations in activities of daily living (ADLs) and instrumental activities of daily living (IADLs) among people age 70 and above with AD.

Activities of Daily Living

As AD progresses, daily activities become harder to manage. Each patient has ups and downs, and some may find simple tasks confusing or challenging while others may not. Most of the people in the advanced stage of AD require help with such basic activities as using the toilet, getting in and out of bed, walking, eating, bathing and dressing. Since bathing, grooming and dressing are usually private activities, the person may refuse help.

Bathing

Some people with AD don't mind bathing, but others may find it to be a frightening, confusing experience. If the person is confused, using the bathroom can be challenging, as the person may perceive bathing as

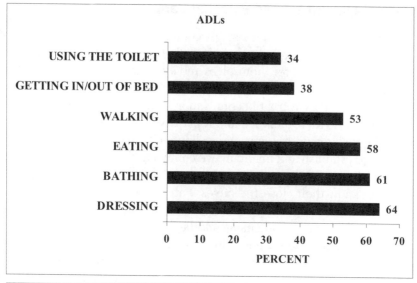

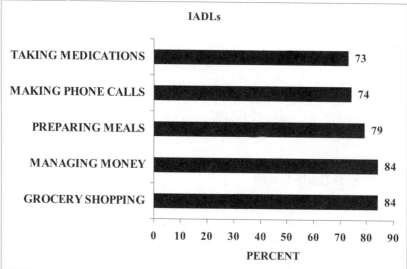

Figure 6.4 Limitations in ADLs and IADLs among people age 70 and above with Alzheimer's.
Source: Analysis of data from the 1993 study of "Assets and Health Dynamic Among the Oldest Old," by National Academy on an Aging Society, 2000.

unpleasant, threatening, or painful. The patient may act in disruptive ways, screaming, resisting, and hitting his caretaker (Alzheimer's Association, 2005b). This behavior occurs because the person doesn't remember what bathing is for or doesn't have the patience to endure the lack of modesty or the cold. Taking care of personal hygiene is often more difficult for relatives than for professional caregivers as the patient may feel less embarrassed if he is being washed by "strangers."

Dressing

For someone who has AD, the simple act of putting items of clothes on can be frustrating. There are many reasons why the person with AD might have problems dressing, including lack of privacy, problems choosing what to wear, not knowing how to dress and undress, getting only some clothes off and other clothes on, and struggling with buttons and zippers (Alzheimer's Outreach, 2007). Too many choices of clothes may be confusing for the person. Other factors may also contribute to problems dressing, such as balance or motor skills difficulties. A person might not be able to recognize her clothes, or she may be unaware of the seasons of the year or be unable to dress quickly under pressure.

Toileting

People with AD commonly experience loss of bladder or bowel control for many reasons. They may lose their ability to recognize natural urges telling them when to go to the bathroom, may forget where the bathroom is located or what to do when in the bathroom, or may be adversely affected by medical problems, physical conditions, or environmental factors (Alzheimer's Association, New York City Chapter, 2007a). Other causes include constipation and dehydration resulting from improper nutrition. Understandably, because toileting is a very personal and private matter, assistance with toileting is distressing for both the person with dementia and the caregiver.

Eating

Eating can be a challenge for people with AD. A person may have a poor appetite, lose interest in food, forget to eat, or forget that he has already eaten (Alzheimer's Society, 2007d). He may not recognize when he is hungry, may forget how to use a fork and spoon, or may forget how to chew and swallow. There may be problems with badly fitting dentures or sore gums, which make eating uncomfortable. If either of these conditions is resulting in eating difficulties, a consultation with a dentist can be quite helpful. If a person is not very active during the day, she may not feel hungry. In the later stages of AD, people may no longer be able to understand that the food in front of them is there to be eaten, even if they are clearly hungry. Some people with AD want to eat all the time, while others have to be encouraged to maintain a good diet. In the early stages of dementia, some people lose interest in food because they are depressed.

Mobility and Balance

Alzheimer's disease can affect physical coordination and mobility, leading to a gradual physical decline (Alzheimer's Society, 2007a). People in the last stage of Alzheimer's require help with all their daily needs. They lose the ability to get in and out of bed; they cannot walk without assistance; and they cannot sit up without support. Neuromuscular weakness is prominent among people with AD, resulting in an unsteady gait or difficulty keeping balance, which impairs activities of daily life.

Instrumental Activities of Daily Living

People with AD experience subtle changes in complex IADLs, such as managing money, preparing meals, shopping for groceries, taking medications, and making phone calls, long before the disease onsets (Richard, 1997). The most visible manifestation of AD is the progressive inability to perform IADLs—proportional to the severity of the disease—and the subsequent loss of independence. All the associated conditions related to cognitive, behavioral, and physical changes affect a person's ability to continue with IADLs as Alzheimer's progresses to the middle to late stage.

Speech and Communication Problems

Oral and written communication is gradually impaired as AD progresses. At first, a person suffering from AD may be able to understand simple speech, but may have trouble finding the correct words to make a point. Slowly, the person finds it harder and harder to understand complex conversations and metaphors and may forget proverbs. These complications make it difficult for a person with AD to correctly take a phone message, which is often a red flag to family members and the AD sufferer himself that there may be a more serious health issue than just normal aging. Further worsening the condition is the realization that it is increasingly difficult to follow a conversation, which might make the person feel confused and frightened and discourage efforts at communicating.

In the later stages of AD, the individuals cannot complete sentences and may often change subjects or use the same words repeatedly. Individuals with AD will start to add paraphasias—other words—to fill in the gaps into a conversation that they (and their audience) no longer comprehend. Spelling and writing become difficult. A person with late-stage AD may not be able to answer questions, since she doesn't understand what is being asked of her, and she may be overwhelmed by topic changes that usually take place in normal conversations. Eventually, the patient reaches a point where her speech does not make any sense and is mostly babbling, usually bringing the sufferer to withdraw from speaking altogether. In the very late stages of the disease, the sufferer will be unable to communicate very basic needs to her caretakers. Some patients may demonstrate an occasional automatic verbal response, but determining what the patient's needs are ultimately falls on the shoulders of the patient's family members and caregivers.

Incontinence

Incontinence is a common condition that can occur at any stage in AD. As the disease progresses, people suffering from AD lose their ability to control their toileting, and both bladder and fecal incontinence occurs (Wong, 2005). Typically, an individual first develops episodic urinary incontinence that slowly progresses over a period of years to total loss of bladder control. The rapid onset of incontinence suggests a behavioral or medical change. When incontinence occurs as part of Alzheimer's, it is normally for one of the following reasons:

- The patient cannot find his way to the toilet or can no longer clean himself.
- The patient does not realize that the bladder or bowel needs to be emptied– this may be because the correct signals are not being received or sent by the brain, or it may be because the sufferer has become unaware of what the sensations mean.

- The patient cannot move fast enough to get to the toilet in time.
- The patient may not know where the restroom is. This may be because the doors to all the rooms in the house look exactly the same, and the patient cannot remember what is behind each. For others, the toilet is no longer where they expect it to be—in childhood the toilet may have been on another floor of the house and it may be this toilet that they are trying to find.
- The patient may mistake one object for another. To a confused patient, a wastepaper basket may resemble a toilet, and this can result in going to the toilet in the wrong place; it may cause enough delay to make it impossible for the sufferer to reach the real toilet once he does realize his mistake.

Incontinence is often difficult, stigmatizing, embarrassing, and stressful and causes misery to both the person with Alzheimer's and to the caregiver (Kennard, 2006a).

Comorbidities

There is a strong association between medical comorbidities and cognitive status in AD (Doraiswamy, Leon, Cummings, Marin, & Neumann, 2002). Most people with Alzheimer's die not of the disease itself but of a secondary illness. Patients with AD frequently have comorbid medical conditions such as cardiovascular disease, infection, pulmonary disease, renal insufficiency, arthritis, and diminution of vision and hearing. As the disease progresses, people with AD develop infections quite frequently, particularly urinary tract infections and pneumonia. It is well documented that pneumonia is the most common cause of death among people with AD.

In advanced AD, people may lose all ability to care for themselves. They may have difficulty eating, become incontinent, or be unable to take a walk and find their way back home (Mayo Clinic, 2007a). These inabilities can increase the risk of additional health problems.

Pneumonia

Difficulty swallowing food and liquids may cause people with Alzheimer's to inhale some of what they eat and drink into their airways and lungs, which can lead to pneumonia.

Infections

Urinary incontinence may require the placement of a urinary catheter, which increases the risk of urinary tract infections. Untreated urinary tract infections can lead to more serious, life-threatening infections.

Falls and Their Complications

People with Alzheimer's may become disoriented, increasing their risk of falls. Falls can lead to fractures. In addition, falls are a common cause of serious head injuries, such as bleeding in the brain. Surgery to repair injury from a fall carries risks, as well. For instance, prolonged immobilization—which may be necessary to recover from injuries related to a fall—increases the risk of pulmonary embolism, which can be life-threatening.

Terminal Stage

In the terminal stage of AD, control of physiologic functions is lost. A person in this stage of AD has few or no verbal abilities, does not recognize family or caregivers, is incontinent and usually nonambulatory, and often demonstrates agitated behaviors such as resistiveness, moaning, or shouting (Sloane, 1998). Problems related to the terminal stage of AD are presented in detail in chapter 11.

7 Prevention and Treatment of Alzheimer's Disease

Current research and advances brings us closer to managing and eventually defeating Alzheimer's disease.

National Institute on Aging

A diagnosis of Alzheimer's disease (AD) can come as a shock. When a person is diagnosed with a chronic disease like AD, individuals and their family members usually leave the physician's office with an uneasy feeling. It is life-changing for both the individual diagnosed with AD and the family. The individual and his family members have many difficult questions in their minds that are specific at the onset of the disease. It is imperative that the physician, the individual, and caregivers become a team in the management of the illness. Physicians have a strong leadership role in their patients' care (Ham, 1997). In persons with AD, this role should extend far beyond the usual medical decisions into emotional, ethical, and financial considerations. The physician should guide the individual and family members about the progression of the disease and provide anticipatory guidance. The physician and other health professionals should educate the individual and the caregiver. A diagnosis of AD should not be looked at as a stigma but as a means to learn more about the illness so that the person can have access to appropriate resources for care, giving structure and dignity to the management.

Caregivers need to understand that the cognitive functions and behavioral symptoms of diagnosed individuals will worsen. The person with AD will need to be part of the team with health care professionals and other professionals to come to the right decisions about appropriate care to the individual. Planning for the future plays an important part in making life better for those living with Alzheimer's (Alzheimer's Association, 2005). Persons diagnosed with AD should have advance directives and health care proxies appointed early on in the disease before significant cognitive decline occurs. Knowing what to expect can help foster ease of mind for all concerned. The physician's goal when prescribing medications and management plans for the persons with AD is to educate the individual and caregivers, facilitating care and removing any hesitation they may have about the treatment plan.

In this chapter we review some evidence-based suggestions for prevention and management of AD. Currently, we do not have definitive cures or preventive measures in our arsenal to combat AD. There are a few studies that support treating certain comorbidities like hypertension and diabetes mellitus; healthy nutrition and certain vitamins and minerals can have an impact on AD. Lifelong learning and an active mind may delay the onset of AD.

PREVENTION OF ALZHEIMER'S DISEASE

Currently, there are no perfect preventive measures that are available for AD. Researchers had developed what looked to be a promising vaccine against Alzheimer's that worked by stopping deposits of beta-amyloid in the brain (Mayo Clinic.com, 2007b). Animal studies were so encouraging that human trials began in 2001. Unfortunately, they soon had to be stopped because some people experienced serious inflammation of the brain, with some recovering fully but others still having cognitive sequelae. However, there are a few theories that are being tested or that may play a role in future research for the prevention of AD. The latest medical research suggests that the best hope for preventing or slowing down AD is to adopt a lifestyle that includes physical and mental exercise and a healthy diet. Further, use of antioxidants, hormone replacement therapy, and nonsteroidal anti-inflammatory drugs along with a few other drugs can help either prevent or slow down Alzheimer's. The following are some of the common recommendations that exist for prevention of AD.

Physical and Mental Exercise

Current evidence shows that people who stay socially and physically active and keep their mind active can delay the onset of AD or stabilize disease progression for some time. As an old adage states, "use it or lose it."

Exercising is good not only for the heart but also for the mind. It is understood that exercising increases blood flow to organs, which includes the brain. Research suggests that increased blood flow to the brain brings nutrients to the brain cells and increases the growth factors in the brain that protect the brain cells from injury. In a study on the effects of exercise on brain power, it was found that subjects who regularly do aerobic exercise perform better on cognitive tests than sedentary individuals of the same age (Hollmann, Struder, Tagarakis, & King, 2007). The authors further concluded that the adjusted physical activity is capable of counteracting age-related changes and performance loss not only in the cardiovascular system but also in the brain. It also has been described that exercise increases nerve cells. It has been shown in many laboratory animal studies that animals that are allowed to perform activities have more growth factors and connections between neurons. Furthermore, it has been shown in humans that average intensity of weekly physical activities and variation in activities are positively and significantly associated with better cognitive performance on processing speed, memory, and mental flexibility as well as performance in overall cognitive function (Angevaren, Vanhees, Wendel-Vos, Verhaar, & Aufdemkampe, et al. 2007). Rolland and associates (2007) established in a study that people who already had developed AD who exercised regularly were able to improve performance on their activities of daily living (ADL) scores. These people also had a slower decline in ADL scores. Furthermore, research also suggests that exercise may reduce risk by as much as 40% and that exercise helps delay progression of Alzheimer's and dementia in people who have begun to develop symptoms (Larson et al., 2006).

It has been shown that people who have a history of at least 8 years of higher level of education tend to have a decreased risk of developing AD and mortality (Qiu, Bäckman, Winblad, Agüero-Torres, & Fratiglioni, 2001). People who maintain their reading, writing, and arithmetic skills may help maintain nerve connections or even increase nerve connections that may delay or even prevent AD. Research has shown that people who have certain talents preserve these skills until very late in the disease (Fornazzari, 2005). As with physical exercise, the more the mind is challenged and the more education a person gets, the more neuron-to-neuron connections a person develops. This may possibly delay the onset of disease or may prevent it. Several studies have found that folks who regularly engage in mentally challenging activities—like reading, doing crossword puzzles, or playing chess to "exercise their minds"—seem less likely to develop dementia later in life.

Nutrition

Different populations show differences in incidence of AD. It has been shown that caloric intake can play a role in mental health. In one animal study, preventing caloric intake above the starvation level helped prevent age-related nerve degeneration (A.D.A.M. Healthcare Center, 2004b). This analogy does not apply to persons with AD who lose weight because they forget to eat or forget to use utensils; this starvation is actually detrimental to brain health.

A number of cohort studies have examined a possible relationship between dietary components and risk of AD and other dementias. In large prospective cohort studies conducted at Rush University Medical Center, as well as cross-sectional studies, higher rates of cognitive decline and/or incident dementia have been associated with higher dietary intake of saturated fats, transunsaturated fats, or cholesterol (Morris, Evans, Bienias, Tangney, & Wilson, 2004). In one study, it was noted that people in China and Nigeria, where total fat intake is less than in the United States, the incidence of AD is 1%, whereas it is 5% in the United States (Rosenfeld, 2000). It has been shown that Japanese people who move to the United States and enjoy the rich, fatty foods common to the U.S. diet have a higher incidence of AD than their distant cousins in Japan. Kalmijn et al. (1997) reported a higher risk of incident AD with higher intake of total fat in more than 5,000 individuals 55 years and older without dementia at baseline who were followed for 2 years. Clinical evidence has suggested that people who carry the ApoE4 gene and whose diet has a relatively high percentage of caloric intake from fat have a higher rate of AD. Luchsinger and associates (2002), in a four-year longitudinal study, found that a higher intake of calories and fats may be associated with higher risk of AD in individuals who carry the apolipoprotein E epsilon4 allele. People should develop healthy eating habits at a very early age and consume diets that emphasize fresh fruits and vegetables and that are low in fat and rich in omega-3 fatty acids.

Antioxidants

There is good evidence that suggests that free-radical production and oxidative damage may be a direct or indirect causative agent for AD development. Free radicals are usually extra electrons on the oxygen molecules that are often produced by the normal metabolism of products in the body. It is these free radicals that can damage cells in the brain and other organs and speed the aging process. Consumption of antioxidants early on in life may delay the aging process and the damaging effects of free radicals. The role of antioxidants in the prevention of dementia has been evaluated in several observational studies with varying results. A large, prospective cohort study reported that higher dietary intake of antioxidants, particularly vitamin C and vitamin E, was associated with a lower risk of AD (Engelhart et al., 2002). There is some evidence that suggests that the consumption of vitamins C, E, and B-12, folate, omega-3 fatty acids, Coenzyme Q, selenium, and certain minerals can help prevent the formation or neutralize the harmful effects of free radicals (Ramakrishnan & Scheid, 2007).

It is advised that the individuals take vitamins according to recommendations and not exceed the recommended dosage. There is no clear evidence that suggests the exact dose of antioxidants that might aid in the prevention of AD. In my practice, I recommend taking 500 mg of Vitamin C, which can be obtained from citrus fruits such as lemons, oranges, and tangerines; 400iu of Vitamin E, which can be obtained from spinach, almonds, peanuts and peanut butter, and sunflower oil; 100 micrograms of B-12, which can be obtained by eating egg whites, red meat, chicken, and fortified foods; 400 mcg of folate, which can be obtained from any green leafy vegetables and fortified foods; and 40–50 micrograms of selenium, which can be obtained from walnuts, brazil nuts, meats, and other fortified foods. One gram of omega-3 fatty acids, including eicosapentaenoic acid (EPA) and docosahexaenoic acid (DHA), can be obtained from eating fatty fish like salmon, mackerel, tuna, and shrimp and from oils like canola and flaxseed oil; 150 mg of Coenzyme Q is available as a supplement. Most vitamins and minerals do not have many adverse side effects but should never be taken in excess with the idea that taking more is better. People need to be cautioned in the usage of vitamins, since a recent meta-analysis showed that the high doses of vitamin E may increase mortality rate, but the evidence in this study was not clear about whether vitamin E was the culprit or whether other risk factors caused the increased mortality rate. Vitamin and mineral supplementation can be expensive, so it should be used only if a healthy diet does not supply an adequate intake.

Male and Female Hormone Replacement Therapy

Epidemiologic studies suggested that estrogen replacement might prevent dementia (LeBlanc, Janowski, Chan, & Nelson, 2001). Estrogen replacement and estrogen-plus-progestin replacement as possible protectors from memory impairment and dementia was evaluated in the Women's Health Initiative (WHI) and WHI Memory Study (WHIMS). It was found that older women who were on estrogen plus progestin actually doubled their risk of developing dementia, and the therapy did not improve or benefit their global cognition (i.e., memory and other basic mental abilities suck as concentration, language skills, and abstract reasoning) (Shumaker et al., 2003). Women who took estrogen alone also did not benefit from the HRT and actually had an increased risk of dementia (Shumaker et al., 2004). Other than the risk of dementia, WHIMS revealed that women on estrogen and progestin had a higher risk of heart attack, stroke, blood clots, and breast cancer than women who took a placebo. Estrogen alone led to an increased risk of stroke and blood clot. After the findings of WHIMS, the U.S. Food and Drug Administration (FDA) recommended that the use of HRT be limited to women with hot flashes and vaginal dryness following menopause and/ or for the prevention osteoporosis in women who cannot tolerate other medications, and then only for the shortest period of time possible (U.S. Food & Drug Administration, 2005b).

Testosterone replacement in some animal studies was found to be helpful in reducing beta-amyloid. Long-term effects and adverse effects are currently unknown. Some experts recommend use of testosterone in elderly men who have low testosterone and also have the ApoE4 gene. Further research is warranted before a broader recommendation can be made. Dehydroepiandrosterone (DHEA) is a testosterone-like hormone that declines with age. Some studies have suggested that replacing DHEA in women can reduce mental decline but not in men. Further research is needed before DHEA can be recommended as a therapy in the prevention of AD.

Nonsteroidal Anti-inflammatory Drugs (NSAIDs)

Research has not shown that NSAIDs have any efficacy in the treatment of AD, but there is some evidence to support this, and further research is being done on drugs like ibuprofen (Advil, Motrin) and naproxen (Aleve) to establish the efficacy of NSAIDs in prevention of AD. Animal study showed that some NSAIDs have properties that reduce the accumulation of beta-amyloid in the brain and in turn reduce the incidence of AD, but further studies are needed to confirm this (Yan et al., 2003). One study found that adults who used NSAIDs for at least two years regardless of dose were 80% less likely to develop AD than were individuals who used these drugs for shorter periods or who did not take them at all (Veld et al., 2001).

Also, a study of elderly identical twins showed that the twin who was taking NSAIDs had a lower incidence of AD than did the twin who did not take NSAIDs (Breitner et al., 1994). NSAIDs can have potentially lethal side effects such as gastrointestinal ulcers and bleeds and renal function impairment. Since there is no clear evidence currently to support a recommendation of a particular dose or type of NSAID to prevent AD, no clear recommendation can be made on their use. Use of low-dose aspirin can be recommended for persons who have risk factors for coronary artery disease (i.e., high blood pressure), diabetes mellitus, and high cholesterol, but this dose has not been proven to prevent AD. Further research is needed to elucidate this matter. Studies using the newer COX-2 inhibitors (Bextra and Vioxx [currently removed from the U.S. market]) were halted due to the drugs' association with adverse cardiovascular effects.

Other Drugs

There is increasing evidence that statin medications may reduce the risk of AD. Statins are drugs like Lipitor, Mevacor, and Pravachol that lower cholesterol. A number of research studies have shown that statins significantly reduce risk of AD. A recent clinical study showed an association between statin therapy and a reduction in the occurrence of AD by as much as 70% (Austen, Sidera, Liu, & Frears, 2003). It further explained that an elevated cholesterol level is a risk factor for the disease. Lipitor, Mevacor, and Pravachol are noted to reduce beta-amyloid, which is deposited in the brains of people with hypercholestrolemia. It was also noted that statins, as they cross the blood-brain barrier, actually worsened AD in people who already had the disease. Further, it was shown that people who did not have elevated cholesterol also benefited from the medications. Currently, studies are under way to establish the efficacy of statins as preventative and treatment measures for AD.

Antihypertensive drugs have been shown to reduce the risk of AD. A specific class of antihypertensive drugs called calcium channel blockers has been shown to have nerve-protective effects. Further research is needed to see whether the lowering of blood pressure is the helpful factor (which may be the case) or whether the actual medication has some protective effects on the brain. It has been demonstrated that having ideal blood pressure (below 140/90) and normal lipids levels reduce all-cause morbidity and mortality.

Ginkgo Biloba

Gingko biloba is a common traditional Chinese medicine that contains antioxidants. It is used to treat circulatory disorders and to enhance memory. The Alzheimer's Society, together with the Cochrane Collaboration, published the largest-ever comprehensive review on the use of Ginkgo biloba for the treatment of dementia. The systematic review identified 33 previous clinical trials of Ginkgo, dating back to 1976 (Press & Alexander, 2007). This new research provides promising evidence that taking Ginkgo biloba can improve memory and overall function for people with dementia. The review, published by the Cochrane Collaboration (Birks, Grimley, & Van Dongen, 2002) concluded that "Ginkgo biloba appears to be safe in use with no excessive side effects compared with a placebo. Many of the early trials used unsatisfactory methods, were small, and we cannot exclude publication bias. But overall there is promising evidence of improvement in cognition and function associated with Ginkgo. Our view is that there is need for a large trial using modern methodology to provide robust estimates of the size and mechanism of the treatment effects."

TREATMENT AND MANAGEMENT

Treatment and management of AD requires a multifaceted approach. As mentioned earlier, no absolute cure exists today for AD, but the disease process can be managed and disease symptoms can be delayed. Care for persons with AD involves medications that function on the pathophysiology of the disease in the brain. It also includes medications necessary, at times, for management of behavioral issues.

Cognitive Management

Currently two classes of medications exist that may slow progression or stabilize AD. The cholinesterase inhibitors (ChEIs) are one class of medication that consists of four drugs—Aricept (donepezil), Reminyl/ Razadye (galantamine), Exelon (rivastigmine), and a rarely used medication called Cognex (tacrine). A second class of medication is N-methyl-D-aspartate (NMDA), a receptor antagonist that currently includes only one drug, Namenda (memantine). The two classes can be used in combination if necessary in persons who have moderate to severe dementia, as they work via different mechanisms (Ramakrishnan & Scheid, 2007).

It has been shown that there is decreased production of acetylcholine transferase, an enzyme important in the synthesis of acetylcholine, in the brains of persons with AD (Press & Daniel, 2007). Acetylcholine is an important neurotransmitter necessary in memory and concentration. Drugs were developed that target increasing acetylcholine in the brain. Medications that were precursors of acetylcholine proved to be ineffective, and the drugs that had agonist effects of acetylcholine carried too many side effects and were deemed intolerable by people with AD. Cholinesterase inhibitors proved to be a better choice because these drugs had better tolerability and worked by preventing breakdown of acetylcholine by cholinesterase.

Aricept (donepezil) is dosed once a day and has become a popular choice for persons with AD. Donepezil is started 5 mg once a day for 4 weeks, then increased to 10 mg daily after 1 month. Adverse effects are mild and transient and include diarrhea, nausea, and vomiting (Cummings et al., 2002). This easy dosing and the mild side effects can help patients' compliance with the drug regimen. One 24-week double-blind placebo-controlled study demonstrated that donepezil clinically improved cognitive and global functioning over placebo. Individuals who were taking donepezil also had modest improvement in their neuropsychiatric symptoms. A drug washout study apparently revealed that once the body was free of the medication, the cognitive improvements disappeared, suggesting the drug has no impact on the course of the underlying disease. The efficacy of donepezil has been shown for up to 5 years.

Reminyl/Razadye (galantamine) is dosed 4 mg twice daily, with breakfast and with dinner, for 4 weeks, then increased to 8 mg twice daily. If tolerance is good and there is clinical benefit, persons can increase dose to 12 mg twice daily. Side effects are mild and include nausea, vomiting, headaches, anorexia, and diarrhea (Cummings et al., 2002). Secondary analysis of randomized control trials has shown that persons taking galantamine have overall better ADL scores than persons in the control group. It has been shown that higher dosages of galantamine, 24 mg to

32 mg, tend to produce greater improvement in cognitive and functional outcomes and in behavioral symptoms. The efficacy of galantamine has been shown for up to 3 years.

Exelon (rivastigmine) is dosed 1.5 mg twice daily and is increased by 1.5 mg twice daily to a maximum dose of 6 mg twice daily. Side effects are anorexia, malaise, headaches, weight loss, nausea, vomiting, and diarrhea. Like other ChEIs for the management of AD, rivastigmine slows cognitive decline and improves function and behavioral symptoms. The treatment with rivastigmine also works for a few years.

Cognex (tacrine) is now considered a second-line agent for the management of AD. Tacrine has a dosing of 10 mg four times a day, increased every 4 weeks to tolerability at a maximum dose of 40 mg four times a day. Tacrine is hepatotoxic; therefore, liver enzyme tests need to be monitored every 2 weeks. Because the medication has daily multiple dosing and requires blood testing, it is the least favored by individuals with AD and by the prescribers.

Namenda (memantine) is the only NMDA receptor antagonist approved for treatment of moderate to severe AD. The medication works by blocking the NMDA receptor and preventing the binding of excitatory neurotransmitter glutamate that is present in cortical and hippocampal neurons (Ramakrishnan & Scheid, 2007). The NMDA receptor is involved in memory and learning. NMDA if excessively exited can become excitotoxic to neurons; therefore, blocking the NMDA receptor by memantine only at times of excessive stimulation can prevent this overstimulation and excitotoxic damage to neurons. Memantine does not interfere with the normal function of the NMDA receptors. Memantine is dosed 5 mg daily, increased by 5 mg every 2 weeks to a maximum dose of 20 mg per day. Doses greater than 5 mg should be taken twice a day. In a study, persons with severe dementia demonstrated reduced deterioration in cognitive function. Studies in persons with mild to moderate dementia also demonstrated the medication's clinical efficacy. Memantine has fewer adverse effects than ChEIs. The most common side effect is dizziness. Confusion and hallucinations have been reported by persons taking memantine, and worsening of confusion and hallucinations is reported in persons who already have these symptoms. Memantine has not shown any statistically significant improvement in persons' behavior or ADL.

In some individuals with AD, use of ChEI, specifically donepezil, in combination with memantine has shown some promise. The combined treatment has revealed improvement in cognition, ADL, behavior, and global outcome over placebo and memantine alone (Grossberg, Dharmarajan, Fillit, & Ringel, 2007).

Cholinesterase inhibitors and memantine are good drugs that can control the progression of AD for some time. It is important to ensure that persons are compliant with the medication and that the adverse effects are not preventing the use of medication. It is also necessary to observe individuals for 6–12 months on medications to note any significant difference in cognitive and functional improvement or stabilization. If individuals are not able to tolerate the medications or if, despite the medication, the disease progression continues at the same rate as prior to the onset of medication, discontinuation of medication should be considered, as there is no benefit to the individual.

Behavior Management

Person with Alzheimer's dementia can have significant behavioral difficulties. These include personality changes leading to passive to aggressive to hostile attitudes, psychotic symptoms, including delusions and hallucinations, and excessive irritability and depression. This subgroup of persons with AD might benefit from antipsychotic medications and mood stabilizing antiseizure medications. Antipsychotics should be used carefully in the elderly as they have been associated with slight increase risk of death in elderly persons with AD. Antipsychotics are not approved by the FDA for behavioral symptoms of dementia but are used for the person's benefit (Cummings et al., 2002). Persons with AD may be depressed or apathetic. Patients who develop AD may have developed major depression 1–2 years prior to their diagnosis of AD. If treated appropriately for depression, these persons may show delayed progression of AD. Apathy should not be confused with depression. Persons who are apathetic show no emotion, have no interest, and lack any enthusiasm; depressed individuals have a sense of hopelessness and truly feel sad. Apathetic persons may benefit from mood stabilizers and antidepressants. Some may suffer from sleep disturbances and can benefit from anxiolytics and other sleep aids, such as Ambien and Lunesta.

Conservative management or nonpharmacological management is the first line in behavioral management in persons with AD and is discussed in detail in chapter 8. If a conservative, nonpharmacologic approach to behavioral management fails, adjunct pharmacological treatment may be necessary. It is crucial that when pharmacological therapy is implemented, persons with AD are started on the lowest dosages and the dosages increased slowly to have the beneficial effect at the lowest dose with minimal adverse effects. Medication should target the specific symptoms, and at times one medication may be able to manage multiple problems. For example, agitation and sleep disorder can be managed by a benzodiazepine. Persons should be evaluated on a regular basis to assess if there is still a need for drugs or if the dosages can be decreased and eventually discontinued. Table 7.1 lists medications used for management of behavioral disorders and their side effects. Table 7.2 lists medications that can be used for sleep disorders and nighttime behavioral disturbances in Alzheimer's patients.

Alternative and Herbal Treatment

There are substances available for the management of AD that are now gaining some support. Ginkgo biloba has antioxidative properties and may help in prevention (as described earlier) and treatment of AD. It also increases blood flow to the brain, increasing oxygen and nutrient delivery. Although it is not definitive, there is promising early evidence favoring use of Ginkgo for memory enhancement in healthy subjects (Mayo Clinic, 2006b). Currently, a specific dose of Ginkgo biloba cannot be recommended because no standard doses are established and active ingredient can vary in products available over the counter. Ginkgo biloba can cause excessive bleeding and therefore cannot be co-administered to persons on anticoagulation therapy. Curcumin is a yellow pigment in curry spice in India that is being researched for treatment of AD. Curcumin is believed to act both as an anti-inflammatory and as a very potent antioxidant. Furthermore, curcumin does more than act as an anti-inflammatory and antioxidant in the brain. It doesn't just prevent the amyloid clumps from causing damage; it actually prevents them from forming into plaques in the first place (Yang, Lim, Begum, Ubeda, & Simmons, 2005). It is also reported that curcumin triggers amyloid plaques to break apart (Ono, Hasegawa, Naiki, & Yamada, 2004). Huperzine A, a product isolated from Chinese club moss, has been used in China for centuries for memory and concentration. It is an acetylcholine esterase inhibitor works similar to the prescription ChEI (Wang & Tang, 2005). Other treatments that can be tried or being researched were mentioned under the prevention section.

Table 7.1

TREATMENT OF BEHAVIOR AND MOOD DISORDERS

ANTIPSYCHOTIC DRUGS

Atypical antipsychotic agents

Recommended uses: control of problematic delusions, hallucinations, severe psychomotor agitation, and combativeness.

General cautions: diminished risk of developing extrapyramidal symptoms and tardive dyskinesia compared with typical antipsychotic agents.

Risperidone (Risperdal)	Initial dosage: 0.25 mg per day at bedtime; maximum: 2 to 3 mg per day, usually twice daily in divided doses.	Comments: current research supports use of low dosages; extrapyramidal symptoms may occur at 2 mg per day.
Olanzapine (Zyprexa)	Initial dosage: 2.5 mg per day at bedtime; maximum: 10 mg per day, usually twice daily in divided doses.	Comments: generally well tolerated.
Quetiapine (Seroquel)	Initial dosage: 12.5 mg twice daily; maximum: 200 mg twice daily.	Comments: more sedating; beware of transient orthostasis.

Typical antipsychotic agents

Recommended uses: control of problematic delusions, hallucinations, severe psychomotor agitation, and combativeness; second-line therapy in patients who cannot tolerate or do not respond to atypical antipsychotic agents.

General cautions: current research suggests that these drugs should be avoided if possible, because they are associated with significant, often severe, side effects involving the cholinergic, cardiovascular, and extrapyramidal systems; there is also an inherent risk of irreversible tardive dyskinesia, which can develop in 50% of elderly patients after continuous use of typical antipsychotic agents for 2 years.

Haloperidol (Haldol), fluphenazine (Prolixin), thiothixene (Navane)	Dosage: varies by agent.	Comments: anticipated extrapyramidal symptoms; if these symptoms occur, decrease dosage or switch to another agent; avoid use of benztropine (Cogentin) or trihexyphenidyl (Artane).
Trifluoperazine (Stelazine), molindone (Moban), perphenazine (Trilafon), loxapine (Loxitane)	Dosage: varies by agent.	Comments: agents with "in-between" side effect profile.

(continued)

Table 7.1

TREATMENT OF BEHAVIOR AND MOOD DISORDERS *(continued)*

MOOD-STABILIZING (ANTIAGITATION) DRUGS

Recommended uses: control of problematic delusions, hallucinations, severe psychomotor agitation, and combativeness; useful alternatives to antipsychotic agents for control of severe agitated, repetitive, and combative behaviors.

General cautions: see comments about specific agents.

Trazodone (Desyrel)	Initial dosage: 25 mg per day; maximum: 200 to 400 mg per day in divided doses.	Comments: use with caution in patients with premature ventricular contractions.
Carbamazepine (Tegretol)	Initial dosage: 100 mg twice daily; titrate to therapeutic blood level (4 to 8 mcg per mL).	Comments: monitor complete blood cell count and liver enzyme levels regularly; carbamazepine has problematic side effects.
Divalproex sodium (Depakote)	Initial dosage: 125 mg twice daily; titrate to therapeutic blood level (40 to 90 mcg per mL).	Comments: generally better tolerated than other mood stabilizers; monitor liver enzyme levels; monitor platelets, prothrombin time, and partial thromboplastin time as indicated.

ANXIOLYTIC DRUGS

Benzodiazepines

Recommended uses: management of insomnia, anxiety, and agitation.

General cautions: regular use can lead to tolerance, addiction, depression, and cognitive impairment; paradoxic agitation occurs in about 10% of patients treated with benzodiazepines; infrequent, low doses of agents with a short half-life are least problematic.

Lorazepam (Ativan), oxazepam (Serax), temazepam (Restoril), zolpidem (Ambien), triazolam (Halcion)	Dosage: varies by agent.	See general cautions.

Nonbenzodiazepines

Buspirone (BuSpar)	Initial dosage: 5 mg twice daily; maximum: 20 mg three times daily.	Comments: useful only in patients with mild to moderate agitation; may take 2 to 4 weeks to become effective.

ANTIDEPRESSANT DRUGS

Recommended uses: see comments on specific agents.

General cautions: selection of an antidepressant is usually based on previous treatment response, tolerance, and the advantage of potential side effects (e.g., sedation versus activation); a full therapeutic trial requires at least 4–8 weeks; as a rule, dosage is increased using increments of initial dose every 5–7 days until therapeutic benefits or significant side effects become apparent; after 9 months, dosage reduction is used to reassess the need to medicate; discontinuing an antidepressant over 10 to 14 days limits withdrawal symptoms.

NOTE: Patients with depression and psychosis require concomitant antipsychotic medication.

Tricyclic antidepressant agents

Desipramine (Norpramin)

Initial dosage: 10 to 25 mg in the morning; maximum: 150 mg in the morning.

Comments: tends to be activating (i.e., reduces apathy); lower risk for cardiotoxic, hypotensive, and anticholinergic effects; may cause tachycardia; blood levels may be helpful.

Nortriptyline (Pamelor)

Initial dosage: 10 mg at bedtime; anticipated dosage range: 10 to 40 mg per day (given twice daily).

Comments: tolerance profile is similar to that for desipramine, but nortriptyline tends to be more sedating; may be useful in patients with agitated depression and insomnia; therapeutic blood level "window" of 50 to 150 ng per mL (190 to 570 nmol per L).

Heterocyclic and noncyclic antidepressant agents

Nefazodone (Serzone)

Initial dosage: 50 mg twice daily; maximum: 150 to 300 mg twice daily.

Comments: effective, especially in patients with associated anxiety; reduce dose of coadministered alprazolam (Xanax) or triazolam by 50%; monitor for hepatotoxicity.

Bupropion (Wellbutrin)

Initial dosage: 37.5 mg every morning, then increase by 37.5 every 3 days; maximum: 150 mg twice daily.

Comments: activating; possible rapid improvement of energy level; should not be used in agitated patients and in those with seizure disorders; to minimize risk of insomnia, give second dose before 3 P.M.

Mirtazapine (Remeron)

Initial dosage: 7.5 mg at bedtime; maximum: 30 mg at bedtime.

Comments: potent and well tolerated; promotes sleep, appetite, and weight gain.

(continued)

153

Table 7.1

TREATMENT OF BEHAVIOR AND MOOD DISORDERS (*continued*)

SSRIs

Recommended uses: may prolong half-life of other drugs by inhibiting various cytochrome P450 isoenzymes

Fluoxetine (Prozac)	Initial dosage: 10 mg every other morning; maximum: 20 mg every morning.	Comments: activating, very long half-life; side effects may not manifest for a few weeks.
Paroxetine (Paxil)	Initial dosage: 10 mg per day; maximum: 40 mg per day (morning or evening).	Comments: less activating but more anticholinergic than other SSRIs.
Sertraline (Zoloft)	Initial dosage: 25 to 50 mg per day; maximum: 200 mg per day (morning or evening).	Comments: well tolerated; compared with other SSRIs, sertraline has less effect on metabolism of other medications.
Citalopram (Celexa)	Initial dosage: 10 mg per day; maximum: 40 mg per day.	Comments: well tolerated; some patients experience nausea and sleep disturbances.
Fluvoxamine (Luvox)	Initial dosage: 50 mg twice daily; maximum: 150 mg twice daily.	Comments: exercise caution when using fluvoxamine with alprazolam or triazolam.

PHENETHYLAMINE

Venlafaxine (Effexor)	Initial dosage: 37.5 mg twice daily; maximum: 225 mg per day in divided doses.	Comments: highly potent; also inhibits norepinephrine reuptake.

LITHIUM

Recommended uses: for anticycling; can also be used to augment antidepressant drugs.
General cautions: at higher lithium dosages, elderly patients are prone to develop neurotoxicity.

Lithium   Initial dosage: 150 mg per day.   Comments: blood levels of 0.2 to 0.6 mEq per L
                                                                    (0.2 to 0.6 mmol per L) are generally adequate
                                                                    and are usually achieved with dosage of 150 to
                                                                    300 mg per day.

ELECTROCONVULSIVE THERAPY

Recommended uses: may be required in patients who are at risk of injuring or starving themselves, patients who are severely psychotic, and patients who cannot tolerate or do not respond to antidepressants.

Source: "Guidelines for Managing Alzheimer's Disease: Part II," June 15, 2002, *American Family Physician.*
Copyright © 2002 American Academy of Family Physicians. All rights reserved. Reprinted with permission.

Table 7.2

PHARMACOLOGIC TREATMENT OF INSOMNIA

DRUG	DAILY DOSAGE (MG)	PEAK ACTION (HOURS)	HALF-LIFE (HOURS)	ADVERSE EFFECTS AND CONSIDERATIONS	FDA APPROVED?
NONBENZODIAZEPINES					
Zolpidem (Ambien)	5–10	0.5	2–3	Abdominal pain, rebound insomnia; controlled-release formulation better for sleep maintenance; FDA pregnancy risk category B (not controlled-release formulation); CYP3A4-dependent metabolism.	Yes
Zaleplon (Sonata)	5–10	0.5	1	Better for sleep maintenance; altered color perception; CYP3A4-dependent metabolism.	Yes
Eszopiclone (Lunesta)	2–3	1	4–6	Unpleasant taste (8%–24%), amnesia, hallucinations, worsening depression; CYP3A4-dependent metabolism.	Yes
MELATONIN RECEPTOR AGONIST					
Ramelteon (Rozerem)	8–16	0.3	2–5	Suicidal ideation, dizziness, headache, increased prolactin levels; contraindicated with fluvoxamine and liver failure; CYP3A4-, CYP1A2-, and CYP2C9-dependent metabolism.	Yes
ANTIHISTAMINES					
Diphenhydramine (Benadryl)	25–50	1–3	8	Anticholinergic, CNS depression/stimulation; FDA pregnancy risk category B.	Yes
Doxylamine (Unisom)	12.5–25	2–3	10	Anticholinergic, CNS depression/stimulation; FDA pregnancy risk category A.	Yes
Hydroxyzine (Vistaril)	25–100	2	3–7	Anticholinergic, CNS depression/stimulation.	No

ANTIDEPRESSANTS					
Amitriptyline	25–100	2–4	17–40	Anticholinergic, morning sedation, daytime somnolence, accidents, cardiac toxicity, sexual dysfunction, serotonin syndrome (SSRI interaction), exacerbates restless legs syndrome and periodic limb movement; CYP2D6-dependent metabolism.	No
Trazodone (Desyrel)	5–150	0.5–2	8	Same as above.	No
Mirtazapine (Remeron)	15–45	1.2–1.6	20–40	Anticholinergic, dyspnea, edema, hyper- or hypokinesia, increased appetite. Rare: facial edema, delusions, hallucinations, seizures, abdominal pain, back pain, agranulocytosis.	No
BENZODIAZEPINES					
Triazolam (Halcion)	0.125–	1–2	1.5–5	Rapid onset, short half-life; anterograde amnesia, rapid eye movement sleep rebound; CYP3A4-dependent metabolism.	Yes
Estazolam	1–2	2 (0.5 to 6)	10–24	Rapid onset, intermediate half-life; daytime sleepiness.	Yes
Temazepam (Restoril)	7.5–30	1.2–1.6	3.5–18.4	Medium onset, intermediate half-life; daytime sleepiness, less effective sleep induction.	Yes
HERBS AND SUPPLEMENTS					
Melatonin	0.5–10	1	0.5–2	Sleep disruption, daytime fatigue, headache, dizziness, irritability.	No
Valerian root	200–1,000	1	Not known	Daytime sedation, hepatotoxicity.	No

Source: "Treatment Options for Insomnia," August 15, 2002. *American Family Physician.* Copyright © 2002 American Academy of Family Physicians. All rights reserved. Reprinted with permission.

LATEST RESEARCH

Every day, advances in technology and in our understanding of the patho-physiology of AD bring us closer to better treatments for AD. Agents that are being developed show some promise. Investigations are ongoing for agents that increase nerve growth factors that stimulate activity in the brain. Drugs undergoing synthesis include drugs that can increase the production of acetylcholine in the brain. Concentrated research is being conducted on drugs that decrease or block the enzymes that lead to the production of beta-amyloid. Chelators, such as Clioquinol (iodochlor-hydroxyquin), is a drug that inhibits the binding of zinc and copper ions to beta-amyloid, promoting dissolution of beta-amyloid. This has been demonstrated in mice models, and human trials are under way. Research is being conducted on other antioxidants and on other drugs that will eventually lead to better drugs or even possibly a cure for AD.

8

Caring at Home for People With Alzheimer's Disease

Caring for a person with Alzheimer's disease at home is a difficult task...basic activities of daily living are often hard to manage for both the person with Alzheimer's and the caregiver.

National Institute on Aging

Alzheimer's disease (AD) has significant and life-changing effects on both the person diagnosed with AD and the caregiver involved. For many families, caring for their loved ones at home is the first choice—it is generally less costly and can be a rewarding experience. More than 80% of those with AD are older than 65, which means that the person with AD will likely be cared for by an elderly spouse or by adult children. A spouse might himself be frail or in poor health, and adult children must care for their own families, making caregiving an overwhelming and challenging task, as well.

Caring for an elder with AD can be particularly frustrating and overwhelming. It is one of the most difficult types of caregiving. Each day brings new challenges, as the changing levels of ability and new patterns of behavior are the only constant. When pressures worsen over time, many caregivers suffer from stress, depression, and illness, and family crises can occur. With support from family, friends, and outside resources, such as home health assistance, a caregiving companion, or a homemaker, caregiving at home can remain a viable option.

According to the National Institute on Aging (2007a), one of the biggest struggles caregivers face is dealing with the difficult behaviors of the person they are caring for. Dressing, bathing, eating—basic activities of daily living (ADLs)—often become difficult to manage for both the person with AD and the caregiver. Having a plan for getting through the day can help caregivers cope, and many caregivers have found it helpful to use strategies for dealing with difficult behaviors and stressful situations.

Caring for people with AD will differ depending on the person's symptoms and the progression of the disease (WebMD, 2007a). Soon after the diagnosis, it will be necessary to get started on making changes that help provide a sense of well-being and physical safety for the person diagnosed with AD. Things that were taken for granted before, such as home safety and socializing, will now require some planning. Simple adjustments made to the residence can provide significant safety benefits for a person with AD who lives at home. General safety precautions, which we will describe in this chapter, can be implemented to improve the quality of life for people with AD and minimize the potential for accidents.

After the diagnosis, all family members face emotional challenges and must cope with mortality, fear, and other emotional issues. Despite the emotional difficulty, it is extremely important that family members and caregivers begin advanced planning to avoid problems at later stages. Important issues—long-range planning for legal and financial matters, planning for individual's care and end-of-life issues, medical management of symptoms, maintaining the sense of well-being (i.e., safety, socializing, fun), managing troublesome behaviors (i.e., wandering or aggressiveness), and placement in a facility if caregiving becomes unmanageable at home—must be discussed and decided upon. Keep in mind that it is important to involve the person with AD in the planning process, particularly during the early stages of disease, when they are still able to make informed decisions about their care.

FALLS IN PEOPLE WITH ALZHEIMER'S DISEASE

Assessment of Fall

Falls and injuries are common safety hazards for people with AD. Individuals with AD are twice as likely to experience a fall as are those without AD (Tideiksaar, 2007). Studies show annual falls incidence are as high as 60% among people with dementia (Shaw & Kenny, 1998). The main causes of falls in older people include their slower reaction time and less efficient balance systems due to age; health problems such as Parkinson's disease, arthritis, foot problems, and dizziness; visual impairments; and environmental factors such as poor lighting, slippery floors, and cluttered paths. Medications are also a significant risk factor for falls. Drug effects and reactions can affect cognition and balance, thus contributing to falls. The most common drugs associated with fall risk include those that act on the central nervous system, such as sedatives and tranquilizers, and benzodiazepines. Taking more than four medications at one time or taking psychoactive medications may predispose older adults to falls. Other medications commonly associated with falls are anticoagulants, antiepileptics, antihypertensives, anti-Parkinsonian agents, diuretics, narcotic analgesics, and vasodilators.

Dementia can increase the risk of falling by impairing judgment, gait, visual-spatial perception, and the ability to recognize and avoid hazards (Buchner & Larson, 1987). People with AD may have an impairment in their sensory-processing abilities (e.g., lack of visual spatial awareness), which can affect the way one reacts to a situation or approaches a task. A person with AD also has difficulty with depth perception. This is seen when a person moves up a staircase. Changes in depth perception or trouble with visual-spatial relations can result in misinterpreting the environment and missing a step (Lach, 1998). Hearing impairment in people with AD also puts them at a high risk for falls. Even if there is no hearing problem, people with AD have difficulty processing auditory information, and their reaction time slows down.

Some people with AD have apraxia, or trouble coordinating movements and walking (Lach, 1998). People with AD develop neuromotor changes and cognitive impairment so severe that they lose the ability to ambulate. This loss usually happens over the course of many months and, sometimes, several years. During this time, people with AD remain at high risk of falling. Ironically, forced immobilization not only significantly reduces quality of life but actually increases falls and injuries. This happens because inactivity results in loss of muscle strength and balance, which can lead to falls.

A fall can be a life-changing event that may lead to disability, loss of independence, or death. About 35% of people 65 and older fall each year (Hausdorff, Rios, & Edelberg, 2001), and 10%–20% of those falls result in serious injuries, at least half of which are fractures (Sterling, O'Connor, & Bonadies, 2001). Falls are the key incident in the pathogenesis of hip fracture. More than 90% of hip fractures occur as a result of falls, with most of these fractures occurring in persons over 70 years of age (Capezuti, 1996). Hip fractures are associated with a remarkable decline in functional status. More than 50% of older persons who survive hip fractures are discharged to a nursing home, and nearly half of these people can still be found in a nursing home 1 year later (Coogler & Wolf, 1999). Hip fracture survivors experience a 10%–15% decrease in life expectancy and a meaningful decline in overall quality of life. One-fourth of elderly persons who sustain a hip fracture die within 6 months of injury (Fuller, 2000).

The fall-related morbidity rate associated with AD is significant. Seventy to 85% of people with cognitive impairment and dementia fall each year, approximately twice the rate expected in cognitively normal older people (Shaw, 2002). In addition, persons with cognitive impairment and dementia are at an increased risk of serious injury and have a poorer prognosis once a fall has occurred than do normal older people who fall. Residents of long-term facilities with AD are less likely to make a satisfactory recovery from injury. About 25% people with AD who fall sustain fractures, with hip fractures being the most common (Tideiksaar, 2007). The main factors specifically implicated in falls in the elderly AD population are postural instability, medication, neuron-cardiovascular instability (e.g., orthostatic hypotension, carotid sinus hypersensitivity), and environmental hazards. Other significant factors that contribute to falls in people with AD are disturbed balance and transfers related to mobility (i.e., inability to maintain stability during postural changes); impaired ambulation (i.e., a small-stepping and shuffling gait); and a cautious gait (i.e., flexed posture, slowness of walking, and uncertainty of foot placement).

Assessing the risk of falls is an important starting point to reduce their occurrence. Risk assessment is used to identify persons with AD who are most likely to fall. Relevant risk factors for falls in people with AD include previous falls, severely impaired cognitive status, disturbed vision and hearing, muscle weakness, unsteady gait and balance, posture, use of multiple medications, incorrect use of ambulatory aids, and environmental hazards. A thorough assessment of people with AD and their environment as a part of a caregiver's education can reduce the risk of falls. There are two fall assessment tools commonly used in the medical community:

1   Dementia-Specific Fall Risk Factors Assessment—used to identify those risk factors that most apply to the advanced dementia person (Figure 8.1)

Place a check by all conditions present. Each of these factors independently increase fall risk. The more factors occurring simultaneously the higher the fall risk.

General	Mobility
☐ New Admission or transfer to another unit	☐ Ambulatory and active
☐ Fall(s) within last 30 days	☐ Ambulatory but weak/debilitated
☐ No trauma	☐ Using assistive device: walker, cane, other _____
☐ Injury _____	☐ Unable to use assistive devices properly
☐ Bowel and/or bladder incontinence	☐ Nonambulatory
☐ Low body mass	☐ Self-propels wheelchair
☐ Seizures	☐ Increased reliance on proprioception to maintain balance (i.e., as evidenced by removing footwear when ambulating)
☐ Episode of Acute Illness	

Cognition	Neuromotor Changes
☐ Depression	☐ Rigidity present: ☐ Arms ☐ Legs ☐ Neck ☐ Torso
☐ GDS Stage 6	☐ Rigidity induced by bed/chair alarm sounds
☐ GDS Stage 7	☐ Decreased grip strength
☐ Change in cognitive level from GDS/FAST stage _____ to _____	☐ Loss of protective reflexes
☐ Poor reasoning/judgment placing self in unsafe situations	☐ Impaired recovery balance
☐ Unable to recognize ambulation deficits	☐ Impaired arm outstretching /extension
☐ Unable to tolerate wearing eyeglasses	
☐ Unable to tolerate wearing hearing aid(s)	
☐ Unable to verbally communicate needs	
☐ Unable to comprehend bed or chair alarm	

Altered Gait & Balance	Vision Changes
☐ Start hesitancy and freezing	☐ Decreased depth perception
☐ Shuffling	☐ Decreased peripheral vision
☐ Scissoring	☐ 1 sided visual neglect _____ Left _____
☐ Non-continuous walk with hesitation	
☐ Deviates from straight path	
☐ Difficulty making turns	
☐ One or both feet scrape ground surface	
☐ Unable to step over obstacles	

(continued)

Figure 8.1 Dementia-specific fall risk factors assessment.
Source: "Geriatric Resources Inc." Retrieved June 2007, from http://www.geriatric-resources.com/

☐ Unable to navigate around obstacles

☐ Reduced walking speed

☐ Unsteady standing balance

☐ Uses furniture to maintain standing or walking balance

☐ Sinks to feet when ambulating

☐ Postural sway
  ☐ Forward   ☐ Left Side
  ☐ Right Side   ☐ Backward

☐ Unstable rising from seated positions

☐ Unstable getting out of bed

☐ Unstable sitting balance

☐ Unable to sit up

☐ Unable to perform unassisted chair/bed transfers

☐ Feet slide away on ground during transfers

Behavior

☐ Self-stimulatory wandering

☐ Restless pacing

☐ Resistive to ADL care

☐ Anxiety, agitation

☐ Sleep disturbance

☐ **Monitor closely 1st week of stay:** Dates _____ to _____

☐ Times of day fall risk increases: From _____ to _____

☐ **Physical Therapy screening/evaluation requested**

☐ **Wear protective device(s) :** *NOTE: Plan for 7 days to get resident able to tolerate wearing device(s) consistently. If multiple devices indicated, introduce 1 device a week.*

☐ Hip protector(s):	☐ Left Hip	☐ Right Hip	
☐ Knee pad(s):	☐ Left Knee	☐ Right Knee	
☐ Elbow pad(s):	☐ Left Elbow	☐ Right Elbow	
☐ Wrist splint(s):	☐ Left Wrist	☐ Right Wrist	
☐ Thick foam helmet	☐ Left Hip	☐ Right Hip	
☐ Hip protector(s):			

☐ **Footwear adaption:** NOTE: Slippers can worsen shuffling gait and aggravate poor steppage height

  ☐ Footwear to increase proprioceptive input

    ☐ Thin hard-soles

    ☐ Leather-type soles

    ☐ Non-slip tread socks

  ☐ Slip-resistant soles

  ☐ Wearing of non-slip tread socks to bed

  ☐ Barefoot

Figure 8.1 Dementia-specific fall risk factors assessment. (*continued*)

☐ **Assistive Device Use**

☐ Cane: Type

☐ Standard Pick-up Walker (dangerous if cannot sequence)

☐ Gliding Walker

☐ Rolling Walker

☐ Quad Cane

☐ Walker: Type

☐ Standard

☐ Wheeled

☐ Merry Walker/Alzheimer's-specific

☐ Other _____

☐ **Alternatives:** Stabilizing object to walk with & push (e.g., wheelchair, sturdy baby stroller): _____

☐ Wheelchair to self-propel with legs

☐ Wheelchair for transport

☐ Bed Alarm

☐ Chair Alarm

☐ Other _____

☐ **Specialized Programming:** Identify when, duration, frequency and discipline responsible for any selected

☐ Structured daily activity programming _____

☐ Scheduled daily rest period(s) _____

☐ Allow to sleep any time is able (Goal: Will sleep 4-6 hours in a 24 hr period.)

☐ Wear high fall risk identifier (i.e., bracelet, special sox, special symbol or special vest) to ensure staff kept visually alerted/reminded

☐ Exercise program

☐ Accompanied walking _____

☐ Physically assisted walking _____

☐ Dancing _____

☐ Exercise to maintaining/enhancing flexibility (particularly neck, ankles and joints) _____

☐ General strengthening exercise _____

☐ Lower extremity strengthening exercise (e.g., stationary bicycling) _____

Figure 8.1 Dementia-specific fall risk factors assessment. (*continued*)

☐ Glider, rocking chair or rocking wheelchair Ad lib _____

☐ Vitamin D & calcium supplements

☐ Sunlight exposure (synthesizes vitamin D & calcium): Frequency _____

☐ **Adaptive Seating**

    ☐ Contrasting colored toilet seat

    ☐ Raised toilet seat

    ☐ Mobility Restrictive Seating/Devices: Rest Enablers Also Considered Physical Restraints (Listed Least to Most Restrictive): Define Times when using:

        ☐ Wedge cushion

        ☐ Slanted seats

        ☐ Deep-seated, soft-cushioned chair

        ☐ Recliner

        ☐ Bean bag chair
        Will reduce ability to shift weight and increases risk for pressure sores in persons with low body mass.

        ☐ Tray/table over chair/seat

        ☐ Wheelchair roll bar

        ☐ Lap-buddy

        ☐ Waist belt

        ☐ Self-release waist belt

        ☐ Vest restraint

        ☐ Other _____

☐ **Ambulation Modifications**

        ☐ Level surfaces only

        ☐ With gait belt

        ☐ With ___ person(s) assist

        ☐ With alternating rest and ambulation periods; Specify _____

☐ Seated when engaged in ADLs

☐ **Incontinence Care**

    ☐ Scheduled toileting _____

    ☐ Night care

        ☐ Scheduled toileting: _____

        ☐ Change incontinent product and turn every 2 hours

        ☐ Change incontinent product and turn every 3-4 hours
        To reduce sleep deprivation that further increases fall risks: Use only if resident is incontinent, ambulatory, is able to shift body weight independently and has no skin breakdown.

☐ Other Interventions

Figure 8.1 Dementia-specific fall risk factors assessment. (*continued*)

2   Safety Assessment Scale for People with Dementia Living at Home (Table 8.1)—designed by a Canadian team of researchers to help caregivers make a more objective assessment of the risk of domestic accidents. With this new tool, caregivers have an instrument that allows them to precisely determine the level of care and services needed to make sure that more people with memory and cognitive deficits can safely stay at home for a longer period of time. When evaluating the results of the assessment, caregivers can intervene to diminish potential risks. This scale has been validated in French and in English in three Canadian provinces, Quebec, Alberta, and British Columbia.

Prevention of Falls

One of the most important goals for providing in-home care for people with AD is to improve home safety, which involves identifying potential problems in the home and offering possible solutions to help prevent accidents. Identifying potential risk factors and developing preventive strategies for falls will have a significant impact in maintaining a person with AD's quality of life. When a caregiver is aware of fall prevention in people with AD, many falls can be avoided. The following guidelines can help to minimize the risk of falls in people with AD.

Mobility

Physical activity is one of the most important and effective ways to prevent falls in people with AD. Being inactive results in loss of muscle strength and balance and increases the risk of falls. Stand-alone physical activity interventions that target fall-related risk factors lower falls risk by 12% and reduces the number of falls by 19% (U.S. Department of Health and Human Services, 2003). Different types of exercises affect balance and posture. Gait, strengthening, and balance exercises are reported to reduce risk of falls in the elderly. Tai chi offers a low-cost, low-impact solution toward improving older persons' physical functions and also addresses their fear of falling. For older adults, exercise programs of moderate intensity that last longer are better than short programs of high intensity. Individualized programs established by a professional are more effective than those created without supervision. If caregivers can observe mobility during daily activities, they can pinpoint possible

Table 8.1

S.A.S. SAFETY ASSESSMENT SCALE FOR PEOPLE WITH DEMENTIA LIVING AT HOME (SHORT VERSION)

1 **Caregiver and living arrangements**
   a This person lives on his/her own.   Yes [1] No [0]
   b This person is alone at home.   Always [4] Most of the time [3]
                                              Occasionally [2] Never [1]

2 **Smoking**
   This person leaves cigarette burn   Yes [1] No [0]
   marks on the floor, furniture, or
   clothing.

3 **Fire and burns**
   a The stove on/off buttons are   On the front of the stove [1] On
     located...   the top of the stove [2] Behind the
                                              hot plates [3]
   b This person is capable of turning   Yes [1] No [0] Doesn't know [1]
     on the stove him/herself.
   c This person cooks his/her own   Always [4] Most of the time [3]
     food.   Occasionally [2] Never [1]
   d This person forgets a pan on the   Very often [4] Often [3] Sometimes [2]
     stove.   Never [1]
   e The heating system uses...   electricity [1] natural gas [2]
                                              wood [3]

4 **Nutrition**
   a This person receives meals-on-   More than once a day [1] Once a
     wheels or other prepared meals.   day [2]
                                              A few times a week (2 to 6 times a
                                              week) [3] Once a week or less [4]
   b This person's meals contain foods   Always [1] Most of the time [2]
     from different food groups   Occasionally [3] Never [4]
     (dairy products, meat or fish,
     cereals, fruit and vegetables).

5 **Food poisoning and toxic substances**
   This person can tell the difference   Yes [1] No [0]
   between food that is fresh and food
   that is spoiled.

6 **Medication and health**
   a This person takes, on a regular   1 to 3 medications [2] 4 to 6
     basis...(Prescribed medication   medications [3]
     only)   7 medications or more [4] Does not
                                              take any medication [1]

Table 8.1

S.A.S. SAFETY ASSESSMENT SCALE FOR PEOPLE WITH DEMENTIA LIVING AT HOME (SHORT VERSION)

b	This person takes medication to help him/her sleep or relax.	Yes [1] No [0]
c	Does this person suffer from any physical health problem?	None [1] Minor [2] Moderate [3] Severe [4]
d	This person accepts treatment for his/her physical health problems.	Yes [0] No [1] Does not apply [0]

7 Wandering and adaptation to changing temperature

a	This person gets lost in familiar surroundings.	Very often [4] Often [3] Sometimes [2] Never [1]
b	Has this person ever gotten lost?	Yes [1] No [0]
c	Can this person find his/her way home?	Yes [1] No [0]
d	Does this person dress appropriately according to the changing temperature, both indoors and outdoors?	Yes [1] No [0]

Score   /47

Source: "S.A.S. Safety Assessment Scale," by CLSC Côte-des-Neiges, 2001. Retrieved October 2007, from http://www.alzheimersupport.com/articles/1567.pdf. Reprinted with permission from CLSC Côte-des-Neiges.

problems with standing, walking, ADLs, and transfers. Caregivers should encourage residents with AD to wear snug-fitting shoes (not too tight) with a low heel and a slip-resistant sole, rather than loose-fitting slippers or socks.

Medications

Reviewing and modifying medications on a regular basis can significantly reduce fall rates. Reducing the number and type of medications, specifically cardiovascular and psychotropic drugs, can also reduce fall rates. Gradual withdrawal of psychoactive drugs can be particularly effective, but long-term compliance might become a problem. Successful programs will need a strong counseling component to improve compliance.

Medication use is perhaps the most preventable or reversible risk factor associated with falls. Have an appropriate clinician conduct a "brown bag" medicine review of all current medications. Most important, observe an individual on new medications, looking for side effects that may lead to falls.

Assistive Devices and Protective Equipment

Assistive devices and protective equipment can make living with AD easier. For example, ambulation aids such as canes and walkers are of great benefit in helping to maintain safe ambulation in people with AD. In some cases, however, the wrong type of ambulatory devices can create a fall hazard. Consult a physical therapist for proper evaluation.

A clinician should instruct the caregiver in the proper use of the assistive device, and, in turn, the caregiver should regularly assess and monitor whether the individual under care is properly using her ambulation aid. In addition, transfers aids, such as side rails, can be used as an assistive device to support bed transfers in persons with AD who have poor balance. The electronic pressure pad with monitor is the most versatile type and works well in transferring to or from a bed, chair, or toilet. The pads electronically detect the absence of pressure, which sends an electronic signal to the monitor and sets off an alarm. Electronic surveillance systems—aka fall alarms—are particularly helpful in monitoring high-risk individuals with AD. These systems consist of position sensors attached to beds or chairs or an individual's body part and alert caregivers of potentially dangerous resident movement. Hip protectors are devices designed to ease the impact of a fall on the hip bone and prevent hip fractures. The padded devices are worn under clothing like underwear and are designed to absorb energy in the event of a fall. For those who may be prone to falling due to memory loss, these are very effective in preventing fractures. Hip protectors have been shown to be effective in reducing hip fractures in older people without AD. In the event of a fall, the inconspicuous hip protector pads redistribute the impact, significantly reducing the risk of injury, further damage, or pain.

Environmental Changes and Modification

Home modifications offer the potential for persons with AD to have greater independence. While considering environmental changes and modifications, it is important to remember that changes can be disruptive for people with AD and may produce anxiety that can intensify cognitive deficits. Environmental modifications must therefore be kept to a minimum. It is recommended to modify only those features that clearly benefit safe mobility and decrease the risk of falls. If several changes are needed, introduce them one at a time. Another factor to consider is that intellectual impairment may make learning a new task impossible for an individual, and she may become frightened of new gadgets. After implementing modifications, always test to ensure that the alteration is safe and beneficial. Since mobility changes over time, it is also recommended that caregivers periodically reassess the need for new modifications or updating existing modifications. The following section describes environmental modifications that may benefit a person with AD and assist the caregiver in providing safe care at home.

HOME SAFETY ROOM BY ROOM

The following are general guidelines listed area by area to promote safety at home for people with AD. The material has been partially excerpted from "Home Safety for People With Alzheimer's Disease" (National Institute on Aging, 2007b) and "The Rush Manual for Caregivers" (Rush University Medical Center, 2004) and then modified.

A thorough home safety evaluation and recommendations for prevention can be performed by physical or occupational therapists who are professionally trained in safety assessment. After the potential safety problems have been identified, home modification should be performed.

Entrance and Exit

- Keep steps sturdy and textured to prevent falls in wet or icy weather.
- Consider having a ramp with handrails leading into the home rather than steps.
- Keep steps or ramp in good repair, without loose or uneven boards.
- Mark the edges of steps with bright or reflective tape.
- Eliminate uneven surfaces or walkways that may cause a person to slip.
- Make sure that the visitors can be seen prior to entering the house or apartment.

- Make sure entrance and exits are well lit and free of clutter. Light sensors that turn on lights automatically as a person approaches the house are available.
- Make sure the lock works.
- Make sure the lock can easily be opened for an emergency exit.
- Make sure that there is an emergency exit plan and more than one fire escape route.
- Restrict access to a swimming pool by fencing it off with a locked gate, covering it, and keeping it closely supervised when in use.
- Prune bushes and foliage well away from walkways and doorways.

Kitchen

- Make sure the doorway is accessible.
- Install childproof latches on storage cabinets and drawers designated for breakable or dangerous items. Lock away all household cleaning products, matches, knives, scissors, blades, small appliances, and valued china.
- Remove knobs from the stove, or install automatic shut-off switch.
- Remove artificial fruits and vegetables or food-shaped kitchen magnets that might appear to be edible.
- Remove or secure the family "junk drawer." A person with AD may eat small items such as matches, hardware, erasers, and plastics.
- Insert a drain trap in the kitchen sink to catch anything that might otherwise become lost or clog the plumbing.
- Consider dismantling the garbage disposal. People with AD may place objects or their own hands in the disposal.
- Remove and hide sink stopper to avoid accidental overflow.

Living Areas

- Keep the walking pathways uncluttered.
- Make sure windows and doors can be opened easily and locked securely.
- Secure electrical and telephone cords out of the way to prevent tripping.
- Adapt the telephone by changing the small buttons to larger push buttons to ease dialing. Have frequently called and emergency numbers programmed into speed dial or tape these numbers to the phone receiver. Keep a portable or tabletop phone where it can be accessed in case of a fall.

- Place decals at eye level on sliding glass doors, picture windows, or furniture with large glass panels to identify the glass pane.
- Do not leave the person with AD alone with an open fire in the fireplace. Consider alternative heating sources. Remove matches and cigarette lighters.
- Keep the controls for cable or satellite TV, VCR, and stereo system out of sight.

Bedroom

- Make sure the doorway is accessible.
- Make sure the light is accessible from the bed.
- Keep clothing in the closet and dresser easily reachable.
- Use an intercom device to alert to any noises indicating falls or a need for help.
- Remove portable space heaters. If portable fans are used, be sure that objects cannot be placed in the blades.
- Be cautious when using electric mattress pads, electric blankets, electric sheets, and heating pads, all of which can cause burns. Keep controls out of reach.
- Use transfer or mobility aids, if needed.
- When the person with AD is at risk of falling out of bed, place fall mattress next to the bed, as long as this does not create a greater risk of accident.
- Use a "trapeze" bar that can be installed if person with AD has difficulty getting out of bed, or get a hospital bed.

Bathroom

- Make sure the doorway is accessible.
- Use a tub bench or tub chair and a handheld showerhead to make bathing easier.
- Install a safety frame, raised toilet seat, or grab bar.
- Install grab bars in the bathroom and tub area.
- Put toiletry items in a locked drawer.
- Remove electrical appliances from the bathroom to reduce the risk of electrical shock.
- Do not leave a severely impaired person with AD alone in the bathroom.
- Remove the lock from the bathroom door to prevent the person with AD from getting locked inside.

- Place nonskid adhesive strips, decals, or mats in the tub and shower. If the bathroom is uncarpeted, consider placing these strips next to the tub, toilet, and sink.
- Use washable wall-to-wall bathroom carpeting to prevent slipping on wet tile floors.
- Use a foam rubber faucet cover (often used for small children) in the tub to prevent serious injury should the person with AD fall.
- In the shower, tub, and sink, use a single faucet that mixes hot and cold water to avoid burns.
- Adjust the water heater to 120 degrees to avoid scalding tap water.
- Insert drain traps in sinks to catch small items that may be lost or flushed down the drain.
- Remove cleaning products from under the sink, or lock them away.
- Remove small electrical appliances from the bathroom. Cover electrical outlets. If men use electric razors, have them use a mirror outside the bathroom to avoid water contact.

Stairways

- Install solid handrails on both sides of stairways, especially in the steep stairwell.
- Maintain adequate lighting at the top and bottom of the stairs.
- Make sure the carpet is secured.
- Put rough texture treads on steps with a smooth surface.
- Keep the steps free of clutter.
- If stairs are difficult, it may be helpful to arrange most of the activities on the lower level of the house.

General

- Remove scatter rugs and throw rugs throughout the house.
- Use night-lights in different parts of the house.
- Store flammable liquids in a locked cabinet in the garage or outside unit.
- Store prescription or nonprescription drugs in a locked cabinet.
- Provide sturdy items to lean against along a main path.
- Keep walking areas clear.
- Use furniture to block dangerous areas.

- Tape down electrical cords.
- Remove or secure in a safe area, guns, power tools, and electrical and motor-operated equipment.
- Reduce glare.
- Supervise smoking, and keep lighters, matches, and cigarettes in your possession.
- Display emergency numbers and your home address near all telephones.
- Use an answering machine when you cannot answer phone calls, and set it to turn on after the fewest number of rings possible. A person with AD often may be unable to take messages or could become a victim of telephone exploitation. Turn ringers on low to avoid distraction and confusion. Put all portable and cell phones and equipment in a safe place so that they will not be easily lost.
- Install smoke alarms and carbon monoxide detectors in appropriate places; check their functioning and batteries frequently.
- Install secure locks on all outside doors and windows.
- Hide a spare house key outside in case the person with AD locks the caregiver and family members out of the house.
- Avoid the use of extension cords if possible by placing lamps and appliances close to electrical outlets. Tack extension cords to the baseboards of a room to avoid tripping.
- Cover unused outlets with childproof plugs.
- Place red tape around floor vents, radiators, and other heating devices to deter the person with AD from standing on or touching a hot grid.
- Make sure there is adequate lighting throughout the house.
- Keep all alcohol in a locked cabinet or out of reach of the person with AD. Drinking alcohol can increase confusion.
- Keep plastic bags out of reach. A person with AD may choke or suffocate.
- Lock all power tools and machinery in the garage, workroom, or basement.
- Remove all poisonous plants from the home. Check with local nurseries or poison control centers for a list of poisonous plants.
- Make sure all computer equipment and accessories, including electrical cords, are kept out of the way. If valuable documents or materials are stored on a home computer, protect the files with passwords. Password-protect access to the Internet, also, and

restrict the patient's amount of online time without supervision. Consider monitoring the computer use of the person with AD, and install software that screens for objectionable or offensive material on the Internet.

■ Keep fish tanks out of reach. The combination of glass, water, electrical pumps, and potentially poisonous aquatic life could be harmful to a curious person with AD.

■ Elevated bed heights and soft mattress surfaces promote balance loss during transfers. Appropriate bed heights can be achieved by replacing thick mattresses with thinner ones. Mattresses should be firm enough to support balance during transfer out of bed. The floor surface along the bed should be slip-resistant to support safe transfers.

■ All chairs used by individuals with AD should have arm rests, which provide leverage and balance support during transfers. Arm rests can also compensate for low seat heights. A cushion can be added to increase the height of low-seated chairs. The stability of chairs is crucial for safety.

CAREGIVING FOR ALZHEIMER'S INDIVIDUALS

The following section on caregiver guidance has been partially excerpted from "Caregiver Guide: Tips for Caregivers of People With Alzheimer's Disease" (National Institute on Aging, 2007a) and "The Rush Manual for Caregivers" (Rush University Medical Center, 2004) and then modified.

Physical exercise, proper nutrition, good general health, and socialization are important for people with AD (WebMD, 2007a). However, people with AD have special needs, which can pose unique challenges for their caregivers. Depending on his level of independence, the person with AD may need help with personal care activities, including eating, bathing, shaving, and toileting. To assist with these activities, caregivers need knowledge, skill, and patience. Unfortunately, caregiving can become so demanding and all-consuming that it makes caregivers vulnerable to problems of their own (Russell, Benedictis, & Segal, 2007). It is important for caregivers to understand and act according to their own physical and emotional limitations. They need to plan daily activities to help provide structure, meaning, and a sense of accomplishment for the person with Alzheimer's. It is always best to establish a routine with which the person can become familiar. As functions are lost, adapt activities and routines to allow the person with Alzheimer's to participate as much as possible (WebMD, 2007a).

Bathing and Personal Hygiene

The physical and mental impairment associated with Alzheimer's can make bathing a frustrating experience for a caregiver. For the person who has Alzheimer's, it's easy to feel confused and overwhelmed by simple daily routines such as bathing and grooming. A caregiver should try to determine the reason a person seems afraid, stressed, or resistant to bathing. Once a reason has been determined, a caregiver will be in a better position to manage the bathing routine. Frequency of washing and bathing is a personal preference; a complete bath may not be needed every day, so one option is to alternate a sponge bath with a more complete bath or shower. If the person continues to resist the idea of bathing, a caregiver can distract him for a few moments and then try again when his mood may have changed. If a person is used to taking a shower in the morning or a bath at night, try to maintain that routine. If there are constant problems with washing, seek support and get another family member or a friend to do it.

A depressed person with AD might have lost her desire to bathe. In this case, the caregiver should associate washing with a fun activity, such as going to a restaurant or visiting friends. This may prompt the person to wash. Try to make it enjoyable and relaxing to wash, rather than forcing the person. Use praise and encouragement when the person is freshly bathed. A person with AD might feel embarrassed and uncomfortable about getting undressed in the presence of a caregiver. Also keep in mind that a person may refuse to take a bath with an unfamiliar caregiver of the opposite sex. In this situation, the caregiver must respect the person's dignity by doing small conscientious gestures, such as keeping portions of their body covered. Not understanding the bathing process may also leave person with AD angry and frustrated. The person may know they need to wash but may have forgotten what to do. Gently remind the person of the required steps as he washes himself.

The entire bathing process should be simplified so that the person can do as much as possible. A shower or stand-up wash may be easier than a bath, but keep in mind that showers are often more dangerous and frightening to people with AD than baths. If the person has not been used to a shower, it may seem alarming, and it is then best to avoid that method of washing. If you must use a shower, install grab bars and use a tub seat. A person with AD may be overly sensitive to running water or changes in water temperature. Keep in mind that the person may not be able to judge temperature. A caregiver should always check the temperature of the water in the bath or shower and never leave a person alone in the bath or shower.

Safety and comfort are important when bathing a person with AD. Bathrooms can be wet and slippery; therefore, use grab rails, nonslip mats, or a bath chair. Avoid using bubble bath or bath and shower oils that could make the tub or shower stall slippery. If the person is heavy or can offer little help, special equipment may be needed. Keep the bathroom warm, comfortable, and well lit. Be directive at bath time by using such phrases as "Your bath is ready." In this way, the person will focus on each step of the task instead of whether or not she needs or wants a bath. Gently coach the person during each step of the bath, reminding her of the areas that need washing. Keep in mind that you may need to complete part of the bath or shower yourself. However, get the individual to participate as much as possible.

Dressing

Physical appearance is critical to a person's sense of well-being and self-esteem. Dressing is a simple way of keeping people with AD active and helping them retain their sense of independence and self-esteem. For the person with AD, the simple act of putting on clothing can be frustrating, and changing from day to night might cause distress. Caregivers should manage dressing difficulties one by one.

There are many reasons why people with Alzheimer's might have problems dressing. They may have problems with balance or motor skills that are needed to fasten buttons or close zippers. They might have forgotten how to dress, may not recognize their own clothes, and may not understand the need to change clothes. A caregiver needs to give easy-to-understand instructions and make simple clothing selections, so the person with AD can dress herself for as long as possible. Lay out clothes in the order the person will put them on. Then, assist her through each step of the dressing process. If appropriate, give the person an opportunity to select favorite outfits or colors. If the person insists on wearing the same clothes every day, try to launder these clothes often or get duplicates of favorite outfits.

The person with AD may be troubled by a lack of privacy, a cold room, poor lighting, or loud noises. A caregiver needs to make sure the atmosphere is calm and warm and must respect the person's privacy. Doors and blinds should be closed, and, if needed, the person can be covered with a towel or bathrobe. Encourage the person to do as much as possible on her own. Too much pressure to get dressed quickly can cause anxiety, so a caregiver should allow plenty of time for dressing. Keep in mind that some items of clothing are easier to put on than others.

The key thing to remember when selecting clothes for a person with Alzheimer's is that simplicity will lead to success in getting dressed. A caregiver should choose comfortable and loose-fitting clothing that is easy to put on and remove. Many caregivers find that cardigans or tops that fasten in front are more comfortable and easier to work with than pullovers. Fabrics should be lightweight and flexible and feel soft and comfortable on the person's skin. Pressure tape or Velcro can be used as a substitute for buttons, snaps, and hooks. To avoid tripping and falling, make sure that clothing length is appropriate. To give the person's feet adequate support, encourage wearing regular shoes instead of slippers. Slip-on shoe styles with elasticized inserts on the top are easy to put on and remove. A caregiver should ensure that the person with dementia is comfortable with the clothes selected and involve them in the selection process.

Grooming and Shaving

People with dementia may forget that it is time to comb their hair or shave. They may have forgotten how to do such grooming activities as combing and brushing hair or shaving. They may forget the purpose of items like nail clippers, a razor, or a comb. A caregiver should encourage a person with AD to keep the same grooming routine every day. Lay out grooming and shaving supplies in clear view, and allow enough time for grooming and shaving activities. Encourage the person to do as much of these activities as possible without help. Give verbal or visual cues with grooming, and use short and simple instructions. A person with AD might resist grooming activities and may get distracted by people, clutter, or noise or be deterred by poor lighting and a lack of privacy. Caretakers should set the room at a comfortable temperature for grooming and shaving with adequate light and privacy. The environment should be calm and without distractions.

Keep hair in a low-maintenance style. At the beauty shop or a barber, encourage the experience, unless it becomes overwhelming. If this happens, ask the barber or hairstylist to come to the person's home. Use electric shavers instead of hand razors. Don't force a person to comb his hair and shave, but rather try distracting the person if there is resistance.

Eating

Some symptoms of AD, including confusion and lack of energy, can be worsened by poor nutrition. It is important for people with AD to have a proper nutritious diet and plenty of healthy fluids. Unfortunately, providing the person with nutritious meals and snacks is a problem for many caregivers. People with AD often forget if they have eaten or why it's important to eat. Eating can be hard for people with Alzheimer's. Some forget how to use utensils. Some may want to eat all the time, while others have to be encouraged to eat. A person with AD may not ask for food, particularly as the disease progresses.

Caregivers should make meals an enjoyable social event. Meals should be served in a quiet, calm place, and encouragement and praise should be offered during the meal so that people with AD look forward to the experience. Use rough-textured foods such as toast or sandwiches made on toasted bread to stimulate the person's tongue and encourage chewing and swallowing. The caregiver may have to remind the person how to eat. Consider suggesting the use of a spoon instead of a knife and fork. Bowls are easier to use than plates, and spoons are easier than forks. Adaptive equipment—plate guards or silverware with specially designed handles— is available for individuals who have difficulty holding or using utensils.

Alzheimer's disease may compromise an individual's visual and spatial abilities, making it tough to distinguish food from the plate. To accommodate this, choose foods with colors that contrast with the color of the plate. Putting only one item on the plate at a time can help keep meals pleasant and simple. Finger food is easier to manage and not as messy. Remind the person to eat slowly, and be aware that the person may not be able to sense hot or cold and may burn her mouth on hot food or liquids.

As the disease progresses, physical problems may arise, such as not being able to chew properly or swallow. Sometimes, a person with Alzheimer's has little sensation of food in the mouth. A caregiver can remind the person under care to chew by gently moving the person's chin. Another way to stimulate chewing is to touch the person's tongue with a fork or spoon and lightly stroke. A light stroke on the throat can remind him to swallow. Liquids can be thickened for easier swallow. A person may clench his jaw tightly and refuse to let a caregiver put a utensil near his mouth. This person may not understand or remember what to do with food. The caregiver may need to serve different portions of food at a time to make eating easier. The caregiver may need to allow for more time and offer more assistance at mealtime. Cut food into bite-size portions. Use bendable straws or lidded cups for liquids. In the later stages of AD, the caregiver might have to feed the person under care or mash or liquefy all food. If the person has difficulty swallowing, a consultation with a speech-language pathologist should be scheduled.

A person with AD needs to be monitored for early behavior changes, such as increased snacking, drastic shifts in food likes and dislikes, dramatic weight fluctuations, or bowel problems. Weight loss is a common and serious occurrence in people with AD, and it is caused by a combination of problems, such as depression, forgetting to eat, and poor food intake. A caregiver should provide close supervision at mealtime to keep the person under care on task with eating. Offering foods that are calorie dense can help, and favorite foods should be served as much as possible. Provide food 24 hours a day instead of just at meal or snack times. When the person is eating well, try to get her to eat as much as you can. Offer second portions. High-calorie and high-protein snacks that offer many calories and a lot of protein in a small amount of food can be offered between meals. Keeping healthy snacks and finger food in plain sight all day may encourage eating. If weight loss continues, nutritional supplements may be needed. Keeping an accurate weight record is essential for the care of persons with dementia.

People with AD often hide food, given the opportunity. Hiding items seems to come from a feeling of insecurity coming from the person's memory difficulty, hearing and vision loss, and a general feeling of loss of control over life. Such people become suspicious of others and accuse caregivers of "not feeding me." They may also fear that others are taking food or hiding food items and fear that they may starve to death. A caregiver should check wastebaskets before emptying them, and it might be wise to completely remove wastebaskets from the individual's room. Always check possible hiding places for food, such as pockets in shirts, slacks, and skirts, and even shoes. In this situation, a caregiver should acknowledge the person's suspicions and offer help. A caregiver should not confront the person or try to reason with him about his beliefs.

Toileting

Alzheimer's disease affects every part of a person's daily routine, including bowel and bladder control. As AD progresses, problems with incontinence often surface, and people with AD may have accidents, soiling on themselves. A person with dementia may lose the ability to recognize when to go to the toilet or what to do when in the bathroom. If incontinence is a new behavior, the first and most important step a caregiver can take is to identify the possible reasons for this loss of control. It could be due to medical reasons. For example, the person could have a urinary tract infection, constipation, or a prostate problem, or it could be the result of an illness such as diabetes, stroke, or Parkinson's disease. Certain medications, such as tranquilizers, sedatives, or diuretics, can contribute to incontinence. Certain beverages, such as coffee, colas, and tea, might produce a diuretic effect and contribute to urinary incontinence. Incontinence can also be caused by stress or movement. For example, the person may release urine with a sneeze, cough, or laugh. A caregiver can withhold fluids if a person with AD starts to lose bladder control, of course keeping in mind that the person might become dehydrated. It is important to remember that dehydration can create a urinary tract infection, which can lead to incontinence.

Environmental factors can also contribute to incontinence. For example, the person may not be able to find the bathroom, or the bathroom may be too far to reach in time. The person may be afraid of falling, or there may be obstacles in his path, such as chairs or throw rugs. Weak pelvic muscles in a woman could cause uncontrollable loss of urine.

Once the cause or causes of incontinence are determined, there are strategies that may help to prevent these incidents, which will save extra work for the caregiver and embarrassment for the person with AD. A caregiver should schedule bathroom breaks every 2 hours, before and after meals and before bedtime, and should allow the person adequate time in the bathroom. Restlessness or tugging on clothing may signal the need to use the bathroom. A sign on the door that says "Toilet" or a picture of a toilet may be helpful.

Clothing should be easy to open or remove. Replace zippers and buttons with Velcro. Choose pants with an elastic waist. Although some caregivers purchase protective pads, you might also want to add an extra layer of protection to regular clothing by lining the backs of skirts or pants with a terrycloth material. Praise toileting success, and offer reassurance when accidents happen; avoid blaming or scolding the individual. Stimulation of urination by giving the person a drink of water or running water in the sink might help avoid accidents. A bedside commode or urinal may be helpful if getting to the bathroom is a problem, especially at night.

Medications are available that can treat incontinence in certain cases. As with any other medication, medications used to treat incontinence can cause side effects, such as dry mouth and eye problems.

HOME SAFETY BEHAVIOR BY BEHAVIOR

A number of behavior problems may accompany AD as the disease progresses, but not every person will experience the disease in exactly the same way. As the disease advances, particular behavioral changes can create safety problems. Should these behaviors occur, the safety recommendations may help reduce risk of injury. We now discuss a few of these recommendations in some behavioral problem areas.

Communication

People with AD develop communication problems, which tend to become increasingly severe as time goes on. They may struggle to find the right words to express themselves or forget the meaning of words and phrases (Alzheimer's Outreach, 1996). People with AD may rely on gestures as their verbal skills decline. When people with AD have trouble finding the right words to communicate their thoughts, they may describe an item instead of naming it or substitute words that have a similar sound or meaning. Questions may be left unanswered because the person cannot understand what is being asked of her, and keeping a sentence going often proves too difficult for the sufferer. Difficulties with communication can be distressing and frustrating for the person with AD and for the caregiver, as well. It takes lots of patience to communicate with individuals who forget names, struggle for the words they want to use, never finish a sentence, or repeat the same phrase over and over. There are several strategies that can be used to enhance communication with Alzheimer's individuals.

A person communicating with a person with AD needs to remain calm and gain the listener's attention before beginning to speak. Approach the person from the front, and speak distinctly using short, simple, and familiar words. Visual communication is very important, and facial expressions and body language add vital information to communication

(WebMD, 2007b). Speak at a normal rate, not too fast or too slow. Use pauses to give the person time to process what is being said. If the person with AD has difficulty understanding what is said, find a different way of saying it. If he didn't understand the words the first time, it is unlikely he will understand them a second time. Shouting, arguing, and using negative body language—raised eyebrows, sighs, impatient foot tapping—will only make the situation worse. Try to reduce background noise coming from the TV or radio when communicating, as these noises make it harder to hear and can distract the listener. Give one-step directions. Ask only one question at a time. Identify people and things by name, avoiding pronouns.

When listening, pay attention to the person, and try to understand what is being said. Try to understand the words and gestures the individual is using to communicate. Encourage the person to continue to express her thoughts, even if she is having difficulty. Be careful not to interrupt. Avoid criticizing, correcting, and arguing. In addition, remember that the presence, touch, gestures, and attention from caregivers can communicate acceptance, reassurance, and love to a person with AD (WebMD, 2007b). In all cases, treat the individual with dignity and respect. Don't speak down to the person or speak to others as if she were a child or weren't present.

Driving

Driving is a symbol of independence, competence, and control. As normal people get older, their eyesight worsens and their reaction times lengthen, making driving a dangerous activity. People with AD are even worse off since AD affects judgment, reaction time, and problem-solving abilities, which are critical to driving. Research suggests that even mild AD is associated with an increased risk of accidents (U.S. News & World Report, 2007). AD can also cause physical and sensory problems that increase the risk of being involved in a car accident.

Some people in the early stages of dementia retain the ability to drive, but this ability can be easily lost. Research shows that people with AD drive, on average, 2.5 years following diagnosis, but that certainly does not mean that everyone with AD should, as the disease affects people in different ways and some more quickly than others (Kennard, 2006b). Many believe that people should not be allowed to drive after a diagnosis of AD, and results from studies conducted at Johns Hopkins University (Lucas-Blaustein, Filipp, Dungan, & Tune, 1988) and at the National Institute on

Aging (Friedland et al., 1988) support the belief. The American Academy of Neurology recommends that people not drive if they have even mild AD—when memory loss is noticeable and complex activities are impaired (Dubinsky, Stein, & Lyons, 2000). It is often up to caregivers to determine when it becomes unsafe for individuals with AD to drive. To standardize the assessment of when a person with AD should or shouldn't drive, the American Academy of Neurology has developed guidelines on driving and AD (Dubinsky, Stein, & Lyons, 2000). Some aspects of a person's day-to-day behavior, such as coordination and ability to judge distance and space, to engage in multiple tasks, to stay alert to what is happening nearby, to make decisions, and to solve problems, can indicate whether a person has lost the skills needed to drive safely. This problem can be difficult to handle, so a caregiver should approach the individual with care. The discussion about stopping driving should be gentle, and a recommendation should be made to use public transportation instead. If the person continues driving and it remains a problem, consider selling the automobile. This way the person with AD won't be continually reminded of the car. If there are other cars in the household, consider making the keys hard to find. At times, it may be necessary to consult with health care professionals or the drivers licensing authority.

If someone wants to be tested to determine whether it is still safe for her to drive, she can seek local resources such as rehabilitation programs, hospitals, AAA, or motor vehicle departments. Asking the physician for a referral is often helpful. Although it is unlikely that results will be reported to licensing authorities, it is important to ask the person conducting the test. It is important to remember that a person with AD has a progressive disease. That means he may pass a safety test, only to begin to have problems several months later. Re-testing may be necessary.

Smoking and Drinking

Cigarette smoking with AD increases the risk of fire and is unhealthy. A person with AD may not realize the dangers related to smoking. A caregiver should always supervise the person when smoking or try to discourage smoking altogether. Make sure that the clothes worn and the furniture in the house are fire-resistant. Consider installing a smoke alarm, which can alert caregivers of any danger. People with dementia have been known to forget about smoking if cigarettes and ashtrays are removed from sight. Trying to make people with AD stop smoking may make them tense and irritable. There is also an ethical question about the person's right to continue to enjoy something that he has enjoyed in the past, whether or not it is bad for him.

A drink in company may be a pleasant way for a person with AD to relax. Monitor the quantity of alcohol, as the person may have forgotten how much he has had. People with dementia can appear more confused after a drink, so the amount may need to be limited. Another factor to remember is that alcohol doesn't mix well with certain medicines (U.S. Food & Drug Administration, 2005a). Keep alcohol out of reach and out of sight to help control alcohol consumption. And, just as with smoking, the caregiver needs to balance the issue of the person's right to enjoy a pleasurable activity against the risk.

Sleep Problems

Many older adults have problems sleeping, but people with AD have an even harder time. People with AD can get disorientated in time and no longer recognize the difference between night and day (Alzheimer's Disease International, 2004). Individuals with Alzheimer's may reverse their sleep-wake cycle, causing daytime drowsiness and nighttime restlessness, which can disturb the family. People with AD may wander through the house at night, waking caregivers and possibly endangering themselves. This can be the most exhausting problem for the caregiver. These sleep disturbances often increase as AD progresses. Eventually, people with Alzheimer's may nap off and on during the day and night. Every hour may have periods of wakefulness and periods of light sleep. These naps replace the deep, restorative sleep most people enjoy at night.

A caregiver's first priority is to establish a routine that will keep the person with AD busy. If possible, follow the same sleep and wake schedule the person maintained during her working years. Limit daytime napping, and, if a nap is needed, make sure it's short and not too late in the day. Have the person under care take the nap on the couch or in a recliner, rather than in bed. Reserve the bed for nighttime sleep. If a person has trouble sleeping at night because he has stayed in bed too long in the morning, wake him up earlier. Do not feed the person a large meal in the evening, and, after the day's activities, keep the evening fairly quiet and relaxed. As bedtime approaches, make the person as comfortable as possible, with a warm and inviting bedroom. If practical measures fail to improve matters, an individual with AD may need to use sleeping pills in order to cope, but these should generally be avoided if possible. Consult a physician for advice on the best course of action.

Some people with Alzheimer's have other associated health problems that may affect their sleep. Sleep apnea is a condition where a person stops breathing for 10 to 30 seconds at a time while she is sleeping. These short stops in breathing can happen up to 400 times every night (American Academy of Family Physicians, 2007). The nonbreathing periods may make the person wake up from deep sleep and if a person is waking up all night long, she may not be getting enough rest from sleep. Restless legs syndrome is a neurological disorder characterized by unpleasant sensations in the legs and an uncontrollable urge to move when at rest in an effort to relieve these feelings. As a result, most people with restless legs syndrome have difficulty falling asleep and staying asleep. Left untreated, the condition causes exhaustion and daytime fatigue. Many people with Alzheimer's also suffer from depression, which can disrupt sleep patterns. A urinary tract infection is an acute infection that can make a person with AD so uncomfortable that she cannot sleep properly. In many situations, these associated problems respond well to treatment.

Wandering

About two-thirds of demented people have a history of wandering (Sink, Covinsky, Newcomer, & Yaffe, 2004). Wandering away from home causes tremendous stress for the family and at its worst may result in serious or fatal injury. Precautions should be taken to prevent wandering.

The most useful strategies for managing wandering include aggressively treating sleep problems to prevent nocturnal wandering; providing increased activity, chores, and stimulation during the day; taking the person on frequent walks during the day; or providing a secure area in which the individual can wander. Remember that places that look safe to some might be dangerous for the person with Alzheimer's. For this reason, the home environment should be assessed for possible hazards, such as fences and gates, bodies of water (i.e., swimming pools), dense foliage, tunnels, bus stops, steep stairways, high balconies, and roadways where traffic tends to be heavy. The following recommendations might help a caregiver prevent or minimize wandering:

- Prevent persons with AD from leaving home without the knowledge of the caregiver.
- Place identification on persons with dementia. A discrete identification bracelet or locket is preferred that includes the person's name, telephone number, memory problem, and medical condition.

Some experts even recommend putting identification on the person's dentures or attaching a sensor to the individual's ankle or wrist. In addition, bright-colored clothing may be helpful or marking on clothes with a sew-on or iron-on label, permanent marker, or reflective material. Identification may also be placed on the person's shoes, eyeglasses, and keys.

■ Place locks out of the normal line of vision—either very high or very low on doors. In addition, a double-bolt door lock is recommended, but it is important to keep the key handy for emergencies.

■ Use a childproof doorknob that prevents the person with Alzheimer's from opening the door.

■ Consider electronic buzzers, infrared electronic eye alarms, or chimes on the doors.

■ Camouflage some doors with a screen or curtain, or put a two-foot square of a dark color in front of the doorknob.

■ Put hedges or fences around the patio or yard.

■ Place locks on gates.

■ Keep car keys out of sight or temporarily disable the car by removing its distributor cap. Although most wandering takes place by foot, some individuals with AD have been known to drive as far as 300 miles—sometimes in an automobile that belongs to someone else.

■ Place visual barriers, such as a stop sign on the door or a large black rectangle on the floor in front of the door, or hide the doorknob with a strip of cloth. These have been shown to decrease the likelihood that a wanderer will go through the door.

■ Provide the person with AD with a Medic-Alert bracelet. She should not wear expensive jewelry or carry large sums of money.

■ Notify the local police department if a person with AD is at risk for wandering. Many jurisdictions have specific programs to facilitate identification of wanderers by police officers.

■ When the person is found, avoid confrontation and showing anger—speak calmly, with acceptance and love. It is not the person's fault, but a problem associated with dementia.

Repetitive Behavior

Repetitive behavior is among the most common and burdensome of the behavioral and psychological symptoms of AD (Cullen et al., 2005). This type of behavior evokes a general feeling of insecurity in people with AD. Repetitive behavior includes saying things over and over again, asking the same question again and again, and repeating certain actions frequently. AD can make a person forget what she has said or done from one moment to the next, which leads to these repetitive actions. These behaviors can be very upsetting and irritating for the caregiver. Rather than answering the question again and again, it may be helpful to say that everything is fine and try to make the person more secure. It might help to write the answer down. If the same question comes up again, the caregiver can direct the person to a written answer. Try to distract the person by changing the subject or giving hugs, if appropriate.

Clinging

The person with AD is living in a world where nothing makes sense any more and where anything could change. A caregiver may be the only stable feature in what has become a constantly changing world. It is therefore not surprising that such people become extra-dependent on their caregivers and follow them everywhere, even to the toilet. This clinging behavior may be caused by an environment that is overwhelming for the person with AD (National Institute on Aging, 2007b). If he is scared or confused, he will likely seek out and stay with a familiar, reassuring caregiver. If the person with AD clings to and follows the caregiver around, it can test the limits of the caregiver's patience. Not only does the person require the caregiver's constant attention, but the caregiver is also deprived of even a moment's privacy. It can also be difficult for a caregiver to relax when she senses that the person under her care is always waiting for her next move. It is important to do something about this before it starts to wear the caregiver down and to help the person with AD feel more secure.

Whenever the caregiver leaves a person with AD, it is important that he tell the person under his care that he will come back. If necessary, a caregiver can write this information down for the person. Another method is to provide the person with AD with something to occupy her attention while the caregiver steps away. Another method is to use a sitter so that the caregiver has time to relax without having to worry about the person with AD. Such breaks help the caregiver cope with caring for someone with AD.

Losing Personal Items

People with AD often lose many items, placing them in inappropriate places. This behavior is caused by insecurity, combined with a sense of loss of control and of memory (Alzheimer's Disease International, 2004). Poor memory and misperceptions about the environment may lead to frustration and agitated behavior. What often happens is that when items go "missing," the person will hide them in a place to prevent them from disappearing again. She then forgets about this hiding place. In some cases, the person with AD will accuse the caregiver and others of taking the missing objects. It is vital to respond to the accusations without confrontation or anger. The first step is to agree with the person that the item is lost and help find it. It is pointless getting into an argument over the loss and will only upset all parties involved. If the caregiver looks carefully, she will probably find the hiding place, so check these first in the search for the missing item. The caregivers should make sure to keep copies or spares of important items, such as keys, glasses, and documents. Finally, always check waste baskets before emptying them; this prevents accidental loss of items.

Hallucinations, Illusions, and Delusions

As dementia progresses in persons with AD, the disruption in the brain can result in the person experiencing hallucinations, illusions, and/or delusions. These symptoms occur in as many as 50% of persons with AD. *Hallucinations* come from within the brain and involve hearing, seeing, or feeling things that are not really there. *Illusions* differ from hallucinations; in this case, the person with AD is misinterpreting something that actually does exist. *Delusions* are persistent thoughts that the person with AD believes are true but that, in reality, are not.

The most common hallucinations are visual, and they frequently constitute the so-called phantom boarder syndrome in which the individual believes that an unseen person is living in the home. A delusion is a false belief. The person may believe that he is under threat of harm from the caregiver. To the person, this delusion is real and causes fear and distress and may result in self-protective behavior. An illusion for those with AD means that they misinterpret common, everyday events, so a shadow on the wall may look like a person, or a design in the carpet might be perceived as an object.

If the hallucinations, illusions, and delusions do not cause problems for the caregiver and family members, they may be ignored. But, it is important to seek a medical evaluation if a person with AD has ongoing disturbing behavior or if the behavior becomes dangerous. Often, these symptoms can be treated with medication. Medical treatment of these behavioral disorders associated with AD was discussed in chapter 7. The following behavior management techniques may be helpful.

If a person with AD has a hallucination, illusion, or delusion, respond in a calm, supportive manner. Do not dismiss the validity of what the person has just seen, but distract the person by drawing attention to something real in the room, like music, a conversation, or a drawing, or by looking at photos or pictures or counting coins. Do not confront a person with AD if she becomes aggressive. Instead, reassure the person with kind words and a gentle touch. A gentle tap on the shoulder may turn the person's attention toward the caregiver and reduce the hallucination, illusion, or delusion. Suggest that the person come with you on a walk or sit next to you in another room. Frightening feelings often subside in well-lit areas where other people are present. Explore the reality of the situation with the person. Ask the person to point to the area where she sees or hears something. To a person with AD, a glare from a window may look like snow, and dark squares on a tiled floor might look like dangerous holes. Hallucinations can be associated with poor vision, so it is worth a trip to the opticians for a checkup.

Environmental adaptations also may be helpful. Check the environment for noises that might be misinterpreted, for lighting that casts shadows, or for glares, reflections, or distortions from the surfaces of floors, walls, and furniture. Paint walls a light color to reflect more light. Use solid colors instead of a patterned wall, since it is less confusing to an impaired person. Large, bold prints may also cause confusing illusions. Keep rooms well lit to ensure that the person is not misinterpreting what is going on around them. Dimly lit areas may produce confusing shadows or make it difficult to interpret everyday objects. Reduce glare by using soft light or frosted bulbs, partially closing blinds or curtains, and maintaining adequate globes or shades on light fixtures.

Sometimes, looking at a mirror, a person with AD thinks that he is looking at a stranger. Remove or cover mirrors if they cause a person with AD to become confused or frightened. Vary the home environment as little as possible to minimize the potential for visual confusion. Keep furniture in the same place. Check for noises that might be misinterpreted, such as noise from a television or an air conditioner. Avoid violent or disturbing television programs. The person with AD may believe the story is real. Ask if the person can point to a specific area that is producing the confusion. Perhaps one particular aspect of the environment is being misinterpreted.

Sexual Relationship/Inappropriate Behavior

Sexual desire and the need for intimacy change when someone has AD and may affect people in varying ways. One person may have an increased interest in sex, while another may have no interest. Physical illness may cause the person with AD to lose interest in sex or make sexual intercourse difficult or painful. Reactions to medications may also reduce sexual desire. The person may forget her marital status and begin to flirt or make inappropriate advances toward members of the opposite sex. The person may forget how to dress or take his clothes off at inappropriate times and in public places. The person may become unreasonably jealous and suspicious and may think that his spouse has a boyfriend and accuse the spouse of going to see him. A person with AD may make sexual advances to a stranger who resembles a former spouse, lover, or companion. Depression is common among people with AD, which can also reduce interest in sex, both in the persons with AD and in their spouse or loved one.

Some caregivers report that they experience changes in sexual feelings toward their loved one after providing daily caretaking actions. For some couples, sexual intimacy continues to be a satisfying part of their relationship, but AD may alter one's attitude toward it. The relationship changes as a spouse's role within the relationship adjusts to meet the demands of Alzheimer's. Taking care of an impaired partner takes the healthy spouse into new and uncharted waters.

A number of action steps can be taken to address this problem. First of all, the spouse should try not to overreact and never forget that it is the disease taking effect. Gentle cuddling and holding may be mutually satisfying and will let the spouse know if the person with AD is able or inclined to engage in further intimacy. It is wise to be patient. The person may not respond in the same way as before or may seem to lose interest. The opposite may occur, too. The person may make excessive demands for sex or behave in a manner that makes the other partner feel uncomfortable. If this is a problem, the other partner may consider sleeping in a separate bedroom. Whether this becomes a permanent feature is a difficult decision to make, but it might be necessary. If needed, consult a psychologist or counselor, who can provide advice and guidance.

Distracting a person with AD with another activity is a useful way of diffusing an uncomfortable sexual situation. If the person removes his clothing, then calmly, quickly, and gently discourage the behavior and encourage another activity. Look for a reason behind the behavior. Keep in mind that if the person exposes himself, he may simply need to go to the bathroom. If the person begins to take off his clothes, he may want to go to bed. If the person is engaging in unusual sexual behavior, carefully remind him that the behavior is inappropriate. Then, lead the person to a private place or try to distract with another activity. Try not to get angry with the person or laugh and giggle at the behavior. In most cases, anger and ridicule may cause negative reactions. Adjust the person's clothing. Consider putting the person's trousers or dress on backward. Or provide the person with pull-on pants with no zipper. Increase the level of appropriate physical contact. Give the person plenty of physical contact in the form of stroking, hugging, and rubbing. In many cases, the person is anxious and needs reassurance through touch and gentle loving communication. Adjust to changes in sexual desire.

Violence and Aggression

From time to time, persons with AD may become angry, aggressive, or violent. Hitting the caregiver or throwing things are some examples, as is destroying things, although this is rare. For persons with AD, it is not a personal attack on anyone but a part of the illness. There are many reasons why a person with AD may feel angry. The person may not like being helped with things she used to do on her own, or she may simply be frustrated by her inability to do certain things. Aggressive behavior among people with AD is also associated with depression, delusions, and hallucinations and might even be associated with constipation. These short-term behavior changes happen for a variety of other reasons, as well, such as a sense of loss of social control and judgment, loss of the ability to express negative feelings safely, and loss of the ability to understand the actions and abilities of others. People with AD may feel humiliated and frustrated when they are placed in a situation where they have to accept assistance, especially with intimate tasks such as bathing and toileting. When their independence and privacy are disrupted, they may react angrily.

Aggressive behavior may come without warning and make a caregiver feel very apprehensive. Violence and aggression often become a problem for a caregiver who might feel a mixture of emotions, such as disbelief, embarrassment, guilt, and shame. Care should be taken to defuse verbal aggression before the situation escalates. It is worth finding and avoiding the causes of certain hostile reactions. Once the caregiver figures out what situations trigger catastrophic behavior, he may be able to work out ways of avoiding them.

If the person with AD feels angry, aggressive, or violent, stay calm and try not to show fear or alarm. A caregiver may consider agreeing or apologizing with an angry or aggressive individual to avoid further argument. Another way to defuse verbal aggression is to play dumb. Encourage independence by allowing the person to do as much for himself as possible, even if it takes longer and is not as efficient. If aggressive behavior is very frequent, consult a physician. It may be necessary to consider using some form of medication, and this will need to be done with careful monitoring.

Depression

Dementia is a disabling disease, and it is understandable that a person with AD would feel depressed at times. Depression is very common among people with AD. It is estimated that 20%–40% of people with AD suffer from clinically significant depression (Mayo Clinic.com, 2007c). Research has also revealed that depression can lead to AD. A person with AD who has a lifetime history of depression has increased plaques and tangles in the brains and undergoes more rapid cognitive decline, according to a study published in the *Archives of General Psychiatry* (Rapp et al., 2006).

Alzheimer's disease and depression have many symptoms that are alike, making it difficult to tell the difference between them. Depression may cause or worsen memory loss and other cognitive impairments, and if a person has AD, the impact is greater. A person with AD may have difficulty articulating sadness, hopelessness, guilt, and other feelings caused by depression. Depression causes loss of interest in once-enjoyable activities and hobbies. Social and emotional withdrawal is common in people with AD who suffer from depression. Depression with AD can affect one's daily routines and interest in food, resulting in a decline in health.

The good news is that with treatment, depressive symptoms in persons with AD generally have an excellent prognosis. In fact, depression is probably one of the most common causes of excess disability in persons with AD that can be treated. Treatment does not improve cognitive functioning, but it does dramatically improve functional status and quality of life. A regular exercise program can also help depression.

If a person with AD is depressed, it is essential to provide more love and support during these periods. Schedule a predictable daily routine, taking advantage of the person's best time of day to undertake difficult tasks, such as bathing. Make a list of activities, like painting, singing, cooking, making collages, or visiting people or places that the person enjoys, and schedule these activities more frequently—no matter how small, they are stimulating. Acknowledge the person's frustration or sadness, while continuing to express hope that he or she will feel better soon. Celebrate small successes and occasions. Find ways that the person can contribute to family life and be sure to recognize his contributions. At the same time, provide reassurance that the person is loved, respected, and appreciated as a member of the family, and not just for what he can do now. Discuss with a physician supportive psychotherapy and/or counseling. Review chapter 7 for the pharmaceutical approach to treating depression in people with AD.

THE CAREGIVER'S BURDEN

Caring for someone with AD can be one of the most challenging and demanding tasks a caregiver can undertake. The slow and inevitable decline in memory, the loss of other cognitive abilities, possible behavioral problems, and the need for assistance with daily tasks presents a tremendous burden. Many have described caring for a person with AD as the reverse of raising a child. Persons with Alzheimer's lose their ability to perform one task after another. They give less feedback and fewer rewards as time goes on and ultimately require as much care as an infant. Caregiving can become so demanding and all-consuming that it makes caregivers vulnerable to problems of their own.

Caregiver stress is an epidemic in this country. As many as one-fourth to two-thirds of caregivers report physical or mental health problems that are the result of caregiving (National Respite Coalition, 2000). A survey by the National Family Caregivers Association (2000) found that 61% of caregivers experience depression; more than 50% experience sleeplessness; and more than 25% experience headaches and stomach disorders. Further, according to the Alzheimer's Association (2004), more than 80% of Alzheimer caregivers report that they frequently experience high levels of stress, and nearly half say they suffer from depression. Furthermore, family caregivers who provide care 36 or more hours weekly are more likely than noncaregivers to experience symptoms of depression or anxiety (Cannuscio et al., 2002). For spouses, the rate is six times higher; for those caring for a parent, the rate is twice as high.

According to the Alzheimer Society of Canada (2007), the following are the 10 warning signs of caregiver stress. Caregivers who regularly experience these conditions should seek help from their physician, says the Alzheimer's Association.

1 *Denial* about the disease and its effect on the person who has been diagnosed.
2 *Anger* at the person with Alzheimer's; anger that people don't understand; anger about treatment options.
3 *Social withdrawal* from friends and activities that once brought pleasure.
4 *Anxiety* about facing another day and what the future holds.
5 *Depression* that begins to break your spirit and affects your ability to cope.
6 *Exhaustion* that makes it nearly impossible to complete necessary daily tasks.
7 *Sleeplessness* caused by a never-ending list of concerns.
8 *Irritability* that leads to moodiness and triggers negative responses and reactions.
9 *Lack of concentration* that makes it difficult to perform familiar tasks.
10 *Health problems* that begin to take their toll, both mentally and physically.

Caregiving for someone with AD is a complex and exhausting task. Depression, empathy, exhaustion, guilt, and anger can wreak havoc on even a healthy individual. When faced with caring for someone with Alzheimer's, many people find that the experience is stressful and can cause burnout. Quite often, caregivers themselves begin to show signs of mental disorder and ill health. In addition to the 10 warning signs already mentioned, there are few more important issues for caregivers. Let's discuss them in detail.

Frustration

Caregivers feel frustrated because they cannot change the progression of the illness. A build-up of frustration can lead one to feel irritable, angry, or depressed. Caregivers suffer from these feelings more than persons with AD, who often have little awareness of lost capacities.

Loss of Identity

Caregivers are left with people who don't recognize them and can't remember their history together. Caregivers may lose a sense of who they are, because their loved one is no longer able to validate their shared experiences.

Burnout

Burnout is a state of physical, emotional, and mental exhaustion that may be accompanied by a change in attitude, from positive and caring to negative and unconcerned. Caregivers may feel constant exhaustion and increase their use of alcohol or stimulants. They may find it hard to relax, experience changes in sleeping patterns, and suffer from scattered thinking and increasing thoughts of death. Many caregivers also feel guilty if they spend time on themselves, rather than on their ill or elderly loved ones.

The Caregiver Burden Scale

Numerous questionnaires have been developed to quantify the largely subjective domain of caregiver burden. The Zarit Caregiver Burden Scale (1988) is the most widely used measurement tool and is used clinically to numerically calculate the burden experienced by caregivers of people with AD (Table 8.2).

Caring for Caregivers

A caregiver is the most important person in the life of someone with AD. So, maintaining good health is important for a caregiver, not only for personal reasons. There are things caregivers can do to help maintain their health and well-being. The Alzheimer Society of Canada (2007) offers 10 ways to reduce caregiver stress.

1   *Learn about the disease.* Knowing as much as possible about the disease and care strategies will prepare the caregiver for the Alzheimer journey. Understanding how the disease affects the person will help the caregiver to comprehend and adapt to the changes.

Table 8.2

CAREGIVER BURDEN SCALE

The following questions reflect how people sometimes feel when they are taking care of another person. After each question, circle how often you feel that way: never, rarely, sometimes, frequently, or nearly always. There are no right or wrong answers.

	NEVER	RARELY	SOMETIMES	FREQUENTLY	NEARLY ALWAYS
1. Do you feel that your relative asks for more help than he or she needs?	0	1	2	3	4
2. Do you feel that because of the time you spend with your relative, you do not have enough time for yourself?	0	1	2	3	4
3. Do you feel stressed between caring for your relative and trying to meet other responsibilities for your family or work?	0	1	2	3	4
4. Do you feel embarrassed over your relative's behavior?	0	1	2	3	4
5. Do you feel angry when you are around your relative?	0	1	2	3	4
6. Do you feel that your relative currently affects your relationship with other family members or friends in a negative way?	0	1	2	3	4
7. Are you afraid about what the future holds for your relative?	0	1	2	3	4
8. Do you feel your relative is dependent on you?	0	1	2	3	4
9. Do you feel strained when you are around your relative?	0	1	2	3	4
10. Do you feel your health has suffered because of your involvement with your relative?	0	1	2	3	4

11. Do you feel that you do not have as much privacy as you would like, because of your relative?	0	1	2	3	4
12. Do you feel that your social life has suffered because you are caring for your relative?	0	1	2	3	4
13. Do you feel uncomfortable about having friends over, because of your relative?	0	1	2	3	4
14. Do you feel that your relative seems to expect you to take care of him or her, as if you were the only one he or she could depend on?	0	1	2	3	4
15. Do you feel that you do not have enough money to care for your relative, in addition to the rest of your expenses?	0	1	2	3	4
16. Do you feel that you will be unable to take care of your relative much longer?	0	1	2	3	4
17. Do you feel you have lost control of your life since your relative's illness?	0	1	2	3	4
18. Do you wish you could just leave the care of your relative to someone else?	0	1	2	3	4
19. Do you feel uncertain about what to do about your relative?	0	1	2	3	4
20. Do you feel you should be doing more for your relative?	0	1	2	3	4
21. Do you feel you could do a better job in caring for your relative?	0	1	2	3	4
22. Overall, how burdened do you feel in caring for your relative?	0	1	2	3	4

Total score: _____

Scoring Key: 0–20 = little or no burden; 21–40 = mild to moderate burden; 41–60 = moderate to severe burden; 61–88 = severe burden.

Source: "Relatives of the Impaired Elderly: Correlates of Feelings of Burden," by S. H. Zarit, K. E. Reever, and J. Bach-Peterson, 1980, *Gerontologist*, *20*, p. 651. Copyright © The Gerontological Society of America. Reproduced by permission of the publisher.

2 *Be realistic about the disease.* It is important, though difficult, to be realistic about the disease and how it will affect the person over time. Once a caregiver is realistic, it will be easier to adjust to the prognosis.

3 *Be realistic about yourself.* Caregivers need to be realistic about how much they can do. What do they value the most? A walk with the person being cared for, time alone, or a tidy house? There is no "right" answer; only the caregiver knows what matters most to him and how much he can do.

4 *Accept your feelings.* When caring for a person with AD, the caregiver will have many mixed feelings. In a single day, she may feel contented, angry, guilty, happy, sad, embarrassed, afraid, and helpless. These feelings may be confusing, but they are normal. Recognize that as a caregiver, you are doing the best you can.

5 *Share information and feelings with others.* A caregiver should share information about the disease with family and friends. This can help loved ones understand what is happening and better prepare them to provide help and support that a caregiver inevitably needs. It is also important for the caregiver to share her feelings and have someone with whom she feels comfortable talking about her feelings. This may be a close friend or family member, someone the caregiver met at an Alzheimer support group, a member of the caregiver's religious community, or a health care professional.

6 *Be positive.* The caregiver's attitude can make a difference to the way he feels. If you are a caregiver, try to look at the positive side of things. Focusing on what the person can do, as opposed to the abilities lost, can make things easier. Try to make every day count. There can still be times that are special and rewarding.

7 *Look for humor.* While AD is serious, a caregiver may find that certain situations have a bright side. Maintaining a sense of humor can be a good coping strategy.

8 *Take care of yourself.* A caregiver's health is important and should not be ignored. If you are a caregiver, eat proper meals and exercise regularly. Find ways to relax and try to get the rest you need. Make regular appointments with a doctor for checkups. You need to take regular breaks from caregiving. Do not wait until you are too exhausted to plan this. Take time to maintain interests and hobbies. Keep in touch with friends and family so that you won't feel lonely and isolated. These things will give you the strength to continue providing care.

9 *Get help and support.* A caregiver will need support that comes from sharing thoughts and feelings with others. This could be individually, with a professional, or as part of an Alzheimer support group. If you are a caregiver, choose the form of support that you are most comfortable with.

10 *Plan for the future.* Planning for the future can help relieve stress. While the person with AD is still capable, review his financial situation and plan accordingly. Choices relating to future health and personal care decisions should be considered and recorded. Legal and estate planning should also be discussed. Think about an alternate caregiving plan in the event that a caregiver is unable to provide care in the future.

Continuum of Options

Being an Alzheimer's caregiver is never easy. No matter how efficiently and effortlessly a caregiver takes care of an individual with AD at home, the caregiver needs to schedule times when he or she can take regular breaks. If a caregiver needs a break, there are a number of options for caring for an individual with AD. The cost of caring for someone with AD is severe and is discussed in the next chapter.

Family Members and Friends

Many American spouses currently care for their husband or wife at home, which can be physically and mentally stressful for the caregiver-spouse. Sometimes adult children help their parents cope with the extra responsibilities. Most people with AD don't like to leave their homes when they are experiencing confusion or forgetfulness. They prefer the routine and familiarity of home and will become angry and resistant to out-of-home care. Sometimes an aging parent or parents move in with their adult children. Relocating can cause stress and irritability and can even result in reduced mental or cognitive functioning, since the safety and familiarity of home and the sense of belonging and ownership are lost. Have other family members or friends provide care.

Hired Help

There are many cases in AD care where additional help is brought in. For example, there are many companion agencies that provide paid helpers who care for people with AD and their spouses. An affordable hired caregiver for some hours daily or weekly can be very helpful for a caregiver-family member. There are also products that can be purchased to make the house a safer environment.

Respite Care

In-home services offer a wide range of options, including companion services, personal care, household assistance, and skilled nursing care to meet the specific needs of those involved. Respite care facilities provide overnight, weekend, and longer stays for someone with Alzheimer's or a related dementia so that a caregiver can have longer periods of time off. These facilities provide meals, help with activities of daily living, offer therapeutic activities to fit the needs of residents, and ensure a safe, supervised environment.

Adult Day Services

Adult day services provide a planned program that includes a variety of health, social, and support services in a protective setting. Some programs are specifically designed for people with AD. These programs are generally available during daytime hours, usually weekdays only. Staff lead various activities, such as arts and crafts, music programs, and support groups. Adult day care also provides opportunities for education and takes into consideration the older adults' favorite hobbies, interests, and needs. Most provide a lunchtime meal, and some offer transportation to and from home.

Home Health Services

The most common assistance involves personal care such as bathing, dressing, grooming, and assistance with eating and going to the bathroom. Some agencies also provide help with meal preparation and household chores. Most provide nursing care that may include monitoring of medications and assistance with wound care and medical equipment. Most agencies also provide rehabilitation therapy including physical and occupational therapy and help with speech and language pathology.

Coping With the Holidays

The activity and festivities of the holiday season can be overwhelming and pose special challenges for many AD caregivers and people with AD.

The fast pace during the holidays and the change in routine can be especially disruptive for people with AD. For caregivers, holiday memories from before the loved one's diagnosis may darken what usually is a joyful season. A caregiver's concerns about how an individual's condition may disrupt family's plans can overshadow the simple pleasure of celebrating the holidays. One of the first things a caregiver should do is realize that the holidays may not be the same as in the past and adjust her expectations. Focusing on making the holidays as enjoyable as possible will lighten the situation, as well. Consider inviting a limited number of visitors to the house, and keep the meal simple. Schedule the meal at a time when the individual with AD is at his best. Avoid crowds, changes in routine, and strange surroundings that may cause confusion or agitation. Maintain the individual's normal routine as much as possible in order to limit disruption and confusion. Try to include the individual in some of the preholiday preparation activities, giving him a small job that you know he can handle. Including the individual helps him feel useful, and the caregiver can accomplish the tasks she is working on as well. Ask for help and support from family members and friends in preparing the holiday celebration.

Tips for Caregivers

Caring for people with dementia is a time-consuming and demanding responsibility because Alzheimer's affects an individual's behavior, daily functioning, and personality. There is no prescribed course to follow in this emotional Alzheimer's caregiving journey. Each situation is different. A few simple guidelines might help caregivers in caring for people with AD at home:

- Treat the person as an adult, not a child. Treat the person in the way you would wish to be treated.
- Do not remind a person that her memory is bad.
- Keep the home environment consistent, quiet, and restful. Utilize familiar pictures, possessions, music, and reminders of prior interests.
- Avoid overcrowding. Small celebrations and one-to-one interactions may be more meaningful and more successful.
- Plan daily activities to help provide structure, meaning, and a sense of accomplishment.
- Stay calm and be patient. Never argue with someone who has dementia.

- Reduce any demands on the person and make sure he has an unrushed and stress-free routine.
- Never force the individual to do something. Be flexible. Walk away, calm down, and try the task again later.
- Allow the person to complete as many things as possible by herself, even if the caregiver has to initiate the activity.
- Simplify tasks and routines. Provide gentle reminders and encouragement, and offer constant praise and reinforcement when tasks are accomplished.
- Reassure the person with a calm voice and a gentle touch.
- Remember that physical exercise, proper nutrition, good general health, and socialization are important.
- Engage in gentle, regular exercise and mild physical activity.
- Keep activities familiar and satisfying, and keep instructions simple.
- Choose the best times to do activities according to the part of the day when the person is usually at her best.
- As functions are lost, adapt activities and routines to allow the person with Alzheimer's to participate as much as possible.
- Find and use familiar routines. Use old habits and skills to identify a routine that is pleasant and comfortable.
- Remember that humor helps. There are moments that can be enjoyable and memorable.
- Accept and validate the person's view of reality. Do no confront these views and feelings. Allow his reality to exist.
- Reminiscence is very valuable. Accept and enjoy this opportunity while you can.
- Never use the phrase "you know what you are doing" with someone with dementia.
- When a person is agitated, restless, or irritable, keep in mind that she may be experiencing pain or have a urinary tract infection.
- Provide "cues" for desired behavior.
- Divert behavior and attention when the going gets tough.

It is important for the caregivers to receive counseling and support for themselves. In fact, one study showed that when the caregivers took part in a support program, the persons with AD that they cared for delayed being institutionalized by a year (Mittelman, Ferris, Shulman, Steinberg, & Levin, 1996).

9

Long-Term Care of People With Alzheimer's Disease

Even with the help of support services, meeting the needs of the person with Alzheimer's disease can be overwhelming...consider alternate caregiving options.

Alzheimer Society of Canada

People with Alzheimer's disease (AD) can live from 3 to 20 years after the onset of symptoms (Administration on Aging, 2007, September). The average duration of AD is 8 years, during which afflicted persons progress from a stage of mild memory loss to a stage where 24-hour supervision is required, and finally to a stage of total dependency (Figure 9.1). Many people with AD do well at home during the early stage of the disease and can be cared for by family and friends. As the disease progresses, individuals with AD require increasing amounts of assistance, constant care, and supervision. For example, the AD individual's need for help with activities of daily living (ADLs)—bathing, dressing, transferring, toileting, and eating—increases. Alzheimer's disease also causes behavior changes in individuals, causing them to become increasingly aggressive, easily agitated, disoriented, and disruptive. They may even have hallucinations and delusions. Meeting the changing needs of a person with AD can be overwhelming for a caregiver. Even with the help of support services, caregivers often feel physically, emotionally, and financially drained.

MAKING THE DECISION FOR LONG-TERM CARE

At the point where the need for increased personal care and supervision is more than can be provided for at home, families usually consider long-term-care (LTC) nursing or assisted-living facilities. Long-term care may include medical assistance, such as administering medication or performing rehabilitative therapy. But, more typically, it involves personal care (e.g., help with bathing and eating) and supervision (e.g., protecting persons from wandering away or inadvertently injuring themselves). Unlike health services for acute conditions, LTC focuses on managing ongoing conditions over time. With LTC, the emphasis is on enhancing a person's ability to function and to enjoy an acceptable quality of life, rather than on curing a condition.

Moving an individual with AD from a home to an LTC facility is a big change that affects the entire family. In order to determine if the time has come for an individual with AD (or any form of dementia) to live in an LTC facility, family members should consider two factors. First, consideration must be given to the caregiver's own physical and mental state. Depression incidence in adult caregivers may range from 14% to

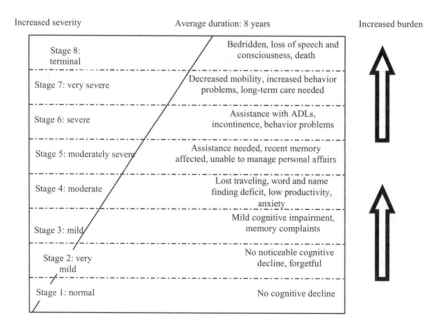

Figure 9.1 Increased severity of symptoms and burden with progression of disease.

47%, and anxiety disorders affect another 10% (Dura, Stukenberg, & Kiecolt-Glaser, 1991). Caregivers of the persons with AD often suffer from stress-related illnesses and neuropsychiatric symptoms. A study conducted by Pillemer and Suitor (1992) found that one-fifth of 236 caregivers experienced violent feelings and feared they might physically hurt their loved one. One-third of these caregivers reported that they had actually engaged in violent behavior. The second consideration is the physical and mental state of the individual with AD. When a person with AD becomes physically abusive and the caregiver's safety is at stake, or the person with AD wanders from home, jeopardizing his or her own safety—placement in a facility should be seriously considered. Table 9.1 compares the reasons and concerns leading a caregiver to place an individual with AD at an LTC facility, or continue caring for them at home.

Caregivers can also use a worksheet to assess whether or not they should place a loved one in a facility. By completing Table 9.2, a caregiver

Table 9.1

DECIDING WHETHER TO PUT A RELATIVE IN A NURSING HOME

REASONS TO CONSIDER PLACING A PERSON WITH AD IN A NURSING HOME	REASONS TO CONSIDER KEEPING A PERSON WITH AD AT HOME
■ Person's behavior has become dangerous or disruptive to caregiver and household. ■ Caregiver's own health is at risk. ■ The burden of caregiving is too great, and the caregiver has no one to help. ■ A nursing home may offer a safer, more controlled situation for person with AD. ■ Person with AD has other medical problems that require skilled nursing care.	■ Family is concerned about the risk of the relative's health declining in a nursing home. ■ Family is worried that the relative will receive less individual attention in a nursing home. ■ Family will feel too much guilt or anxiety about putting the relative in a nursing home. ■ A nursing home costs much more than caring for the relative at home. ■ The facility may have a waiting list if the family has not planned ahead.
Are there other reasons why a person with AD might need nursing home placement?	Are there other reasons why family might consider caring for the relative at home?

Adapted from "Should I Put My Relative With Alzheimer's or Other Dementia in a Nursing Home?" by L. Sabra and R. P. Katz-Wise, 2006, Healthwise, Incorporated, www.healthwise. org. Reprinted with permission. This information does not replace the advice of a doctor. Healthwise disclaims any warranty or liability for your use of this information.

Table 9.2

WORKSHEET TO HELP MAKE A DECISION ABOUT PUTTING A RELATIVE IN A NURSING HOME

Caregiving is negatively affecting my health or well-being or that of my family.	Yes	No	Unsure
My relative has developed medical or behavioral problems that require more care than I can provide.	Yes	No	Unsure
My relative has become a danger to himself, me, or my family.	Yes	No	Unsure
I am healthy enough and physically strong enough to take care of my relative.	Yes	No	Unsure
I can afford to devote most of my time to caregiving.	Yes	No	Unsure
I have other family members and friends who can help with caregiving.	Yes	No	Unsure
I have medical problems that are making it difficult to take care of my relative.	Yes	No	Unsure
There is a long-term care facility in my community that I trust.	Yes	No	Unsure
The cost of nursing home care will be an unbearable hardship.	Yes	No	Unsure

Adapted from "Should I Put My Relative With Alzheimer's or Other Dementia in a Nursing Home?" by L. Sabra and R. P. Katz-Wise, 2006, Healthwise, Incorporated, www.healthwise. org. Reprinted with permission. This information does not replace the advice of a doctor. Healthwise disclaims any warranty or liability for your use of this information.

can get an honest look at how he or she feels about putting an individual in an LTC facility.

New challenges arise after an individual with AD is placed in an LTC facility. Caregivers—particularly the spouse—continue to feel distressed by the suffering and decline of their loved one. Caregivers now must make frequent trips to the LTC facility and adjust to having significantly less control over the care provided to their loved one. Studies have shown that caregivers continue to exhibit symptoms of anxiety and depression comparable to those experienced prior to admission (Schulz et al., 2004).

Planning Long-Term Care

For a person with AD, an LTC facility provides a safe setting where one can maintain as much independence as possible and receive assistance when needed. There is no standard answer for the question What type of care is best? The philosophy of care, appropriate level of care, preferred location, and budget are all important factors that deserve equal consideration. For this reason, planning for LTC can be a difficult process.

Physicians play a vital role in the placement process. A caregiver must seek permission from a physician to place a person with AD in an LTC facility. Physicians, social workers, and members of your local Alzheimer's Association chapter (or another community agency) can help determine the potential needs of an individual with AD. It is important to include the person who needs LTC in the decision-making process whenever possible. This will make the transition to an LTC facility easier for all, because many important decisions will have been made or at least discussed out in the open.

Planning ahead is critical. In the event of a crisis, family members are more likely to be forced into finding a quick fix, which can result in a hasty choice that doesn't solve the patient's long-term needs. Exploring living arrangements and levels of care is a critical step to making the right decision. Keep in mind that some settings are not designed for people with Alzheimer's. And, as an individual's needs change, caregiving options might also need to change. Some settings may not be able to care for a person with AD throughout the course of the disease. In fact, most people require more support and help as the disease progresses.

Fortunately, LTC facilities can provide different levels of care. A family coping with AD needs to learn what to expect from each level of care in order to pick the type of LTC that is most appropriate for their loved one. A wide range of LTC facilities is available in most communities. The next session describes the most common types of LTCs available for people with AD.

ASSISTED-LIVING FACILITIES

Prior to assisted-living facilities (ALFs), nursing homes were the only care facilities available for the elderly. People lived in the expensive facilities, but not all of them needed the extensive level of care provided. As a result, ALFs began to emerge—a type of housing designed for people who needed differing levels of medical and personal care. ALFs—including board and care, group homes, community-based residential facilities, and foster homes—gave the elderly the opportunity to live in a more homelike environment for half the cost of a nursing home.

Assisted-living facilities offer their residents a balance between living independently and living in a nursing home, providing housing but also tailoring services to meet an individual's specific needs and preferences. Assisted-living facilities generally provide a homelike setting and are designed to promote the residents' independence. Living spaces can be individual rooms, apartments, or shared quarters. Services are offered to assist residents with daily living. Assisted-living facilities are a promising option for seniors because they share one philosophy—to promote residents' independence and their right to make decisions about their lives as much as possible.

Not all residents of ALFs need significant care or assistance. Many are there because they want a simpler lifestyle without the worry of maintaining a home and are seeking the companionship of other people their own age. They also may have chosen assisted living over an independent retirement community because they need minor help (e.g., reminders to take medications), they desire a secure environment, or they require minor supervision. They may be able to get this help at other places, but they are preparing for a time when they might need the more intensive care that only an ALF can offer.

Some ALFs specialize in the care of persons with AD, but these types of facilities are few in number and tend to be expensive. Alzheimer's-dedicated facilities are appropriate for those in the mid-to-advanced stages of the disease or those who cannot live alone or be cared for by a caregiver but can still function fairly well on their own. Figure 9.2 presents the percentage of assisted-living residents needing help with ADL.

Alzheimer's-dedicated facilities range in capacity from 6 residents to more than 100, and the average-size facility houses about 60 residents. Accommodations tend to be spartan and functional; usually residents are housed two to a room. What differentiates this type of ALF facility from a residential care home or nursing home is that only dementia patients are accepted. Typically, an individual with AD does not require a lot of medical attention but instead requires supervision and confinement. To respond to these behaviors, Alzheimer's-dedicated facilities offer a care program that is designed to make residents comfortable and secure. For example, Alzheimer's-dedicated ALFs have locked entrance doors to prevent residents from wandering.

Staff members of Alzheimer's-dedicated facilities are usually better trained than those of the average care home, and they have more experience working with dementia patients. The spectrum of services offered by different facilities varies tremendously, which makes the cost vary, as well. Services may offer just a supervisor or 24-hour supervision

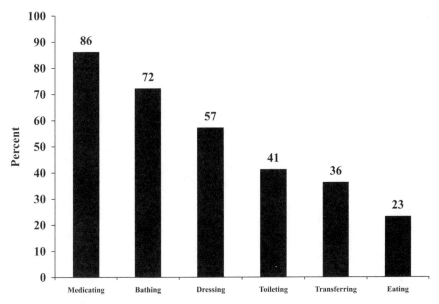

Figure 9.2 Assisted living residents needing help with activities of daily living.
Source: "Residents Leaving Assisted Living: Descriptive and Analytic Results From a National Survey", by C. D. Phillips, C. Hawes, K. Spry, and M. Rose, June 2000, U.S. Department of Health and Human Services. Retrieved October 2007, from http://aspe.hhs.gov/daltcp/reports/alresid.htm

and one meal per day to three meals a day. Other services may include monitoring of medication, personal care (e.g., bathing, grooming, dressing, and toileting), housekeeping and laundry services, limited medical services, and social and recreational activities in a supervised environment. Quality of care and staffing levels also can differ significantly among ALFs, since regulations vary from state to state. Many assisted-living facilities allow home health agencies to come in and offer services for residents. Some states may allow facilities to have a resident nurse or therapist to help with minor medical problems. Some states even allow variances for assisted-living facilities to offer limited nursing home services.

A good match between an ALF and a resident's needs depends as much on the ALF's philosophy and services as it does on the quality of care. It is highly recommended that prior to making a decision on a facility, a family coping with Alzheimer's perform a detailed preadmission evaluation of the ALF. The Assisted Living Federation of America and Elizabeth Parker Welton (2002) recommend several factors to consider when selecting an ALF.

Important Factors to Consider When Selecting an Assisted-Living Facility

At times a crisis may necessitate a rapid decision about long-term care, but it is always good to take the time to make an informed decision about a care facility for a loved one if possible. The best way to do this is to gather as much information as possible, which should involve visits, question-and-answer sessions, and other needs assessments. The goal set in choosing a residence should not be considered met until a setting has been selected in which the prospective resident can feel physically cared for and can thrive emotionally (Welton, 2002).

Atmosphere

Family members involved in the selection process must look at the atmosphere of the facilities and also look at the facilities they visit through the eyes of the person who will be living there (Welton, 2002). How does the prospective resident react when she meets the staff and other residents? Do residents socialize with each other and appear happy? Will the particular personality and culture of that setting support the physical, emotional, mental, and spiritual needs of the prospective resident? Several return visits to the top facilities on the family's list might be necessary to experience the staff and residents in a variety of situations.

Physical Features

A facility's physical setup is also an important factor in decision making. Is the facility well designed for residents' needs? Is the decor welcoming and homelike? Does it include safety features? A facility that is modern and tastefully decorated almost always creates an initial favorable impression (Welton, 2002). However, an aesthetically pleasing setting that is not designed to maximize comfort and ease in functioning may not be a particularly wise choice. For example, a modern and beautifully decorated ALF may not have been designed to be easily navigated by people using walkers or wheelchairs or those whose mobility is impaired by failing eyesight. A bathroom that is too small to permit a wheelchair or walker or that does not have safety rails reflects poor design. Hallways that are long and/or poorly lit without handrails may confuse and overwhelm elderly residents.

Contractual Agreement

A thorough assessment of the agreement is another important consideration. The agreement should cover all the terms that the family and the provider have agreed to, such as costs, services, discharge policies, grievance procedures, and rights and obligations of the resident. It will be important to understand potential future costs for increased levels of care and services, should the resident's physical and/or cognitive functioning decline (Welton, 2002). In most cases, it is reasonable to expect costs to increase over time as functioning declines. Another way to determine the viability of a particular residence is to learn whether each resident has a written care plan (Welton, 2002). Without such a tool, it is possible that the care needs of residents will be unrecognized and therefore unmet. A comprehensive care plan should be created with the help and input of the resident (if possible), family members, physician and health care providers, and any staff members who will have direct contact with the resident. This plan of care must be reviewed and updated periodically as the resident's condition changes. The agreement should state whether and how often health care professionals—nurses, physicians, therapists—come to the facility. The agreement should also specify what kinds of health services will be provided by staff, such as helping with medications, calling in prescriptions to the pharmacy, or arranging for prescription delivery.

Level of Services

More and more ALFs are providing an increased scope of services as their average tenant acuity level has risen dramatically in recent years. The scope of services available in an ALF may vary tremendously depending on state law and regulations and the ALF's philosophy about the level of services provided. The level of services available is an important criterion in selecting an ALF, and the family should determine as specifically as possible the level of care the resident requires and the services that are offered by the ALF to meet that level. Cognitively impaired adults may need assistance in their daily functioning different from that required by other residents of ALFs (Welton, 2002). A family coping with AD needs to make a detailed list of the type of assistance that will be required for its loved one. Further, the number, type, and training of ALF staff members vary from the facility to facility. It is important to know whether the facility staffing pattern will meet the level of care required by the potential resident. A recent government report noted that inadequate staffing in ALFs was a major quality-of-care issue nationwide (U.S. Department of Health and Human Services, 2000).

Choice in One's Living Space

Nurturing the spirit and individuality of residents as they move from their home into a residence is challenging but achievable. A future resident's participation in the choice of a residence and the various options available within that facility will have a direct and vital effect on the quality of that resident's adjustment to his new home (Welton, 2002). The opportunity to have a choice in one's living space is an important way to empower new residents. Most facilities offer private as well as double-occupancy rooms. Cognitively impaired individuals may not care as much for this particular choice. The family has to make a decision on the basis of the individual's past living habits, whether the loved one prefers privacy or may feel isolated in a unit by herself. Bringing some treasured pieces of furniture and pictures from home will greatly facilitate the transition and simulate familiar surroundings.

Social Activities and Exercises

It is one thing to assist residents with the basics of daily life such as dressing and bathing; that help is guaranteed in a contract with an assisted-living residence. It may be quite another thing to help residents to lead mentally, physically, and socially active lives. Activities are an important way in which social and emotional connections are made in a new setting. A diverse program of planned community activities both within the residence and in the community should be an integrated part of the assisted-living program. Activities such as social events, outings, arts and crafts, and music are important for people with AD. Studies suggest that efforts to improve social support in ALFs help reduce rates of depression among residents. This includes not only providing activities for residents but also encouraging relationship building among residents and between residents and staff. Most facilities plan group activities and exercise classes, as well as regular gatherings for the residents to visit among themselves. There are several ways to get a sense of the quality of group and individual activities at a particular facility. Take a look at what is scheduled for any given week, but it is also important to visit during one of these planned activities to see if residents participate and seem to enjoy doing so. As for more individual attention, find out whether there are any rules against staff spending nonscheduled time with residents. And, during the visits, watch how the staff interacts with residents. The best facilities also help individual residents to participate in these activities to the extent possible and provide alternatives—an assisted walk around the hallways, for example, or a one-on-one chat in a resident's private room—if it's not feasible to participate in a group. A well-balanced coordination of activities both within the residence and in the community allows the resident to feel a sense of belonging in both places (Welton, 2002). Activities are an important way in which social and emotional connections are made in an ALF. In addition, research shows that the presence of animals in the lives of older adults is another important way of nurturing the spirit. A residence that has a dog or cat viewed as the house pet can provide opportunity for constancy and daily love for someone who may be feeling a sense of loss. Many residences allow a small animal to accompany its owner in the move. When discussing this option with the staff, gain a full understanding of how the animal will be cared for.

Health and Well-Being

In addition to providing help with daily activities, ALF staff monitor residents' health. That does not mean that they provide nursing or other active treatment of a medical condition. Rather, it means that they keep track of and help residents with their health aids such as oxygen, providing emergency call systems and checking on residents' well-being during the night. There is, however, a serious lack of health promotion programs for people with AD. Food is also a significant part of life, particularly for people with AD. One of the universally significant ways in which people feel nurtured is through the food they eat. Keeping that in mind, food preparation should include fresh, diverse, and interesting ingredients. Is the dining room visually appealing to encourage residents to linger over their meals there? One of the most important avenues for socialization is dining with other people. It represents a natural opportunity to gather and share the events of the day, and, sometimes, a lifetime. If a resident is feeling too ill to come to the dining room for a meal, can food be delivered to his room? There is growing recognition that the mental health of elderly people is critically related to their physical health and functioning.

The Administration on Aging Guidelines for an Assisted-Living Facility

The Administration on Aging (Administration on Aging Fact Sheet, 2007), a division of the Department of Health and Human Services, provides the following suggestions to help start the search for a safe, comfortable, and appropriate ALF:

- Think ahead. Ask yourself the following questions:
  - What will the resident's future needs be and how will the facility meet those needs?
  - Is the facility close to family and friends? Are there any shopping centers or other businesses nearby (within walking distance)?
  - Do admission and retention policies exclude people with severe cognitive impairments or severe physical disabilities?
  - Does the facility provide a written statement of the philosophy of care?
- Visit the facility, sometimes unannounced, and gather information.
  - Visit at meal times, sample the food, and observe the quality of mealtime and the service.
  - Observe interactions among residents and staff.
  - Check to see if the facility offers social, recreational, and spiritual activities?
  - Talk to residents.
- Research the background of the ALF:
  - Learn what types of training staff receive and how frequently they receive training.
  - Review state licensing reports.
  - Contact the state's long-term care Ombudsman to see if any complaints have recently been filed against the ALF that you are interested in. In many states, the Ombudsman checks on conditions at ALFs as well as nursing homes.
  - Contact the local Better Business Bureau to see if that agency has received any complaints about the ALF.

If the ALF is connected to a nursing home, ask for information about it.

The Alzheimer Society of Canada has also compiled a list of questions to be considered when visiting LTC facilities (Table 9.3).

Table 9.3

ASSESSING A LONG-TERM-CARE FACILITY

AREA OF CONCERN	QUESTIONS TO ASK
Location	Is the facility conveniently located? Will you be able to visit easily? Does public transportation run nearby?
Appearance	Are the kitchen, day rooms, and bedrooms clean and tidy and free from unpleasant odors?
Menus	Is the menu varied, nutritious, and tasty? Can the facility accommodate special dietary needs? Is food available throughout the day? Is snacking possible? Are mealtimes flexible?
Bathrooms	Are they private? Are they clean? Are they easy to find? Are there grab bars and other safety devices present?
Alzheimer-friendly	Are staff specially trained to care for someone with Alzheimer's disease? Is there ongoing staff training about Alzheimer's disease? Is the facility "homelike"? Is there a separate unit for Alzheimer residents? Can the residents walk safely indoors and outside?
Resident-to-staff ratio	What is the resident-to-staff ratio? What proportion of residents have Alzheimer's disease?
Interaction	Do all staff interact with residents on a regular basis and in a friendly and personable manner?
Activities	Are there a variety of meaningful activities for groups and individuals? Are there therapeutic activities, such as music, pets, horticulture? Are there opportunities to socialize? Is there flexibility in the routine?
Visiting	When can you visit? Can you have privacy with the resident? Can you take the resident for outings?
Understanding behavior	Do staff try to understand what residents are communicating through their actions (e.g., a person may pace because he is looking for a family member)? Restraints should not be used without first exploring all alternative ways of responding to a person's behavior. (Restraints may include physical restraints, like a geri-chair; chemical restraints, like sedatives; or restraints to the environment, like a locked door.)
Safety	Are there smoke detectors? Are there slip-proof mats in the baths, grab rails, and so on?

(*continued*)

Table 9.3

ASSESSING A LONG-TERM-CARE FACILITY (CONTINUED)	
AREA OF CONCERN	**QUESTIONS TO ASK**
Quality	Is the facility accredited by an independent body? What were the results of the most recent inspections?
Medical care and continuum of care	Can you continue to use your own doctor or is there a resident doctor? Is there a doctor on call? How often does the doctor visit? Can you meet the doctor? How are medical emergencies handled? Are there situations where the facility will no longer be able to provide care to the person?
Care philosophy	Does the facility focus on individual resident needs? Can it accommodate flexibility in routines? ("My mother has never been a morning person.") Are there regular care planning meetings that include family members?
Individualized care	Is consideration given to individual cultural, religious, or spiritual needs? Are several languages spoken?

Source: Alzheimer Society of Canada, August 2007. Reprinted with permission.

The estimated average length of stay in an ALF ranges from approximately 2.5 to 3 years. Residents who leave typically do so because they need to move to a nursing home for more care or because of death. A 2000 study found that, among those who moved to another setting, the need for more care was the most commonly cited reason for leaving (Figure 9.3). Results total more than 100% because respondents could give more than one answer.

NURSING HOMES

In general, nursing home care is best designed for persons with physical or mental impairments that prevent them from living independently.

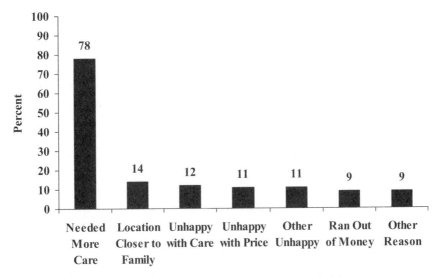

Figure 9.3 Reasons assisted living residents moved to another facility.
Source: "Residents Leaving Assisted Living: Descriptive and Analytic Results From a National Survey", by C. D. Phillips, C. Hawes, K. Spry, and M. Rose, June 2000, U.S. Department of Health and Human Services. Retrieved from http://aspe.hhs.gov/daltcp/reports/alresid.htm.

Nursing homes are expensive and are certified to provide skilled nursing services, when necessary, as well as custodial care. Many older adults are admitted to nursing homes after an AD diagnosis; however, a long stay in a nursing home often results in the individual developing and being diagnosed with dementia after admission to the facility.

Alzheimer's disease is not, by itself, a reason for nursing home admission; most persons with dementia are cared for in the community or in an ALF. The decision to place a person with dementia in a nursing home is complex and is based on patient and caregiver characteristics and the sociocultural context of patients and caregivers (Yaffe et al., 2002). Most studies have developed predictors of nursing home placement primarily according to patient or caregiver characteristics alone. Patient predictors of nursing home placement also include ethnicity (e.g., there is less likelihood of placement for people of African American or Hispanic descent); living situation (i.e., one is more likely to be placed if one has been living alone); dependency in one or more activities of daily living (ADLs); lower Mini-Mental State Examination scores; and the presence of at least one difficult behavior. Caregiver predictors of nursing home placement are older age and a higher Zarit

Burden Interview score. A recent study published in the *American Journal of Psychiatry* (Wilson, McCann, Li, Aggarwal, & Gilley, 2007) reported that people with AD experience acceleration in the rate of cognitive decline after being placed in a nursing home. However, researchers posit that an intermediate placement, such as adult day care, may help lessen the mental changes associated with permanent placement. "The findings suggest that experience in day care [settings] may help individuals with Alzheimer's disease make the transition from the community to institutional residence," said the study author, Robert S. Wilson, PhD, a neuropsychologist at the Rush Alzheimer's Disease Center (p. 914).

Nursing homes provide skilled nursing care up to 24 hours a day. A good nursing home will be able to address a host of needs such as care planning, recreational activities, spirituality, nutrition, medical care, meals, laundry, help with personal needs (such as dressing, bathing, and using the toilet), and other support services. A regular nursing home may not accept individuals with AD whose symptoms are too advanced to be safely accommodated and whose behavior may be disruptive to other nursing home residents. These people may need to move to a nursing home specifically for those with AD. Some nursing homes have special care units to accommodate people with serious behavior problems of AD—designed so that the environment, activities, philosophy of care, and staff training revolve around the special needs of people with Alzheimer's. These units are designed to meet the needs of people with this disease, and they include staffs experienced in dealing with erratic or dangerous behavior. A trained staff and creative programming diminish the use of physical and pharmacologic restraints and focus on preserving the residual skills of individuals with AD. A nursing home is the most expensive type of long-term care facility, but it also may be the most appropriate choice for many people with advanced dementia. The offices of Medicare and Medicaid have an extensive database that can help to locate a good Alzheimer's nursing home. Their database rates the Alzheimer's nursing homes by quality of care, quality of life, nutrition, and safety. The federal government uses surveys to monitor nursing homes. The results of these surveys can be obtained using the Nursing Home Compare tool on the Medicare Web site. It's best to compare facilities within a region to one another. The Web site also provides a checklist for people to use when visiting the different Alzheimer's nursing homes. This form will help clinicians and families keep track of the different nursing homes so that they can evaluate them for the best alternative.

This checklist is available at http://www.alzinfo.org/pdfs/checklist.pdf, and the database of nursing homes can be found at http://www.alzinfo.org/providers/default.aspx?AreaId 3.

Types of Care in Nursing Homes

There are two types of nursing home facilities that can care for an individual with AD: skilled care and long-term care.

Skilled Care

This type of Alzheimer's nursing home provides only care that that requires the services of a physician, licensed nurse, physical or occupational therapist, speech-language pathologist, respiratory therapist, or social worker. These types of nursing homes are also known as "subacute" or "Medicare occupancy." This type of nursing home is generally paid for by Medicare for approximately 100 days, so is not suitable for the long term. Skilled care may also be needed on a long-term basis if a resident requires injections, ventilation, or other treatment of that nature.

Long-Term Care

This type of Alzheimer's nursing home is for those individuals who require a 24-hour, high level of care to insure their safety. Medicare does generally not cover long-term Alzheimer's nursing homes. Clients must have their own resources to fund this level of care, although there are some government programs that may help after resources have been exhausted. If the nursing home does not accept that type government funding, it may be necessary to move to a nursing facility that does.

Ethical Considerations in Nursing Homes

The quality of nursing homes has been perceived as the most troublesome aspect of the U.S. health care system. Monitoring quality of nursing homes has been a long-standing challenge. Despite the federal, state, and local advocacy mechanisms in place to continuously monitor and maintain quality in nursing homes, inadequate quality of care continues to be a serious and pervasive problem. Nursing home abuse and neglect may include minor to serious conditions such as death, physical and sexual abuse, beating, financial exploitation, and serious neglect. This is one of the nation's largest growing problems, particularly as population is aging and more and more elderly are in need of long-term care.

According to the 2001 congressional report prepared for Congressman Henry Waxman, researchers found that between January 1999 and January 2001, more than 30% of nursing homes had at least one reported incident of abuse that could have resulted in harm to a resident, and almost 10% of nursing homes were cited for abuse violations that caused actual harm or placed residents in immediate jeopardy. These nursing homes were cited for almost 9,000 abuse violations during this 2-year period. More than 2,500 of the abuse violations in 1999–2001 were serious enough to cause actual harm to residents or to place residents in immediate jeopardy of death or serious injury. Furthermore, the percentage of nursing homes cited for abuse violations has increased every year since 1996. In 2000, more than twice as many nursing homes were cited for abuse violations during annual inspections than were cited in 1996. The Nursing Home Reform Act of 1987 set new standards for care and established rights of nursing home residents in response to numerous reports of neglect and abuse in nursing homes. A notable impact of the act is a substantial reduction in the unnecessary use of physical and chemical restraints in nursing homes. Recent statistics have shown that 30% of all nursing homes in the United States were cited for nursing home abuse, and many of these cases involve pressure ulcers and inadequate nursing care. Nursing professionals have a legal and ethical duty to prevent the deterioration of a patient's physical, emotional, mental, and psychosocial well-being. Some of the most common situations involve the problems discussed in the following sections.

Pressure Ulcers

According to the Nursing Home Abuse Resource, statistics have shown that 30% of all nursing homes in the United States commit nursing home abuse, and many of these cases involve pressure ulcers. The nursing home should take care to prevent the development of pressure ulcers by proper skin care and hygiene to ensure that skin is kept clean, dry, moisturized, and away from harmful substances. Nursing staff must periodically check a patient who is immobile for any signs of pressure ulcers. They must also be careful not to pull a patient from the bed or wheelchair to avoid shearing that can lead to development of pressure ulcers. Frequent repositioning and turning of a patient is also important to prevent pressure ulcers. Special pressure-releasing devices can also be used to reduce the risk of developing pressure ulcers. Physical therapy should be implemented to promote mobility of patients who are at high risk for developing pressure ulcers. Proper nutrition is also crucial to avoid pressure ulcers. As the nursing home industry continues to experience continued and growing demand for its services and the pool of qualified providers shrinks, residents are at higher risk for developing pressure ulcers.

Malnutrition and Dehydration

Thousands of patients in America's nursing homes are killed by malnutrition and dehydration every year, victims of a silent and largely preventable epidemic caused by a breakdown in basic care. Nearly 14,000 nursing home residents died of malnutrition and dehydration between 1999 and 2002 according to an investigation by Brad Heath of the *Detroit News* (2004), which was based on federal records. A study by the Commonwealth Fund (2000), a private foundation that supports research to promote improvements in health care, found that at least one-third of the nation's nursing home patients may suffer from malnutrition and dehydration. Many of them die because caregivers are too busy or inexperienced to give them the help they need. In addition, patients may find the food unappealing or be reluctant or unable to eat. Because of insufficient staffing at nursing homes, some residents who are unable to eat unassisted are not receiving proper nourishment. The limited staff is simply unable to assist every resident who needs assistance to eat. Improper nutrition or malnutrition can lead to infections, confusion, and muscle weakness, resulting in immobility and falls, pressure ulcers, pneumonia, and decreased immunity to bacteria and viruses. Malnutrition is costly, lowers the quality of nursing home residents' lives, and is often avoidable. The elderly are at an increased risk of dehydration and malnutrition since they often fail to monitor their own intake of food and water. Therefore, the facility must take steps, based on a nutritional assessment, to ensure that the residents receive proper nutrition and hydration to maintain their health.

Falls

Fall-related injuries are a major health threat for nursing home residents. Each year, a typical nursing home with 100 beds reports from 100 to 200 falls (Rubenstein, 1997). Many falls go unreported. Older people who live in nursing homes tend to fall more frequently than older adults who live within the community. As many as three out of four people in nursing homes fall each year, which is twice the rate of falls for older adults living in the community (Rubenstein, Josephson, & Robbins, 1994). Patients often fall more than once. The average is 2.6 falls per person per year (Rubenstein, Robbins, Josephson, Schulman, & Osterweil, 1990). About 35% of fall injuries occur among residents who cannot walk (Thapa, Brockman, Gideon, Fought, & Ray, 1996). Furthermore, about 5% of adults 65 and older live in nursing homes. But people in nursing homes account for about 20% of deaths from falls in this age group (Rubenstein, 1997). Falls in the elderly can be fatal. Approximately 50% of nursing home residents aged 65 and over fall each year, and nearly 1,800 die annually as a result of their falls. About 10%–20% suffer injuries, and 6% sustain fractures.

A majority of nursing home falls occur in the resident's room. Muscle weakness and gait problems are the most common causes of falls among nursing home residents. These problems account for about 24% of the falls in nursing homes (Rubenstein, Josephson, & Robbins, 1994). Hazards in the nursing home also cause 16%–27% of falls among residents. Such hazards include wet floors, poor lighting, incorrect bed height, and improperly fitted or maintained wheelchairs. Furthermore, medications can increase the risk of falls and fall-related injuries. Drugs that affect the central nervous system, such as sedatives and anti-anxiety drugs, are of particular concern. Other causes of falls include difficulty in moving from one place to another (e.g., from the bed to a chair), poor foot care, poorly fitting shoes, and improper or incorrect use of walking aids.

Elderly fall cases are hospitalized longer and experience more severe injuries than younger victims of falls (Nurmi & Luthje, 2002). In fact, older adults are five times more likely to be hospitalized for a fall-related injury than for any other cause (Rubenstein, Josephson, & Robbins, 1994). Severe injuries include fractures (75% of all major injuries), head trauma, soft tissue injuries, and dislocations (Fuller, 2000). These injuries occur in up to 15% of all falls each year. Four percent of all nursing home falls result in a fracture (Hoffman, Bankes, Javed, & Selhat, 2003). One of the most common injuries is hip fracture. Falls contribute to more than 90% of hip fractures, and such fractures occur in 1%–2% of all falls (Fuller, 2000).

It is the responsibility of a nursing home to assess whether a resident's condition places him at high risk for falls. Fall prevention takes a combination of medical treatment, rehabilitation, and environmental changes. Interventions to prevent falls include a thorough assessment of the patient after a fall to identify and address risk factors and to treat the underlying medical conditions (Rubenstein, Robbins, Josephson, Schulman, & Osterweil, 1990). Intervention to prevent falls also requires making changes in the nursing home environment, including but not limited to installing grab bars in the bathroom, adding raised toilet seats, lowering bed heights, and installing handrails in the hallways to make it easier for residents to move around safely. Furthermore, it is important to review prescribed medicines to assess their potential risks and benefits and to minimize use to reduce the risk of fall. The impact of injury from falls can be reduced by providing patients with hip pads that can effectively prevent most hip fractures if a fall occurs (Kannus et al., 1999) and by using devices such as alarms that go off when patients try to get out of bed or move without help (Rubenstein, Josephson, & Robbins, 1994). Exercise programs can improve balance, strength, walking ability, and physical functioning among nursing home residents (Vu, Weintraub, & Rubenstein, 2005).

William Haddon, Jr., developed his conceptual model, the Haddon matrix (Table 9.4), more than three decades ago. He applied basic principles of public health to the problem of traffic safety (1968). Since that time, the matrix has been used as a tool to assist in developing ideas for preventing injuries from falls in nursing homes. This matrix helps to evaluate the possible reasons for and the consequences and control of fall injuries and fatalities in nursing home on the basis of the timeline sequence. Furthermore, Haddon (1970) has also developed 10 basic strategies for injury prevention that apply to different phases and the different factors in the matrix (Table 9.5). These strategies can also be used to systematically fight fall-related injuries and fatalities in nursing homes.

Medication and Reporting Errors

According to a study published in 2005, each month nearly 1 out of every 10 nursing home residents suffers a medication-related injury. The study found that 73% of the most severe injuries—including internal bleeding and death—were preventable, along with many of the others (Gurwitz et al., 2005). These figures, still considered conservative, indicate that the problem of incorrect medication is five times more prevalent than previously believed. The most common problems were confusion, oversedation, hallucinations, or bleeding due to prescribing errors or failure to

Table 9.4

HADDON MATRIX TO PREVENT FALLS IN NURSING HOMES

PHASE	HUMAN FACTORS	AGENT FACTORS	PHYSICAL/SOCIOECONOMIC ENVIRONMENTAL FACTORS
Preinjury phase	1. Impaired visibility 2. Decrease muscle strength 3. Decreased proprioception 4. Stroke 5. Postural hypertension 6. Parkinson's syndrome 7. Heart attack 8. Medication/ drug usage 9. Impaired cerebral perfusion 10. Reduced cognition 11. Decline in neurological ability 12. Hearing problems	1. Body position— potential energy inherent in being in higher position 2. Hardness of the floor on which fall could occur 3. Poor bed design	1. Poor lighting 2. Slick or irregular surfaces 3. Unsafe stairways 4. Loose shoes 5. Trip hazards 6. Poor furniture arrangement
Injury phase	1. Response speed 2. Agility of the body 3. Susceptibility to the fall injury	1. Energy impact on the floor 2. Energy exchange between the human body and hit surface	1. Characteristics (e.g., hardness) of the contact surface
Post-injury	1. Recuperative ability 2. Susceptibility to other possible complications 3. Other conditions complicated by fall	Energy acting on the host	1. Availability of emergency service. 2. First aid ability 3. Medical and surgical care conditions
Total losses/costs	1. Individual morbidity 2. Impact on normal lives	N/A	1. Medical expenses 2. Environment reconstruction 3. Insurance cost 4. Impact on family members

Source: "Using the Haddon Matrix: Introducing the Third Dimension," by C. W. Runyan, 1988, *Injury Prevention,* 4, p. 304. Copyright © BMJ Publishing Group Ltd.

Table 9.5

HADDON'S 10 BASIC STRATEGIES FOR FALL INJURY PREVENTION

1. Prevent the creation of the hazards.	■ Arrange furniture to reduce the likelihood of tripping. ■ Use high-wattage light bulbs.
2. Reduce the number of hazards.	■ Review medications, especially if proprioception ability is affected by the prescribed medicine. ■ Encourage walking on flat ground and avoiding traveling on irregular surfaces as much as possible.
3. Prevent the release of hazards that already exists.	■ Apply soft material (e.g., carpet) to cover the floor. ■ Ensure that common pathways are free from obstacles, including cords, clutter, and family pets.
4. Modify the rate or spatial distribution of release of the hazard from its source.	■ Eliminate environmental hazards (e.g., nonslip strips or rubber bath mats on the bathroom floor; keep the night-light on; wear nonslip slippers, and so on).
5. Separate, in time or in space, the hazard and that which is to be protected.	■ Make sure that any wet spills are cleaned up as soon as possible.
6. Make modifications to be more resistant to damage from the hazard.	■ Wear hip protector.
7. Modify relevant basic qualities of the hazards.	■ Wear shoes with thin soles and high uppers, improving balance and mobility over other styles of footwear. ■ Installing sturdy grab bars on tubs and beds.
8. Improve resistance to damage from hazard.	■ Do strength and balance exercises regularly to keep muscles warm and to keep body mobile. ■ Increase calcium intake to reduce likelihood of a fracture.
9. Begin to counter damage already done by the environmental hazard.	■ Develop fall injuries/fatalities emergency response plan and train nursing home staff.
10. Stabilize, repair, and rehabilitate the object of the damage.	■ Offer movement rehabilitation through physical activity to get the individual walking or using the injury body part again.

Adapted from "The Basic Strategies for Reducing Damage From Hazards of All Kinds," by W. Haddon, 1980, Hazard Prevention, 16.

carefully monitor patients for side effects. The researchers found that psychoactive drugs and anticoagulants caused the most problems.

A nursing home should ensure that its residents are free of significant medication errors. In the event of a medication error, the charting should be reviewed to uncover the cause of the medication error and to help determine if it was a mistake or a manifestation of a chronic problem within the facility. Nurses are legally responsible for applying the five rights of medication administration as a standard of care:

Right Drug. Administration of the wrong drug is the most common error that occurs. Factors that contribute to wrong-drug error include similar labeling and packaging of products, medications with very similar names, and storage of these similar products together. In addition, poor communication is a common cause of administering the wrong drug. When transcribing verbal orders or verifying transcription of orders, a few simple precautions can help avoid errors—always repeat verbal orders, avoid using dosage and product abbreviations, never assume route of administration, never use trailing zeros (write 25, not 25.0), never try to decipher illegible orders, always check the drug label and dose against the doctor's order three times prior to administration, and do not administer any drug if you are unsure of its intended use for your patient.

Right Dose. If dosage must be calculated, always recheck the math and have someone else verify the final dosage. It is important to consider the patient's age, size, and vital signs when deciding if a dose is appropriate. Elderly patients, like pediatrics, are particularly susceptible to slight changes in medication dose.

Right Time. In general, medications must be given one-half hour before or after the actual time specified in the orders. When scheduling administration times, it is important to consider drug-drug and drug-food interactions. Many drugs interfere with absorption of other drugs when given simultaneously. Appropriate spacing of doses also needs to be considered. Bioavailability, the need for consistent dosing around the clock, should also be considered to ensure efficacy of the medication.

Right Route. Many medications can be administered by a variety of routes, such as oral, rectal, intravenous, subcutaneous, intramuscular, or sublingual. The route selected by the prescriber depends on the patient's condition and the speed with which the therapeutic effect will need to occur. The prescribed dosage is based on the route by which the drug is given. In general, oral dosages are greater than injected dosages for the same drug. Errors can occur when a dose intended for oral administration is given by injection. Special caution must be taken with medication given by the intravenous route. Many drugs will cause severe soft tissue injury if the IV becomes infiltrated. It is important to check for blood return prior to administration of any intravenous medication given by direct IV injection or intermittent or continuous infusion. Medications given intravenously have a rapid onset of action. It is necessary to stay with the patient during the first few minutes of any intravenous infusion to assess for signs and symptoms of adverse reaction.

Right Patient. In today's hectic health care environment, it is especially important to confirm a patient's identity prior to conducting any procedure. Many nurses float between units or work part-time. These situations increase the probability of giving medication to the wrong patient. It is imperative to check every patient's ID bracelet prior to giving a medication. Always confirm the patient's name, age, and allergies, and ask the patient to state his name, if appropriate.

Exercises and Activities

Alzheimer's disease results in a progressive deterioration in the ability to perform activities of daily living (ADLs). During the past decade, considerable effort has been applied to develop therapeutic agents to slow the gradual impairment in cognitive function that comes with AD. Slowing the loss of ability to perform ADLs has received less attention. The loss of ADLs is a key determinant of a patient's quality of life, institutionalization, risk of death, and burden for the caregiver and the community. Interventions such as exercise programs have been shown to improve function even in frail nursing home residents (Lazowski et al., 1999) and may yield an important and potent protective factor against ADL decline. Moreover, an exercise program may yield benefits in the management of falls (Buchner & Larson, 1987), malnutrition (White, Pieper, Schmader, & Fillenbaum, 1997), behavioral disturbances, and depression (Taylor et al., 2004)—key problems for people with AD. Exercise programs may be all the more relevant for people with AD living in nursing homes, because they spend a protracted period in the nursing home, with a high rate of functional decline; they are frequently physically inactive (Ballard et al., 2001), and long-term exercise programs are easier to organize in institutions than in the community. Rolland and associates (2007) in their recent study reported that a simple exercise program, 1 hour twice a week, led to significantly slower decline in ADL score in patients with AD living in a nursing home than routine medical care.

Music therapy for people with AD has been also been widely used in long-term-care facilities. It has been proposed that even in advanced stages of dementia, certain levels of musical perception may still be retained in the absence of hearing impairment (Swartz, Hantz, Crummer, Walton, & Frisina, 1989). There is anecdotal evidence that music cognitive ability may be preserved in at least a subset of individuals with dementia, despite deficits in simpler cognitive tasks. Beatty et al. (1997) described preserved musical ability in individuals with dementia who had cognitive deficits, such as loss of language function and inability to dress. In stroke patients, it has been observed that the areas of the brain involved in verbal memory are different from the areas involved in musical memory (Hachinski, 1989). This suggests that patients with a loss of language function secondary to Alzheimer's disease may have preserved musical abilities (Madan, 2005). There are several mechanisms by which music intervention may affect individuals with dementia. For example, music may evoke pleasant memories (Gerdner & Swanson, 2001) or induce relaxation (Alexander, 2001). Several studies have demonstrated that music intervention in elderly persons with dementia improves social behaviors (Koger, Chapin, & Brotons, 1999), enhances language function (Brotons & Koger, 2000), and increases spatial-temporal reasoning (Johnson, Cotman, Tasaki, & Shaw, 1998). There are also several studies showing that music intervention may reduce agitation and aggression among long-term-care residents with dementia (Madan, 2005).

Nursing Home Reform Act

In a 1986 study, conducted at the request of Congress, the Institute of Medicine found that residents of nursing homes were being abused, neglected, and given inadequate care. The Institute of Medicine proposed sweeping reforms, most of which became law in 1987 with the passage of the Nursing Home Reform Act, part of the Omnibus Budget Reconciliation Act (OBRA) of 1987. The basic objective of the Nursing Home Reform Act is to establish quality standards for nursing homes nationwide. It established resident rights and defined the state survey and certification process to enforce the standards. The changes OBRA brought to nursing home care are enormous. Some of the most important resident provisions include:

- Emphasis on a resident's quality of life as well as the quality of care
- New expectations that each resident's ability to walk, bathe, and perform other activities of daily living will be maintained or improved absent medical reasons
- A resident-assessment process leading to development of an individualized care plan; 75 hours of training and testing of paraprofessional staff
- Rights to remain in the nursing home absent nonpayment, dangerous resident behaviors, or significant changes in a resident's medical condition
- New opportunities for potential and current residents with mental retardation or mental illnesses for services inside and outside a nursing home
- The right to safely maintain or bank personal funds with the nursing home; the right to return to the nursing home after a hospital stay or an overnight visit with family and friends; the right to choose a personal physician and to access medical records
- The right to organize and participate in a resident or family council
- The right to be free of unnecessary and inappropriate physical and chemical restraints
- The imposition of uniform certification standards for Medicare and Medicaid homes
- The imposition of prohibitions on turning to family members to pay for Medicare and Medicaid services
- The application of new remedies to be applied to certified nursing homes that fail to meet minimum federal standards

The Omnibus Budget Reconciliation Act set in motion forces that changed the way state inspectors approached all their visits to nursing homes. Inspectors no longer spend their time exclusively with staff or with facility records. Conversations with residents and families are a prime-time survey event. Observing dining and medications administration are a focal point of every annual inspection. Under OBRA, Long-Term-Care Ombudsman Programs have defined roles to fulfill and tools to use in the annual inspection process to nurture the conversations between residents/families and inspectors and life in the nursing home.

Long-Term-Care Ombudsman

Under the Older Americans Act, every state is required to have a Long-Term-Care Ombudsman Program. This program was established in 1975. Funded under the Older Americans Act and in some cases by state funds, the program serves nearly 2.8 million residents in more than 60,000 facilities. In addition to the 53 state ombudsmen, there are nearly 600 local programs with more than 970 paid staff members and 14,000 volunteers. An LTC Ombudsman is an advocate for residents' rights and quality care in nursing homes as well as board and care homes, including assisted-living facilities. The mission of the LTC Ombudsman Program is to advocate for the dignity, quality of life, and quality of care for all residents in LTC facilities. According to California Long-Term-Care Ombudsman (2007), this mission is carried out through six core functions of Ombudsman programs: (1) to receive, investigate, and resolve complaints; (2) to ensure a regular presence at long-term facilities; (3) to address patterns of poor practice; (4) to maximize community awareness and involvement; (5) to influence public policy; and (6) to ensure effective program administration. According to the National Long-Term-Care Ombudsman Resource Center, the mission of the programs is accomplished through the following: resolution of complaints made by or for residents of long-term-care facilities; education of consumers and long-term-care providers about residents' rights and good care practices; promotion of community involvement through volunteer opportunities; provision of information to the public on nursing homes and other long-term-care facilities and services, residents' rights, and legislative and policy issues; advocacy for residents' rights and quality care in nursing homes, personal care, residential care, and other long-term-care facilities; and promotion of the development of citizen organizations, family councils, and resident councils.

Long-Term-Care Community Coalition (LTCCC)

Despite strong legal requirements that nursing homes provide good care and dignified conditions for residents, the nursing home crisis continues. As a result, too many of the most vulnerable citizens suffer needlessly every day because nursing homes fail to provide good care and the government fails to hold them accountable. The LTCCC was created to improve care for the elderly and disabled. Their goal is to ensure that long-term-care consumers are cared for safely and treated with dignity. To accomplish these goals, LTCCC:

- Researches policies, laws, and regulations affecting care for the elderly and disabled
- Advocates for state and national policies to improve care
- Addresses systemic problems in the delivery of long-term care
- Identifies good practices and develops recommendations to improve care and dignity of the elderly and disabled and to offer better conditions to professional caregivers
- Educates and empowers the elderly and disabled to advocate for themselves
- Actively engages government agencies and elected officials in discussion and action on the needed changes

Cost of Long-Term-Care Facilities

It is important to talk about finances before the need for LTC arises. A study estimated that the annual cost of caring for one person with AD in 1998 was $18,408 for mild disease, $30,096 for moderate disease, and $36,132 for severe disease (Leon, Cheng, & Neumann, 1998). However, presently, LTC facilities for Alzheimer's individuals can cost $4,000–$6,000 a month (New York City Department for the Aging, 2007). Since the cost estimates of LTC facilities are significant, delaying long-term-care placement benefits Alzheimer's individuals, their families, and payers. Mittleman and colleagues (2006) reported that the caregiver counseling can help keep AD persons at home for a longer period of time and can delay the need for nursing home placement. They randomized 406 spouse caregivers of community-dwelling persons with AD to either individual counseling with continuous support or usual care. The effect of counseling sessions on delaying time to nursing home placement was measured over a 9.5-year period. Caregiver counseling reduced the number of nursing home placements by 28.3% and delayed overall time to placement by a median of 557 days. The study concluded that the delay was most likely due to beneficial effects on social support, response to patient behavior, and depressive symptoms in the caregiver.

The American Community Survey Report (U.S. Census Bureau, 2006) reveals that the average national cost of care in nursing homes, assisted-living facilities, and the home has steadily increased and has reached new highs that exceed most household incomes in the United States. The rising costs of LTC may, therefore, present difficulties for many Americans should they need to pay for LTC out of their own pockets. A separate national poll conducted by Public Opinion Strategies with input from the Alzheimer's Association found that 75% of Americans have made no LTC plans, and 59% expressed concern about being able to pay for LTC. Almost half of the respondents (44%) incorrectly believe that Medicare or their private health insurance will pay for their long-term-care needs. In actuality, health insurance and the federal Medicare program do not generally cover long-term care.

Following are key findings from the 2007 Cost of Care Survey, broken out by major category.

- Nursing Homes: The average annual national cost of a private room in a nursing home in 2007 was $74,806, or $204 per day, reflecting a 14.8% increase over 2004 rates. This remains the most costly care option. The most expensive per day room rate was found in Alaska ($539), and the least expensive was found in Louisiana ($119).
- Assisted Living: A private one-bedroom unit in an assisted-living facility had an average annual cost of $32,573, a 13% increase since 2004. The most expensive one-bedroom unit was found in Massachusetts ($4,753 per month), and the least expensive was found in North Dakota ($1,609 per month).
- Home Care: The average hourly rate for Medicare/Medicaid-certified and state-licensed home health aides was $25.47 an hour, a cost that translates to $52,977 per year for 40 hours per week.

Financial Burden of Long-Term Care

Long-term care includes a broad range of health and support services that people need as they age or if they are disabled. The majority of these services are personal care, or assistance with activities of daily living. A person with sufficient income and assets is likely to self-pay for the LTC needs. If a person meets functional eligibility criteria and has limited financial resources, or would deplete them paying for care,

Table 9.6

PAYMENT SYSTEM FOR MOST COMMON LONG-TERM CARE

LONG-TERM-CARE SERVICE	MEDICARE	MEDICAID	SELF-PAYMENT
Nursing home care	Pays in full for days 0–20 if you are in a Skilled Nursing Facility following a recent hospital stay. If your need for skilled care continues, may pay for days 21 through 100 after you pay a $128/day copayment.	May pay for care in a Medicaid-certified nursing home if you meet functional and financial eligibility criteria.	Applies if you need only personal or supervisory care in a nursing home and/or have not had a prior hospital stay, or if you choose a nursing home that does not participate in Medicaid or is not Medicare-certified.
Assisted-living facility (and similar facility options)	Does not pay.	In some states, may pay care-related costs but not room and board.	You pay on your own except as noted under Medicaid if eligible.
Continuing-care retirement community	Does not pay.	Does not pay.	You pay on your own.
Adult day services	Not covered.	Varies by state, financial, and functional eligibility required.	You pay on your own except as noted under Medicaid if eligible.
Home health care	Limited to reasonable, necessary part-time or intermittent skilled nursing care and home health aide services, and some therapies that are ordered by your doctor and provided by Medicare-certified home health agency. Does not pay for ongoing personal care or custodial care needs only (help with activities of daily living).	Pay for, but states have option to limit some services, such as therapy.	You pay on your own for personal or custodial care, except as noted under Medicaid, if you are eligible.

Source: "National Clearinghouse for Long-Term Care Information," by U.S. Department of Health and Human Services, 2008. Retrieved February 2008, from http://www.longtermcare.gov/LTC/Main_Site/Paying_LTC/Costs_Of_Care/Costs_Of_Care.aspx.

Medicaid may pay for the care. If a person requires primarily skilled or recuperative care for a short time, Medicare may pay. The Older Americans Act is another federal program that helps pay for LTC services. Some people use a variety of payment sources as their care needs and financial circumstances change. Table 9.6 presents a payment system for most common LTC.

There are variations in costs according to the type and amount of care individuals need, the provider they use, and where they live. The U.S. Department of Health and Human Services (2008) presents the average 2007 costs in the United States as follows:

- $181 per day for a semiprivate room in a nursing home
- $205 per day for a private room in a nursing home

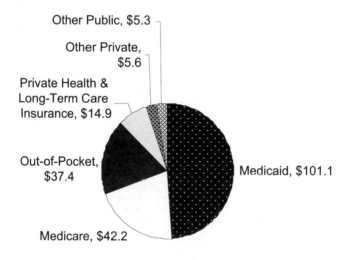

$ in billions
Total= $206.6 billion

Figure 9.4 National spending for long-term care by payer (2005).
Source: Health Policy Institute, Georgetown University, based on the sum of (1) expenditures for nursing home and home health care provided by free-standing facilities, from Centers for Medicare and Medicaid Services (CMS), National Health Expenditures by type of service and source of funds, calendar years 2005–1960, http://cms.hhs.gov/NationalHealthExpendData/02_NationalHealth AccountsHistorical.asp; (2) Medicare and Medicaid expenditures for nursing home and home health care provided by hospital-based facilities, from CMS, Office of the Actuary, National Health Statistics Group (unpublished, 2007); and (3) Medicaid expenditures for home and community-based waiver services, from B. Burwell, K. Sredl, and S. Eiken, Medicaid Long-Term Care Expenditures in FY2005 (Cambridge, MA: Medstat, July 5, 2006, memorandum). Reprinted with permission from Dr. Robert Friedland, Georgetown University.

- $2,714 per month for care in an assisted-living facility (for a one-bedroom unit)
- $25 per hour for a home health aide
- $17 per hour for homemaker services
- $61 per day for care in an adult, day, health care center

About 10 million Americans need LTC—the assistance and services provided to people who, because of chronic illness or disabling conditions, are limited in their ability to perform basic activities (Rogers & Komisar, 2003). Spending for professional LTC services—such as nursing home, home care, and assisted-living services—is substantial. According to the Georgetown University–LTC Financing Project, in 2005 national spending on LTC totaled $207 billion (Figure 9.4). Medicaid is the largest spender for LTC (48.8%) followed by Medicare (20.4%) and private pay (18.1%), which together account for 87.4% of such spending. Most LTC spending is for nursing home care (Figure 9.5).

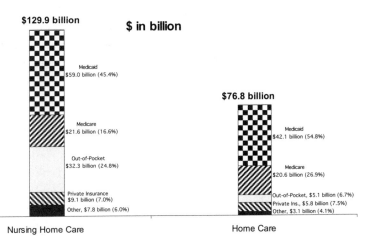

Figure 9.5 National spending for nursing home and home care by payer (2005).
Source: Health Policy Institute, Georgetown University, based on the sum of (1) expenditures for nursing home and home health care provided by free-standing facilities, from Centers for Medicare and Medicaid Services (CMS), National Health Expenditures by type of service and source of funds, calendar years 2005–1960, http://cms.hhs.gov/NationalHealthExpendData/02_NationalHealth AccountsHistorical.asp; (2) Medicare and Medicaid expenditures for nursing home and home health care provided by hospital based facilities, from CMS, Office of the Actuary, National Health Statistics Group (unpublished, 2007); and (3) Medicaid expenditures for home and community-based waiver services, from B. Burwell, K. Sredl, and S). Eiken, Medicaid Long-Term Care Expenditures in FY2005 (Cambridge, MA: Medstat, July 5, 2006, memorandum). Reprinted with permission from Dr. Robert Friedland, Georgetown University.
Note: Private insurance consists of health and long-term-care insurance. Components may not sum to totals because of rounding.

Long-Term-Care Reform

According to a report published by the U.S. Administration on Aging of the U.S. Department of Health and Human Services (2005), LTC reform is happening across the nation, and some states are using systems change as an opportunity to better coordinate across aging and disability networks: The overarching goal of these efforts is to increase access to home and community-based services for people with disabilities of all ages. While the needs of older adults and people with disabilities are distinct, they rely on many of the same long-term support services. The U.S. Department of Health and Human Services (HHS) has adopted an LTC Systems Change Framework that identifies four areas of reform: access, services, financing, and quality. The major trend in states that are restructuring their LTC services is to emphasize in-home and commu-nity-based care rather than institutionalization. This is the result of two pressures: consumer preference and cost containment. Repeated stud-ies have shown that people who need assistance would rather receive it in familiar settings than move to nursing homes. And nursing homes, which take the lion's share of public funds expended on long-term care, are an expensive way to deliver care unless a person actually needs round-the-clock nursing attention. Experts believe that many existing residents of nursing homes, who receive 24-hour-a-day care, could be served in home or community settings if adequate but limited assistance was available (p. 3).

10

Rehabilitation Challenges of People With Alzheimer's Disease

Alzheimer's patients like former President Ronald Reagan, their families and their medical teams, the combination of dementia, the healing of broken bones and the rehabilitation process can present an extraordinary challenge.

New York Times

Alzheimer's disease (AD) generally develops slowly and adversely affects cognitive, emotional, and behavioral function, ultimately leading to physical deterioration and functional dependency. Persons with AD experience difficulties storing new information, and, as a result, they may not benefit from receiving reminders from others or from using notes to aid their recall. Health care professionals have tended to overlook the needs and requirements of Alzheimer's individuals for physical exercises and activity programs. Because of the memory retention problems, many health care professionals feel that majority of the persons with AD have little, if any, rehabilitation potential. Furthermore, besides retention problems, many clinicians also take the "They're just going to get worse anyway" approach in their clinical decision making. Perhaps this is not true that people with AD will not benefit from physical exercises and rehabilitation process. What about the value of making each day a little less foggy, less frustrating, less isolated, less stressful for as long as possible? What about living as fully as possible with whatever time an individual with Alzheimer's has? What about the quality of life? These are some of the ethical issues that can be addresses through a well-designed rehabilitation program.

REHABILITATION

Rehabilitation plays a vital role in the management of this challenging neurodegenerative disease. Rehabilitation gives special consideration to a person's quality of life. People with AD have many of the same health problems and emotional needs as everybody else, and regular balanced exercise programs and physical activities have the same effect on persons suffering from AD as for any population without AD (Arkin, 2006). The benefits of physical exercise for older adults are well documented. However, few studies have been conducted to ascertain the needs and to assess the limitations of people with AD. Studies have shown that exercise is beneficial for people with AD. Along with cardiovascular fitness, increased endurance, and strength, people with AD get added benefits from exercising. Flexibility, balance, and strength exercises have been studied in persons with AD and compared to the effect of medical management alone (Inverarity, 2007). Persons with AD who were treated with both exercise and medical management were less depressed than those who were treated with medical management alone and showed marked improvement in their physical functioning. Physical therapy plays an important role in exercises for persons with AD by tailoring routines to meet the individual needs of each person. According to the National Center on Physical Activity and Disability (NCPAD [Arkin, 2006]), persons with AD derive benefits from exercise programs that are unique to their situation, that is, the ability to gain skill and show regular improvement in physical fitness at a time when they are losing skills in every other arena of life. Such a tangible gain can be a tremendous source of pride, both for the persons with AD and for the caregivers. Regular exercise programs also improve behavioral and psychological symptoms in persons with AD.

Neuromuscular weakness is a prominent symptom among people with AD and typically leads to disability in activities of daily life. Thomas and Hageman (2003), in their study of people with dementia, used moderate-intensity progressive resistance training of the hip extensors, abductors, knee extensors and flexors, and dorsiflexors for up to three days a week over a six-week period. They reported improvement in some areas of muscular capacity (quadriceps and handgrips) along with improvement on most tests of lower-extremity function, such as sit-to-stand, gait, and timed-up-and-go, whereas there were declines in other areas (dorsiflexion and iliopsoas strength). According to the researchers, although strength or functional deficits in all domains were not remediable, the results suggest the potential benefit of a resistance-exercise intervention of longer duration and/or greater intensity on the neuromuscular functioning of people with dementia.

A regular exercise program is recommended for people with AD not only to support physical health but also to improve quality of life and behavioral and psychological symptoms. Recent research findings in this area clearly demonstrate that a major aim of exercise programming is not just to decrease mortality but also to decrease morbidity, that is, to "add life to years" and not just "years to life." A study published by Teri and associates (2003), a recipient of the Alzheimer's Association's Pioneer Award, demonstrated that a regular exercise program combined with caregiver education and training on supervising exercise improved the physical and emotional health of individuals with moderate to severe AD. "Through programs of exercise and caregiver training, such as the one demonstrated in this study, people with Alzheimer's may be able to maintain their physical health and share more positive interactions with their caregivers. That is potentially a big quality of life improvement for patients, caregivers, and family members—in fact, everyone touched by this devastating disease," said Cornelia Beck of the Alzheimer's Association Medical & Scientific Advisory Council (Neurologyreviews.com, 2003).

Bach and associates (1995) carried out a landmark study on the effects of two different therapy strategies on two samples of 22 long-term patients with mild to moderate dementia. The control group received a 24-week functional rehabilitation (FR) program of occupational therapy, physical therapy, and speech therapy. The study group received this program and an additional occupational therapy activity program for 24 weeks. A variety of psychometric tests were carried out at baseline, after 12 weeks, and after 24 weeks by a psychologist who was blind to the group distributions. Both groups showed a significant improvement in cognitive performance, psychosocial functioning, and well-being, with the study group showing significantly higher scores than the control group. The authors conclude that the application of an occupational therapy activity program in addition to FR is significantly more effective than FR alone.

According to the NCPAD (Arkin, 2006), there are a number of challenges to engaging people with Alzheimer's in physical activity programs, including but not limited to these points:

- Even during the very early stage of AD, people with AD have difficulty initiating and maintaining a new behavior or routine on their own.
- Most of them no longer drive independently, making it difficult to get to a gym or health club.
- Caregivers are also often in poor health and are not able to motivate and help a person with AD maintain a physical activity program.
- It's difficult for most early-stage people with AD to keep track of dates and appointments.
- Many persons with AD get lost or disoriented when away from home.
- The ability to read is preserved, but the rapid forgetting that occurs makes the activity generally unsatisfying.
- Most persons with early-stage AD can carry on a coherent one-to-one conversation but will get lost in a complex discussion, particularly if several people are involved.
- The net result of this constellation of symptoms is a loss of confidence and a withdrawal from former activities and relationships. Persons at this early stage will most certainly benefit from an exercise program from the standpoint of enhancing social stimulation, particularly if it is provided one-on-one or in a small, supportive group setting.

According to many health care institutions, it is important to remember that with Alzheimer's rehabilitation, although any skills lost will not be regained, the caregiver team must keep in mind the following considerations:

- In managing the disease, physical exercise and social activity are important, as are proper nutrition and health maintenance.
- The team should plan daily activities that help to provide structure, meaning, and accomplishment for the individual.
- As functions are lost, the team should adapt activities and routines to allow the individual to participate as much as possible.
- It's important to keep activities familiar and satisfying.

■ The team should allow the individual to complete as many things by himself or herself as possible. The caregiver may need to initiate an activity but should allow the individual to complete it as much as he or she can.

■ The team should provide cues for desired behavior (i.e., label drawers/cabinets/closets according to their contents).

■ It's important to keep the individual out of harm's way by removing all safety risks (i.e., car keys, matches).

■ It is important that the caregiver (full-time or part-time) understand and act accordingly to her own physical and emotional limitations.

Functional impairment is a core symptom of AD. As the disease progresses, persons with AD require increasingly more assistance with activities of daily living (ADLs) such as eating, bathing, toileting, and functional mobility, as well as in instrumental activities of daily living (IADLs) such as meal preparation, shopping, and managing one's finances. The most accurate indicator of functional impairment is the decline in performance of ADLs and IADLs. It is critical that assessments of ADLs and IADLs be evaluated in order to ensure that one can make valid judgments based on the results of the assessment. Exercise has been shown to improve function even in frail nursing home residents and may yield an important and potent protective factor against ADL decline (Lazowski, et al., 1999). In a study, 134 persons living in nursing homes with mild to severe AD exercised 1 hour twice weekly, whereas a control group received routine medical care for 12 months. The investigators reported that exercise program significantly slowed, by approximately one-third, the progressive deterioration in the participants' ability to perform ADLs (Rolland et al., 2007).

Differing from physical therapy, occupational therapy primarily focuses upon ADLs and IADLs. Occupational therapy interventions are skilled rehabilitative treatments that help persons with AD achieve independence in all facets of their lives. As AD progresses, persons with AD are expected to have declines in logical thinking, judgment, and problem-solving ability. The confusion and disorientation of mid-stage Alzheimer's bring increasing difficulty with maintaining normal behaviors. Most behavior problems will require the caregiver to modify the home environment and change communication styles, as discussed in chapter 8. Occupational therapy has achieved proven results in addressing many of the behavioral problems associated with AD and dementia and in assisting caregivers with these issues.

In persons with AD, there is slow deterioration of speech and language. During the early stages of AD, an understanding of simple speech often remains intact; however, difficulties in locating and expressing correct word usage can begin very early in the course of the disease. People with AD may experience difficulty in interpreting complex conversations, proverbs, and metaphors. Because of this, it may become very difficult to construct a complex sentence. Language problems may depend on the person's level of fatigue and mood, the time of day, and the emotion behind what she is trying to communicate. As AD progresses, it becomes difficult for persons to complete sentences. Further, persons with AD often move from one subject to another and frequently repeat the same words again and again. Writing and reading can be affected in the early stages of the disease, often as a result of spelling difficulties. There is also an associated lack of interest in the tasks involved; therefore, tasks are very often left uncompleted. The typical AD person has difficulty following a conversation. The realization that they are having such difficulties causes them to become more confused and frightened, thereby worsening the problem. With the progression of the disease, communication problems increase. With the decrease in the ability to locate appropriate words to complete a sentence or to become involved in a conversation, persons with AD may add other words as fillers to the remaining gaps. This usually results in the loss of a conversation's true meaning. Comprehension skills also decrease with the progression of the disease. Eventually, when speech mainly consists of babbling gibberish, people with AD gradually withdraw from talking altogether. In advanced stages of the disease, AD persons are unable to communicate to others even their basic needs.

Writing disorders are an early manifestation of AD, often more severe than difficulties with spoken language. Recent studies suggest that writing may be an aspect of cognition through which we can identify impairments specific to persons with AD (Forbes, Shanks, & Venneri, 2004). They produce shorter and less informative written descriptions of a complex picture. The precise nature and progression of the writing disorder, however, remains unclear. Forbes and associates (2004) assessed the central and peripheral aspects of writing in a sample of minimal, mild, and moderate AD persons and a group of healthy elderly controls on a narrative description task. Comparisons of the two groups indicated that persons with AD suffer from a primary impairment at the semantic level. Even those in the minimal stages of the disease could be differentiated from controls on measures of word finding and information conveyed.

This semantic impairment was coupled with a secondary milder impairment in phonological processing. The prevalence of phonological errors increased, but no shift in error type (plausible/implausible) was identified as the disease progressed. In addition to the central impairments, AD persons evinced damage at the peripheral level. In the more severe stages, they experienced more problems with letter formation and stroke placement and tended to rely upon the more simplistic writing form of print. The researchers concluded that the writing impairments in AD have multiple components and follow the pattern of cortical deterioration reported in the brains of AD persons.

Dysphagia is a common problem in persons with AD. As the disease progresses, persons with AD usually develop serious difficulties in swallowing, resulting in weight loss and aspiration pneumonia. They may resist having food placed in the mouth, fail to manage the food bolus once it is in their mouth, or aspirate when swallowing. Coughing and choking during eating are common signs of aspiration. Early screening and intervention is critical. Evaluation by a speech-language pathologist can be helpful in determining the presence and severity of swallowing dysfunction. Speech-language pathologists can also help in selecting the most appropriate therapeutic modalities to prevent dysphagia complications in persons with AD.

Rehabilitation Goals

Rehabilitation plays a vital role in the nonpharmacologic management of this neurodegenerative disease. There is growing evidence that an early diagnosis and targeted management can preserve function and independence in AD persons. It is designed to restore basic abilities such as dressing and eating and may help to enhance people's ability to take part in meaningful activities within their environment and enjoy family events. Rehabilitation focuses on people's abilities, rather than their disabilities. The foremost goal of the care provided must be to maintain as high a quality of life as possible for as long as possible. People are assessed and treated by an interprofessional team made up of physical therapists, psychiatrists, family physicians, social workers, nurses, occupational therapists, pharmacists, dieticians, and speech-language pathologists. It is this interdisciplinary approach that makes rehabilitation so effective. For this chapter, we will focus on physical therapy, occupational therapy, and speech-language remediation. Depending on specific needs of people with AD, rehabilitation services may include physical therapy, occupational therapy, and/or speech language remediation. The skills of the physical therapist (PT), the occupational therapist (OT), and the speech-language pathologist (SLP) can be used to assess cognition and function and to implement programs that allow people with cognitive impairment to maximize their remaining capabilities and avoid excess disability, improving their quality of life. The goals of physical therapy in people with AD are to rebuild and maintain motor skills and flexibility, decrease falls, and reduce the rate of disease-associated mental decline. The primary focus of occupational therapy is to improve people's abilities to perform activities of daily living and hence to promote independence and participation in social activities. OT can also reduce the burden on caregiver by increasing the person with AD's sense of competence and ability to handle the behavioral problems she encounters. The primary role of treatment by a speech-language pathologist for people with AD is to prolong communication for as long as possible, and at as high a level as possible. The goals of speech-language pathologists are also to assess deficits in swallowing in persons with AD, recommend appropriate consistency of food, and educate caregivers to maintain adequate nutrition and hydration.

PHYSICAL THERAPY

A supervised exercise program is very important for management of AD. It is suggested that a regular exercise program may protect specifically against Alzheimer's as well other forms of mental deterioration and dementia and may produce desirable outcomes to alleviate or slow the process of AD. Maintaining a reasonable level of exercise is important for many reasons, both for overall health and to address issues specific to AD. Exercise can improve mobility and help one maintain independence. In people without AD, moderately strenuous exercise has been shown to improve cognitive functioning, and this could be applicable to persons with AD. It is recommended that for people with AD, exercise be continued for as long as possible. This will help prevent muscle weakness and health complications associated with inactivity. Exercise also promotes a normal day-and-night routine and may help to improve mood and sleep patterns. Although exercise does not stop AD from progressing, persons with AD do receive the emotional satisfaction of feeling they have accomplished something. Regular exercise has psychological benefits such as decreased depression and confusion, as well as an improved capacity for self-esteem and a sense of personal worth. There have been a number of studies in the past suggesting that the supervised exercise program may be as important as mental activity. Arkin (2001) reported in her study of AD that a supervised exercise program can maintain or improve cognitive, language, social, and physical functioning in Alzheimer's patients.

There is enough evidence to confirm that regular and moderate exercise is a potent disease prevention and health promotion resource for the elderly. Data are sparse, but accumulating, that exercise may even have an important role in moderating dementias such as AD. Preliminary evidence supports that exercise may alleviate some of the negative characteristics associated with AD. While the explanations for these early findings are lacking, several promising hypotheses are that exercise (1) stimulates the cortex of the brain; (2) promotes the immune system; and (3) may moderate the arteriosclerotic disease process of the brain (Bonner & Cousins, 1996). If exercise proves to be a positive influence with dementia, the social challenge will be to mobilize cognitively afflicted individuals with practical and humane strategies. Studies suggest that exercise also reduces the risk of developing dementia. Larson and associates (2006) showed that those who exercised more reduced their rate of dementia 38% over those who exercised less. Interestingly, those who started with the lowest exercise levels at baseline had the greatest risk reduction with increased exercise.

The National Center on Physical Activity and Disability states that the physical and mental benefits of exercise are universally recognized but seldom available to persons with early to moderate stage dementia. Difficulty in initiating and maintaining purposeful behavior, coupled with the inability to travel independently, keep most community-dwelling dementia sufferers from accessing organized fitness programs. Overburdened caregivers typically lack the inclination and know-how to structure and supervise systematic exercise sessions.

A balanced exercise program for persons with AD should include activities that improve flexibility, cardiovascular endurance, and strength. It is recommended that for persons with AD who are otherwise in good health, a session might start with a 5-minute walk or a series of stretches, followed by 20 minutes of an aerobic activity, 20–30 minutes of weight training, and from 5 to 10 minutes of stretching. Balance exercises and activities are equally important and should be performed on a regular basis. It is recommended that the program start with simple balance exercises and modified as skill level and balance improves.

The Role of the Physical Therapist

The role of the PT in care for the individual with AD is threefold. First, the PT needs to assist the individual with AD, family, and caregivers with activities that are functional in order to maintain and slow physical decline. Second, the PT needs to assist in changing and enhancing the environmental and physical spaces of care to maintain function. The person with dementia, in order to be most fully functioning, needs a simple, safe environment that enhances mobility and ADLs. Finally, the PT should also assist the caregiver in providing functional, meaningful, pleasant, and safe activities.

The key to managing behavioral problems is accurate assessment and ruling out alternative diagnoses. Common problems that are confused with dementia include delirium and depression. Dementia is defined by a chronic loss of intellectual or cognitive function of sufficient severity to interfere with social or occupational function. Delirium is an acute disturbance of consciousness marked by an attention deficit and a change in cognitive function. Depression is an affective disorder evidenced by a dysphoric mood, but the most pervasive symptom is a loss of ability to enjoy usual activities. Be certain that dementia has been diagnosed. A quick screening that can be used to determine if a person needs further testing for dementia is the Mini-Mental State Exam, described in chapter 5. Also use a functional assessment such as the Barthel ADL Index (Figure 10.1), the Blessed Dementia Scale (Table 10.1), or the Functional Activities Questionnaire (Table 10.2). Scales should assess complex social functions as well as basic ADLs. The PT should directly observe what is being measured in order to be as accurate as possible and to avoid overdependence on reports of caregivers. Caregivers should be questioned about multiple domains of the person's life. The PT assessment should assess the environment for both safety and fall hazards. There are multiple instruments to choose from. Once problematic behaviors are better understood, practical suggestions such as removing objects that may be related to agitation or aggression can be recommended. For example, mirrors should be removed if persons no longer recognize themselves and think strangers are present. Televisions should be removed if persons with AD are confused, thinking the actors or action is authentic. Families should be assisted with designing a predictable environment that is familiar and comfortable. Routines are important behavior stabilizers for persons with dementia. The physical therapist should try to link episodes of agitation or aggression with triggers for these behaviors, whether related

Activity	Scores
FEEDING	
0 = unable	
5 = needs help cutting, spreading butter, etc., or requires modified diet	
10 = independent	———
BATHING	
0 = dependent	
5 = independent (or in shower)	———
GROOMING	
0 = needs to help with personal care	
5 = independent face/hair/teeth/shaving (implements provided)	———
DRESSING	
0 = dependent	
5 = needs help but can do about half unaided	
10 = independent (including buttons, zips, laces, etc.)	———
BOWELS	
0 = incontinent (or needs to be given enemas)	
5 = occasional accident	
10 = continent	———
BLADDER	
0 = incontinent, or catheterized and unable to manage alone	
5 = occasional accident	
10 = continent	———
TOILET USE	
0 = dependent	
5 = needs some help, but can do something alone	
10 = independent (on and off, dressing, wiping)	———
TRANSFERS (BED TO CHAIR AND BACK)	
0 = unable, no sitting balance	
5 = major help (one or two people, physical), can sit	
10 = minor help (verbal or physical)	
15 = independent	———
MOBILITY (ON LEVEL SURFACES)	
0 = immobile or < 50 yards	
5 = wheelchair independent, including corners, > 50 yards	
10 = walks with help of one person (verbal or physical) > 50 yards	
15 = independent (but may use any aid; for example, stick) > 50 yards	———
STAIRS	
0 = unable	
5 = needs help (verbal, physical, carrying aid)	
10 = independent	———
TOTAL (0–100):	———

Figure 10.1 The Barthel index.
Source: "Functional Evaluation: The Barthel Index," by F. I. Mahoney and D. Barthel, 1965, *Maryland State Medical Journal, 14,* p. 62. Reprinted with permission.

to a person-specific or event-specific factor. From the caregiver, find out what the person enjoys doing. Learn more about the "person." Ask about past and present hobbies, joys, frustrations, and problems. For example, have the caregiver complete the Pleasant Events Schedule-AD (Teri & Logsdon, 1991). When something is upsetting and results in a behavioral problem, distracting the person with AD with some "pleasant" activity will lessen or change the undesired behavior. Plan activities according to these personal interests, and observe and modify the environment as needed.

Table 10.1

BLESSED DEMENTIA SCALE

Activity	Score
One point for each, unless otherwise indicated.	

Changes in performance of everyday activities

Inability to perform household tasks	____
Inability to cope with small sums of money	____
Inability to remember short list of items; for example, shopping list	____
Inability to find way about indoors	____
Inability to find way about familiar streets	____
Inability to interpret surroundings; for example, to recognize whether in hospital or at home; to discriminate among patients, doctors, nurse, relatives, other hospital staff	____
Inability to recall recent events; for example, recent outings, visits of relatives or friends to hospital	____
Tendency to dwell in the past	____

Changes in habits

Eating

(0) = cleanly, with proper utensils
(1) = messily, with spoon only
(2) = simple solids (for example, biscuits)
(3) = has to be fed   ____

Dressing

(0) = unaided
(1) = occasionally misplaces buttons, etc.
(2) = wrong sequence, commonly forgetting items
(3) = unable to dress   ____

Sphincter control

(0) = complete control
(1) = occasionally wets bed
(2) = frequently wets bed
(3) = doubly incontinent   ____

Changes in personality, interests, drive

Increased rigidity	____
Increased egocentricity	____
Impairment of regard of feeling for others	____
Coarsening of affect	____
Impairment of emotional control	____
Hilarity in inappropriate situations	____
Diminished emotional responsiveness	____
Sexual misdemeanor (arising de novo in old age)	____
Hobbies relinquished	____
Diminished initiative or growing apathy	____
Purposeless hyperactivity	____
Total:	____

Source: "The Association Between Quantitative Measures of Dementia and of Senile Change in the Cerebral Grey Matter of Elderly Subjects," by G. Blessed, B. E. Tomlinson, and M. Roth, 1968, *British Journal of Psychiatry, 114,* pp. 808–809. Reprinted with permission.

Table 10.2

FUNCTIONAL ACTIVITIES QUESTIONNAIRE

Writing checks, paying bills, balancing checkbook	
Assembling tax records, business affairs, or papers	
Shopping alone for clothes, household necessities, or groceries	
Playing a game of skill, working on a hobby	
Heating water, making a cup of coffee, turning off stove after use	
Preparing a balanced meal	
Keeping track of current events	
Paying attention to, understanding, discussing TV, book, magazine	
Remembering appointments, family occasions, holidays, medications	
Traveling out of neighborhood, driving, arranging to take buses	
Total score	

Dependent = 3
Requires assistance = 2
Has difficulty but does by self = 1
Normal = 0
Never did (the activity) but could do now = 0
Never did and would have difficulty now = 1

Source: "Measurement of Functional Activities in Older Adults in the Community," by R. I. Pfeffer, T. T. Kurosaki, C. H. Harrach, J. M. Chance, & S. Filos, 1982, *Journal of Gerontology, 37,* p. 327. Copyright © The Gerontological Society of America. Reproduced by permission of the publisher.

Tips for Physical Therapists Working With Clients With Dementia

The following section is adapted from a Web site publication by Martha R. Hinman of The University of Texas Medical Branch, Galveston (2004).

When working with clients who have dementia, the PT should maintain a functional focus but realize that the memory deficits will interfere with the client's ability to learn new motor tasks. Thus, the approach to functional training will differ from that used with cognitively intact clients. The acronym FUNCTIONAL is designed to highlight key points that PTs may find helpful when designing a rehabilitation program for individuals with dementia:

Familiarity. This applies to the type of treatment, the treatment environment, and the therapist. Find out what the client used to do for work or as hobbies, and match these functional movements with the type of exercise you want him to perform. For example, if you want to emphasize weight-bearing activity, familiar music may be used to prompt a client to dance. Also determine any interventions that might trigger an undesired reaction. For example, aquatic therapy may be ideal for someone who loved to swim but will be a poor choice for someone who was fearful of water or had a near-drowning experience in the past. Whenever possible, try to treat the person in a familiar environment (the home or hospital room), rather than the physical therapy clinic, and always have the same therapist work with the same client.

Understanding. Use simple language that is very literal and can be clearly understood by the client (e.g., walking machine rather than treadmill). In addition, the therapist must understand the nature of the disease and be ready to abandon one communication strategy if it isn't working and try another approach. The therapist must remain calm and constantly reassure the client to keep him or her from acting out in response to frustration or anxiety.

No distractions. All physical therapy evaluations and treatments should take place in an environment with minimal amount of visual and auditory stimuli that may distract the client's attention from the therapist. If treating a client in his room, close the door to prevent interruptions.

Cues and contact (eye). Individuals with dementia require repetitive cueing, both verbal and nonverbal. The therapist should make eye contact each time he speaks to the client and should reinforce verbal cues with visual ones whenever possible. Small group exercise classes are sometimes useful in reinforcing repetitive exercises because the clients can watch the group leader and other group members perform the activity with them. Brightly colored objects (e.g., scarves, balloons, balls) used in the exercise session may also elicit a better response from this population because people with AD tend to experience spatial and perceptual problems. Likewise, when they are ambulating on steps, the edges should be highlighted with bright paint or tape to accommodate their loss of depth perception. When attempting to minimize wandering and/or prevent falls, it may help to use familiar signs as visual cues. For example, a stop sign on the door may keep people with AD from entering a certain area.

Touch. Individuals with dementia often respond better to physical prompts than to verbal ones. Holding a client's hand and gently guiding it through a motion is more likely to elicit the desired response than describing or demonstrating the motion to the client. The therapist should always ask permission before touching the client and may need to experiment with the type of touch used to find out what the client responds most positively to. For example, clients with dementia are more likely to attend to the gentle pressure of an open hand than to light tapping or touching with a fingertip. Touch may also be used to soothe or calm a client who is agitated. Soft furry animals (real or stuffed) such as cats, rabbits, and small dogs are often helpful therapy aids, particularly for nonverbal clients.

Intact abilities. Teaching a new motor skill to a client with dementia is usually an unrealistic goal. Instead, the therapist must focus on developing and maintaining intact physical abilities. For example, a severely demented client with a hip fracture cannot be expected to learn how to use a walker with restricted weight-bearing status. Thus, a wheelchair is a more realistic option during the immediate post-op period. Remember, it is always easier to adapt the client's environment to meet her altered functional status than it is to retrain the client.

One step at a time. The therapist must realize that clients with dementia cannot process multistep directions and may not be able to complete a task if steps are skipped. For example, when cueing a client to get up from a chair, the therapist may need to give five separate commands such as: "Sit up straight. Place your feet flat on the floor. Put your hands on the armrests. Lean forward. Push yourself up." Likewise, it is usually unwise to combine multiple interventions (e.g., an exercise program and gait training) in the same treatment session.

Never rush. Extra time should be scheduled when evaluating or treating a client with dementia. Cognitive deficits will slow reaction and movement time, and if the client is rushed, motor errors will occur that could compromise the client's safety. Whenever possible, it is better to see the client for multiple, short treatment sessions rather than a single, long session. Clients with dementia tend to fatigue easily, and this will further compromise their ability to attend to the task at hand.

Automatic activities. The best exercises are those that utilize the most primitive, automatic responses. Thus, kicking or tossing a ball is a better way to strengthen leg and arm extensor muscles than lifting a weight. However, small cuff weights (1 to 2 lb.) applied to the wrist or ankles during functional activities such as walking or dancing are an excellent way to strengthen muscle and bone.

Limit choices. When evaluating a client with dementia, avoid using forms or scales that ask the client to rate her pain or to describe her activity level. Questions that require a "yes" or "no" answer are best. Likewise, clients with dementia have difficulty with open-ended treatment questions such as "What exercise would you like to do first today?" Thus, the therapist should be very organized and directive; when giving the client a choice, he should offer no more than two: "Would you rather ride the bicycle or take a walk?" "Would you like to dance to this song or that song?"

OCCUPATIONAL THERAPY

As the disease progresses through the mild to the severe stage, the person loses the ability to think clearly, reason, control his behavior, and communicate. Daily activities for Alzheimer's persons also tend to change with the progression of the disease and become difficult to manage. AD tends to limit concentration and to cause difficulties in following directions. These factors can turn simple activities into daily challenges. Because people with AD may have difficulty completing routine tasks in their day-to-day lives, OT can help individuals and their families to adapt tasks and environments to help promote or maximize independence, safety, and function. The primary focus of occupational therapy is to restore basic abilities such as dressing and eating and may help to enhance a person's ability to take part in meaningful activities within her environment and to enjoy family events. Further, occupational therapy improves persons' ability to perform ADLs and hence promotes independence and participation in social activities and reduces the burden on the caregiver by increasing their sense of competence and their ability to handle the behavioral problems they encounter. Although there is no cure for AD, research shows that occupational therapy and occupational interventions can help cope with the life-altering changes faced by people living with AD, their families, and caregivers.

The following section is adapted from a continuing professional education presentation by Lorie Richards, from The University of Kansas Medical Center (2007).

As people progress through dementia, they become more and more compromised in their ability to carry out basic and Instrumental ADLs. As their abilities decrease, they become less able to process and interpret environmental stimuli (including screening out irrelevant and attending to salient stimuli) and to formulate an action plan that leads to successful task completion. The frustrations of being unable to complete a requested or desired task can lead to behaviors that further interfere with the ability to complete the task, create a risk for safety, and disturb others who share the environment with the individual. The inability to accurately interpret environmental stimuli can also lead to behaviors that interfere with task completion, safety, or disturb others.

As individuals with dementia become increasingly demented, they commonly withdraw from engagement in meaningful occupations. While the importance of human activity to mental health is not a new idea, modern society is just beginning to realize the importance of engagement in occupation to quality of life. Humans are occupational beings, and the lack of meaningful occupations has been associated with poor health, such as maladaptive behavior patterns, depression, and stress-related medical problems. In those with dementia, an abundance of unstructured time can lead to increased behavior problems. The key is to structure the environment, routines, and tasks so that they support the individual's ability to engage successfully in meaningful occupations.

The role of the OT in the care of individuals with dementia is twofold. First, it helps the individual with dementia to continue participating in his required and desired occupations to the best of his ability. Second, it helps the person's caregivers to perform the required and desired occupations and interactions with that individual.

To develop an understanding of the best interventions for minimizing the influence of problem behaviors on the occupational performance of the individual with dementia and those around him or her, it is important that the OT understand when and under what conditions these behaviors occur. Various person-specific and event-specific factors can lead to problem behaviors:

- Overstimulation
- Boredom
- Need for social contact

- Attempting to participate in activities that are beyond the person's cognitive ability
- Forced participation in activities that hold no meaning for the individual
- Physiologic need

Common dementia staging assessments, such as the Global Deterioration Scale or the Clinical Dementia Rating Scale, are limited in their ability to indicate functional difficulties due to cognitive decline. Thus, the OT needs to complete assessments that will delineate occupational performance strengths and problems and the supports and barriers to the performance. The OT needs a full understanding of the person as an occupational being and the interaction of the person, context, and task variables that facilitates or impedes the occupational performance of each individual with dementia. Fully understanding problem behavior requires the use of both performance assessments and self and/or caregiver report assessments, including interviews.

- If the person is capable of giving reliable verbal answers, self-report assessments allows the OT to determine the meanings that the person attaches to various activities. These meanings are determined by the person's culture, social history, lifestyle, and personality. Also, the person's temporal patterns of meaningful activities may be important for understanding her current occupational engagement. Attempting to engage an individual in an activity that holds little meaning for her may result in problem behavior. Even if the activity, such as personal hygiene, is meaningful, the way in which this behavior is carried out or the period during the day when the activity is attempted may have ramifications for behavior.
- For example, if the person comes from a culture in which body modesty is extremely important, having a male caretaker attempt to help a female with a bath could result in problem behavior. Requiring a person to take a bath first thing in the morning when he has never been a morning person, preferring to lounge in the morning and not have social interaction before 10:00 A.M., and usually took a bath in the evening may result in problem behavior. Asking a person to take a bath or shower rather than a sponge bath, when she has never taken a shower or bath due to fear of water from a near-drowning accident as a child is likely to result in problem behaviors.

Gathering reports from the caregiver also leads to insights on the causes and possible solutions to problem behaviors. The OT needs to determine exactly what behaviors are considered problematic to the caregivers, because what are seen as problem behaviors varies from situation to situation and from caregiver to caregiver. This information will help the OT to focus the remainder of the assessment. In addition, as the OT will not be able to observe the individual around the clock, caregivers can be important sources of information about antecedent events that might have a causative role in the production of problem behaviors. It is important to gather information from both formal caregivers (health care professionals) and informal caregivers, such as family and friends. This is especially critical, as these latter individuals often have little or no training in how to interact with their loved one and may be especially impacted by problem behaviors. Finally, after determining when and in what situations the caregivers encounter the problem behaviors, the OT needs to directly observe the individual during those times.

- While there are many structured assessments of ADLs and Instrumental ADLs, most of these will be of little use here because they usually just identify at what level of independence the task is completed.
- What is really needed is the identification of the reasons behind unsuccessful task completion. For this, the OT needs to carefully record the
  - Person's responses to environmental stimuli to determine his cognitive ability to process stimuli and plan adaptive behavior
  - Social interactions
  - Task demands
  - The therapist needs a thorough understanding of the task demands in relation to the person's cognitive abilities. If formal cognitive testing is not available from other health care providers, then the OT may need to administer cognitive assessments to obtain this information.

There are several points to remember when selecting a particular kind of assessment.

- First, understand what the assessment was designed for. Many of the assessments that are found in the literature were designed to discriminate elders with dementia from those without. Thus, they may contain items that are irrelevant for the individual who resides in an institution.

■ Second, know what stage of dementia the assessment is valid for. Some of these assessments may have been designed for those with mild dementia. These assessments may be unable to measure functioning in individuals with moderate and severe dementia because by the time an individual's functional ability and behavior have declined to the point at which they need institutionalization, the items on the assessments are too difficult for that person to complete.

■ Third, it is important to remember that assessments must be appropriate in terms of culture and language for the persons who are performing the assessment. Simple translations of existing English-based measures do not always convey the appropriate cultural concepts.

By the time individuals with dementia enter a long-term-care facility, they are often unable to participate in formal performance assessments. Thus, skilled observation of how they participate in activities and interact with persons and objects in their environment and a careful assessment of the antecedents of both adaptive and problem behaviors is usually the best approach for determining cognitive levels and skills. Several assessments and frameworks may be helpful in this endeavor.

1 A very useful assessment tool that can be used to interview either the person with dementia or significant others or both is the Canadian Occupational Performance Measure (COPM).
   ■ This structured interview asks the interviewee what problems he or she is experiencing in the areas of self-care, productivity, and leisure.
   ■ The person also rates the importance to themselves of the task, their perceived ability to perform that task, and her satisfaction with their ability to perform the task.
   ■ The OT, after identifying the functional problems, can probe each activity deeper to obtain further details on the nature of the performance difficulty.
2 Another caregiver-report questionnaire is the Functional Activities Questionnaire, which emphasizes the cognitive aspects of functional performance.

3   Activity history checklists can be used to identify past occupational patterns of the individual with dementia. As with the COPM, the therapist can ask for details regarding the temporal parameters and settings of each occupation.

4   One such framework is the Cognitive Disabilities Model, which uses observations about attention to sensory cues, sensorimotor associations, and motor actions to categorize individuals into six cognitive levels. Associated with each cognitive level is a description of the functional capabilities at that level and the type of assistance and contextual and task modification that will most likely be required for successful occupational performance.

5   Associated with the Cognitive Disabilities Model are several assessments that assist the OT in determining cognitive level. These include the Cognitive Performance Test (Burns, Mortimer, & Merchak, 1994), the Routine Task Inventory II (Allen, Earhart, & Blue, 1992), and the Allen Cognitive Level Test (Allen, 1982) and its enlarged form.

The Cognitive Performance Test (CPT) is a standardized, performance-based assessment instrument, originally designed for the objective evaluation of function in Alzheimer's disease. This instrument uses six common ADL tasks (dress, shop, toast, phone, wash, and travel), for which the information-processing requirements can be systematically varied to assess ordinal levels of functional capacity. For each task, standard equipment, set-up, and methods of administration are required. A gross level score is determined for each of the six tasks; these scores are then added for a total score and averaged to determine the functional level and mode.

The Routine Task Inventory (RTI) is a standardized list of routine tasks, including dressing, bathing, toileting, and 10 other ADLs. The therapist observes the person carefully to determine what the person pays attention to, what his motor response is, and what verbal performance is happening during the task. For patients with very low cognitive functioning, the Allen Battery has a sensory stimulation kit, which presents a set of stimulations to the patient, who is observed in the same manner—what does the patient pay attention to, what is the motor response, and what is the verbal response to each stimulation.

The Allen Cognitive Level Test (ACL) is a standardized screening tool used mainly by occupational therapists to determine a person's ability to understand instructions and perform tasks. The screening tool is a square piece of leather with holes in it, along with a blunt needle, and some waxed thread and leather lacing. It divides the qualitative capacity to function into 6 levels, with 10 modes in each level. The levels measure with a high degree of sensitivity what a person pays attention to and how the use of this information is expressed in motor and verbal performance.

6   Another approach to understanding the cognitive level of individuals with dementia is based on Piaget's stages of development. The assumption is that the cognitive decline seen in dementia mirrors in reverse the cognitive development stages that Piaget described. The Modified Ordinal Scales of Psychological Development is a structured observation assessment that allows the clinician to categorize individuals with severe dementia into one of Piaget's four developmental stages. It contains lists of behaviors that indicate cognitive functioning at each stage.

7   Recent research suggests that individuals with dementia often have visual spatial processing impairments that are linked to such problem behaviors as wandering and getting lost, in addition to diminished cognitive skills. Thus, paying attention to how the individual with dementia interacts with the space around him should be an important aspect of an occupational therapy evaluation.

Interventions to restore person variables are not the intervention of choice with individuals with dementia. Dementia is a disease in which specific areas of the brain continues to deteriorate.

■ Restorative approaches attempt to restore brain function, often by facilitating other areas of the brain to undertake the functions of the damaged portion, or attempt to teach the individual new strategies for approaching problems. However, individuals with dementia will continue to experience more and more damage as their disease progresses.

■ Because of severe declarative memory impairments, individuals with dementia have shown little ability to learn new strategies. Thus, it is a better use of therapy time to find ways to improve participation in activities than to attempt to restore cognitive function.

■ The best approach for individuals with dementia is to reconstruct the context or the tasks so that these support successful participation in occupations.

- It is critical for the OT to identify the cognitive level and remaining cognitive skills of the individual with dementia in order to match contextual and task modifications to the individual. The understanding is that the environmental and task supports that are found to facilitate occupational performance and decrease problem behaviors will be long-term modifications.

There are multiple intervention strategies for individuals of all disciplines when attempting to reduce the problem behaviors exhibited by someone with dementia. In using these strategies, several points are important to keep in mind.

- One of the key principles is that the OT should ensure that the person with dementia experiences just the right amount and kind of stimulation in order to minimize problem behaviors and facilitate occupational performance.
- Everyone needs environmental stimulation to behave adaptively. As people age, their peripheral sensory systems become less efficient. Thus, fewer good-quality environmental stimuli reach the brain. At the same time, the person with dementia becomes less able to screen out environmental stimuli. Thus, the person with dementia may be experiencing sensory deprivation as well as being easily overstimulated. In addition, the person with dementia is less able to process and attach meaning to stimuli that do reach the brain.
- Many times, problem behaviors occur because the person's time is unstructured. In addition, disrupted sleep patterns have been at least partially associated with increased sleeping during the day. Humans have an inner drive to engage in occupations, yet people with dementia often do not have the cognitive capacity to initiate and structure activities that are meaningful for them.
  - It is the job of the OT to assist in the development of activity programs that offer an appropriate cognitive and psychosocial challenge to the person with dementia. These activities need to be structured to capture the attention and interest of the person with dementia but must be within the person's cognitive ability in order to ensure success.
  - The OT should do this by using his understanding of how to adapt task variables to the person's past occupational patterns and interests and current cognitive functioning.

- The OT can assist in the development of activities that relate to the person's past occupations, sufficiently simplified to ensure success despite the person's cognitive limitations. Such simplifications may include decreasing the number of task-related items in the activity, making the important features of the task more salient, developing cueing strategies that assist the individual in task completion, presenting one part of the task at a time, or asking the person to complete only those parts of the task that he can.
- Humans also have a need to control their environment and what occupations they engage in. While in the past the recommended practice with those with dementia was to remove the requirement of making choices, the current thinking is that a lack of control can also lead to problem behaviors.
  - Thus, allowing the person with dementia to make choices may lead to fewer problem behaviors. However, the choices offered must be within the person's cognitive capabilities. Too difficult a choice could lead to an increase in problem behaviors due to cognitive stress. Also, the choices must be logical. For example, allowing a person to choose when to take a bath might not lead to reduced problem behaviors if the person can't remember that it was his choice when the time comes to take the bath. However, the choice between a shower and a bath at this moment might be well within the person's cognitive capabilities.

Education of Caregivers

Informal caregivers, such as family and friends, as well as staff who do not have expertise in working with persons with dementia, need training in how to prevent and minimize problem behaviors in these individuals. They should be educated about the reasons that problem behaviors occur in general and know the specific antecedents that affect the person in their care. They need training on how to interact with the individuals with dementia. Family members and friends need assistance in planning activities to do with their loved one that provide successful and satisfactory social interaction for both parties. The OT should be involved in planning an educational programs for caregivers, both formal and informal. In addition, the OT should directly assist the friends and family in how to plan visits.

Occupational Therapist: Member of an Interdisciplinary Team

There are many members of the interdisciplinary team whose disciplines overlap with occupational therapy in the assessment and intervention of individuals with dementia. The uniqueness of occupational therapy in these endeavors is that the OT views persons with dementia through the lens of their ability to engage in satisfactory occupational patterns across a variety of time durations. It is important for the OT to understand what the roles of the other interdisciplinary team members are in order for the team to avoid unnecessary duplication of services and to develop well-integrated programs of intervention.

A   Other health care professionals with whom the OT collaborates to assess occupational performance:
  1   Nurses—particularly for ADL activities
  2   Dieticians—for eating behavior
  3   Social workers—particularly for the person's past social and cultural history as it impacts the type of occupations found in the individual's culture and social environment
B   Other health care professionals with whom the OTs collaborate to assess and intervene regarding strengths and barriers to the person's occupational performance
  1   PT—particularly in the realm of motor strengths and weaknesses; may make environmental/task modifications
  2   Psychologist—particularly in the realm of cognitive, affective/emotional, and behavioral strengths and weaknesses; may make environmental/task modifications; may educate significant others
  3   Neuropsychologist—particularly in the realm of cognitive strengths and weaknesses; may educate significant others
  4   Speech pathologist—particularly in the realm of language and cognitive strengths and weaknesses; may make environmental/task modifications; may educate significant others
  5   Pharmacist—particularly in the realm of understanding the influence of the person's medications on the person; may educate significant others
  6   Social worker—particularly in the realm of the person's social and financial resources; may educate significant others

7 Physician—particularly in the realm of understanding the influence of pathology and medications on person variables; may educate significant others

8 Nurse—particularly in the realm of understanding the influence of pathology and medications on person variables; may educate significant others

9 Dietician—particularly in the realm of feeding; may make environmental/task modifications; may educate significant others

10 Activities personnel—particularly in the realm of participation in leisure pursuits; may make environmental/task modifications

Occupational Therapy Interventions

The Allen Cognitive Levels (ACL) is an occupational therapy tool and resource (Allen, 1982). Unlike the traditional dementia staging system, which describes the early, middle, and late stages of the disease, these levels provide a more precise measurement of an individual's abilities and needs. It is scored on a scale of 1–6, where 1 = severe cognitive impairment and 6 = normal cognitive functioning. Each Allen Cognitive Level is generally associated with characteristics or patterns of behavior that are commonly seen within that level. Each level has three components: Attention, Motor Control, and Verbal Performance. Here is a brief summary of each level, including common characteristics or patterns of behavior associated with that level:

Level 6: Independent in daily care, finances, decision-making skills. Can learn new information.

Level 5: Independent in daily care; assistance may be needed with finances, decision making, and organizational skills. Subtle problems with memory may be noted. Can learn new information.

Level 4: Physically independent with daily care; assistance needed to initiate/monitor quality of care. Increased assistance needed with all cognitive skills. Notable problems with memory are noted. New information can be retained only after much repetition. Transitional stage for supervision. By the end of this level, most individuals will require supervision to ensure their safety and assistance to complete care with quality.

Level 3: Assistance with all daily care is needed. Full assistance required with all cognitive skills, including initiating, sequencing, judgment, problem solving, and decision making. Significant memory impairment is noted. Unable to learn new information. Difficulty with language skills are observed.

Level 2: Dependent on others for daily care. Significant impairment of all cognitive skills. Loss of language skills. Decrease in motor and visual/perceptual skills. No longer recognize familiar people or objects.

Level 1: Totally dependent on others for all care. Generally bedridden. All basic needs met by caregiver.

The ACL recognizes the existing abilities of an individual with dementia. By identifying the individual's abilities, caregivers can work to highlight or emphasize those abilities, allowing the individual with dementia to remain engaged in day-to-day activity and to maintain their skills. When the ACL score is interpreted by an OT, accurate and appropriate care strategies can be selected to enhance the quality of life for the individual and to ease the work of the caregiver. Table 10.3 provides occupational therapy interventions based on the cognitive limitations in people with AD.

Tips for Occupational Therapists Working With Dementia Clients

The following section is adapted from a Web site publication by Elicia Dunn Cruz of The University of Texas Medical Branch, Galveston, (2004).

The OT uses a variety of approaches during intervention with clients who have dementia. The goals of therapy include maintaining, restoring, and improving occupational performance; promoting health and quality of life; and easing caregivers' burdens (American Occupational Therapy Association, 1994). In the early stages of dementia, clients may be able to learn or relearn self-care or other forms of occupational performance, particularly if they benefit from medications that aim to slow the progression of dementia. Most clients, however, will not be able to learn or relearn skills. The clients' cognitive deficits necessitate compensatory strategies that promote their performance of daily life tasks despite their cognitive impairments.

Compensatory strategies for cognitive impairment improve or maintain occupational performance within the person's remaining capabilities

Table 10.3

OCCUPATIONAL THERAPY INTERVENTIONS BASED ON THE COGNITIVE LIMITATIONS

LEVEL	LIMITATION	INTERVENTION
Six	■ Normal functioning in routine daily activities	■ Intervention is not necessary
Five	■ Unable to manipulate symbols or use abstractions ■ Unable to retain information to be used at a later date ■ Writing and reading comprehension and math skills are impaired	■ Concrete, manual task-oriented activities ■ Encourage the individual to pursue activities ■ Minimal supervision is required ■ Support groups and networking
Four	■ Has significant impairment ■ Does not notice mistakes or solve problems ■ Unable to make plans beyond the immediate situation ■ Unable to remember directions for use at a later time ■ Adapting to change is difficult ■ New learning cannot occur ■ Depression, anxiety, and agitation are common	■ Structure and scheduled essential ADLs ■ Slowly introduces adaptive equipment for safety ■ Activities must be simple and familiar, two–three step, error-proof, and action-oriented and have predictable results ■ Yard work, domestic chores, sports and dance activities, board games, puzzles, video games, and walks, simple crafts are acceptable ■ Memory aides, large calendars, notebook, daily schedule of ADLs, system to organize and secure personal possessions may be helpful
Three	■ Disorganized thinking ■ Aware that actions are producing an effect on the environment but does not understand and can't predict what effect a given action might have; hides valuables, puts soup into coffeepot, plays with radio dials ■ Learning is not possible	■ Repetitive action activities that have predictable effects on the environment ■ Familiar one-step, repetitive, action-oriented activities that have predictable effects ■ Suggested activities include sports activities (basketball, golf, biking, swimming, weight, catch); folk and ballroom dancing; household maintenance activities (hosing, gardening, washing cars, chopping wood, mowing lawns, sweeping and mopping floors, vacuuming, hammering nails, sawing wood); kitchen activities (mixing batters,

washing and drying dishes, washing vegetables, chopping vegetables, cleaning countertop); creative and manual arts activities (painting, sculpting, drawing, needlework, simple hemming and mending); eye-hand coordination (sewing cards, manipulation tasks such as nuts and bolts, jars and lids, cutting, tracing, crafts); games (paper-pencil puzzles, "Hi-Q," dominoes, card games); aerobic exercise (routines demonstrated by instructor) (exercycles, rebounding trampoline)

- Keep environment routine and predictable
- Avoid sensory overload
- Make posters listing the steps involved in ADLs (making coffee, sandwich, brushing teeth, getting dressed)

- Familiar one-step, visually demonstrated repetitive gross-motor actions
- Suggested activities are similar to those in Level 3, but they are carried out with less awareness and attention (vacuum the same section of the carpet incessantly, polish the same spot), folding laundry, chopping vegetables, polishing furniture, catching a ball, rebounding tennis balls, dancing, knitting
- Simplify more complicated self-maintenance activities into step-by-step process, and provide one item at a time
- Alter items to simplify the task (pull-on vs. buttons, cut meat)
- Do not expect accuracy
- Maintain a predictable routine
- Encourage ambulation
- Understands simple sentences, one question at a time
- Relies on visual cues to verify existence of objects; keep doors open and frequently used objects and treasured possessions visible

Two

- Engages in purposeless body movements (aimless pacing, constant undressing, bizarre behaviors—sitting backwards on the toilet and driving it like a car)
- Unaware that actions can affect one's environment
- Ignores objects and people

(continued)

267

Table 10.3

OCCUPATIONAL THERAPY INTERVENTIONS BASED ON THE COGNITIVE LIMITATIONS

LEVEL	LIMITATION	INTERVENTION
		■ Use pictures to label drawers ■ Provide sensory stimulation 　Gustatory—favorite flavors and spices; aromatic teas 　Olfactory—aftershave, hand lotion, flowers, potpourri, cooking odors 　Tactile—house pets, loving touch, massage, lotions, foot and hand soaks, favorite fabrics and textures in bedclothes, blankets, sheets. 　Visual—keepsakes in view, fish tanks if familiar 　Auditory—favorite vocal and instrumental tapes and records, family voices 　Kinesthetic—rocking chairs, porch swings, walking, exercise, hammocks, car rides
One	■ Initiates no spontaneous activity ■ Except for carefully presented and highly familiar sensory stimuli, external stimuli are experienced as meaningless ■ New and unfamiliar stimuli increase agitation and confusion ■ Grooming, dressing, and bathing must be done by others, and the individual may need to be fed, told to chew, or allowed to eat with fingers	■ Continue to stimulate sensory channels, but emphasize highly familiar sensations ■ Use one-word commands ■ Keep environment (e.g., people, objects, and sensory stimuli) consistent and familiar ■ Introduce change very slowly ■ Family members and close friends should visit one at a time ■ Strange sounds, sights, tastes, odors, or medications need to be explained ■ Communicate on an emotional level

Adapted from *Alzheimer's Disease: Activity Focused Care* (2nd ed.), by C. R. Hellen, 1998, Burlington, MA: Butterworth-Heinemann.

by changing the way the task is performed or the environment in which it is performed. Occupational therapy intervention must focus on the people who will actually implement various compensatory strategies, including clients and their caregivers, be they formal (paid) or informal (unpaid, such as family). Compensatory strategies should result in improved daily life satisfaction for both the client and the caregiver. Often, it is assumed that therapists must aim to facilitate independent performance among clients with dementia. It is important to recognize, however, the value of shared occupational performance (or interdependence), in which a caregiver assists with task performance in a way that meets the needs of and promotes satisfaction among both the client and the caregiver. For example, clients may be able to dress themselves in the morning with a good deal of verbal cues and physical prompts. However, the time and energy that it takes to facilitate this "independent" dressing may result in the client and caregiver avoiding other necessary or desired tasks, such as sitting down to a good breakfast. Thus, it might benefit such clients and caregivers to share the chore of dressing so that they have time and energy for other desired activities. Therapists should discuss clients' and caregivers' wishes in order to negotiate an ideal plan for independent and shared occupational engagement. This plan should address current and anticipate future needs.

Occupational therapists have employed a variety of ways to compensate for memory or learning deficits and to promote satisfying occupational performance. Abreu's *quadraphonic approach* is a theoretical model that nicely synthesizes a variety of intervention approaches (1990). It can be applied in efforts to teach independent performance or to teach clients and caregivers strategies for shared occupational performance. Her model incorporates practice, feedback about performance, and environmental modifications that are based on the clients' and caregivers' needs. *Practice* involves repetitious performance of desired behaviors, followed by *feedback* about the client's performance. Most clients with dementia will not benefit from practice or feedback because of their cognitive deficits. However, OTs can use these specific approaches when training caregivers to assist with or promote clients' occupational performance. The therapist has the caregiver practice new skills, such as assisting with dressing or bathing, after which the therapist and caregiver discuss what worked and did not work during the activity. The therapist also provides helpful feedback about the caregivers' actions and how these actions are related to performance outcomes.

The use of *environmental modifications* is critical to task success and to satisfaction with performance. Modification can be made in the

Table 10.4

MODIFICATIONS TO PROMOTE OCCUPATIONAL PERFORMANCE

MODIFICATIONS BY THERAPIST/CAREGIVER	MODIFICATIONS IN THE OCCUPATION, TASK, AND EXERCISE ITSELF	MODIFICATIONS BY THE CLIENT
■ Change verbal and body language, concreteness of instructions, physical cues or reassurance ■ Change tone of voice ■ Change type of feedback (verbal, written, pictures, photos, physical) ■ Change when and how often feedback is given ■ Change how feedback is explained ■ Change own expectations and biases (alter own value judgments about ideal/necessary performance)	■ Change sensory modalities challenged during a task (i.e., decrease tactile, auditory, or visual distractions) ■ Change amount of workload (i.e., set up task to limit number of steps, lay out needed objects, label cabinets and drawers) ■ Change complexity of task (i.e., simplify the number of objects, the number of steps, the number of instructions, the form of instructions, the type of instructions or feedback) ■ Change pace/speed of task ■ Change duration of task	■ Change awareness levels (arouse prior to task performance) ■ Change safety challenges ■ Change need for error detection & correction ■ Change the social environment ■ Change postural readiness prior to task performance ■ Change organizational strategies prior to task performance ■ Change medication or its timing

Adapted from *The Quadraphonic Approach: Evaluation and Treatment of the Brain Injured Patient,* by B. C. Abreu, 1990, New York: Therapeutic Service Systems. Reprinted with permission.

client's approach to the task, in the therapist's or caregiver's approach, and in how the occupation, task, or exercise is set up or performed (Abreu, 2000). Table 10.4 lists specific modifications that may be made to the context in order to promote occupational performance.

SPEECH-LANGUAGE PATHOLOGY

Management of persons with dementia and dysphagia can be very complex. People with dementia may exhibit changes in behavior during meals, changes in the physiology of swallowing, and changes in cognitive or language function that affect their ability to understand or implement treatment strategies (Logemann, 2007). They may also exhibit sensory loss that affects both their ability to eat and swallow and their ability to use treatment strategies. Clinicians must evaluate all aspects of the person's function in relation to their swallowing and eating ability and also place the results of this evaluation in the context of the person's cognitive problems and ability to apply and use therapy strategies.

Speech-language pathologists, in the past, generally did not provide service to persons with AD; however, the profession's practice has recently changed. Since the implementation of speech and language services for this population, speech pathologists have contributed to the evidence regarding speech and language behaviors in individuals with AD. The speech and language abilities of people with AD, particularly in the early and middle stages of the disease, remarkably resemble those of a person with aphasia. Further, the speech of persons with AD is often described as "empty," as it contains a high proportion of words and utterances that convey little or no information (Almor, Kempler, MacDonald, Andersen, & Tyler, 1999). Once the similarities between AD speech and aphasia were documented, the questions that remained were whether persons with AD could benefit from the same pragmatic language therapy as aphasia patients. Furthermore, people with AD may initially present with an agnosia for food and a swallowing apraxia, resulting in prolonged holding of food in the oral cavity (Logemann, 1998). Other physiologic changes in the swallow may compound to the point that the person cannot eat or drink enough to maintain adequate nutrition and hydration (McHorney & Rosenbek, 1998).

The following section is adapted from a continuing professional education presentation by Susan Jackson of The University of Kansas Medical Center (2007).

Overview of Language

Language makes humans unique. It is the primary form of communication. In dementia, language and thus communication deteriorate over time. Communication nonetheless persists, such as refusal to eat, screaming, elopement attempts, repetitive questioning, and/or accusatory remarks. Although the term *problem behaviors* may be descriptive of this set of behaviors, each behavior reflects a communicative gesture, whether appropriate or inappropriate. SLPs are experts in communicative disorders. They are qualified through their education and training to assess and treat the communicative disorders in dementia. The information presented addresses the assessment of communication strengths and weaknesses in dementia and management strategies.

The Role of the Speech-Language Pathologist in the Assessment and Management of Behavioral Disturbances in Dementia

Assessment of Communication Strengths and Weaknesses

Assessment involves identification of communication strengths and weaknesses. Appropriate assessment tools are crucial so that both weaknesses and strengths are revealed. Since all behaviors (even negative ones) have some communicative value, SLPs are in a good position to determine the cause of the negative behaviors and make recommendations for reducing such behaviors. It is reasonable to assess the communicative skills of someone with dementia every 6 months.

Communication Strengths in Dementia

- Desire to communicate
- Retention of remote memory
- The ability to read aloud
- Social niceties
- Procedural memory
- Continued recall of grammar, syntax, phonology of language

Communication Deficits in Dementia

- Empty content
- Perseveration
- Lack of cohesion or coherence
- Use of concrete language
- Increased or decreased talkativeness
- Diminished auditory and reading comprehension, especially in terms of higher level language (e.g., metaphor, sarcasm, inferences)

Negative Communication Behaviors

All behaviors have some communicative value—even "negative" ones. The challenge for the care provider is to find the meaning in these negative behaviors and then figure out a way to decrease them, perhaps either by substituting a more acceptable behavior, by providing stimuli that compete with the negative behavior, or by changing the environment/behavior of others so that that it is more supportive of the person with dementia. The following is a short list of behaviors that many would consider negative:

- Screaming, moaning, repeatedly shouting, "Help me! Help me!"
- Asking the same question over and over again
- Throwing food, refusing to eat
- Emptying the contents of an entire chest of drawers
- Entering other people's rooms and ransacking them
- Urinating on the floor of a bedroom

Underlying Reasons for Communication Deficits in Dementia

- Memory problems
  - Problems with episodic memory (memory for events, e.g., what you did on your 21st birthday)
  - Problems with semantic memory (conceptual memory, e.g., what you know about a birthday—cake, balloons, presents)

Other Barriers to Communication

- Reduced opportunity to communicate
- Having nothing to communicate about
- Hearing loss (on the part of the person with dementia and also on the part of the communication partners)
- Negative effects of drugs on communication
- Cultural differences

Management

There are a number of techniques that can be tried to improve communication with persons with dementia. Several of these techniques are described here.

- Individuals with dementia will experience a decline in communicative ability over time. Thus, the goal of treatment is not to return them to their previous skill levels but to maximize their residual communicative abilities and to help them compensate for areas of deficit. Since decline is ongoing, the treatment plan should be changed as the pattern of communicative strengths and weaknesses changes.

■ In managing communicative disorders in dementia, strategies focus either on facilitating a particular skill (e.g., improving the ability to recall information over longer intervals of time) or on compensating for weak skills (e.g., creating a picture and sentence memory booklet for a person who cannot recall the events that happened over the past week).

■ As dementia progresses, the burden of communication falls more and more to the intact communication partner. The majority of the management strategies described in the module are aimed at communication partners rather than at the persons with dementia.

Language Boards

These boards contain phrases from another language phonetically translated into English.

■ Phrase in English: How are you?
■ Phrase in French: Comment ça va?
■ Phrase in French phonetically translated into English: Caw maw suh vuh?

They are designed to be used by nursing home staff with residents whose first language isn't English so that the person with dementia hears phrases spoken in his native language. Mattern and Camp (1998) reported that "In observations in which the staff member used Russian phrases, the subject responded in a compliant manner and with pleasant affect more often than when spoken to in English" (p. 3). Use of these language boards compensates for poor auditory comprehension of English.

FOCUSED Program for Caregivers

■ This training program consists of seven strategies (Ripich, Ziol, & Lee, 1998):
  1 Face-to-face to attract attention
  2 Orientation to topic of conversation
  3 Continuity or maintenance of the topic
  4 Unsticking for overcoming communication blocks
  5 Structured in how questions are formed
  6 Exchange ideas, needs, and feelings during conversation
  7 Direct in the types of verbal messages

- Use of these strategies compensates for the communication deficits of the person with dementia. Ripich (1994) has provided this training to nursing assistants and family members of persons with AD.
- After training, nursing assistants showed a significant improvement in attitude toward persons with AD, improved knowledge of AD, and greater knowledge of communication strategies (Ripich, 1994). After training, family members showed increased knowledge of AD and increased communication satisfaction with their family member who had AD (Ripich, Kercher, Wykle, Sloan, & Ziol, 1998); in the same study, some differences between White and African American caregivers emerged: only African American caregivers showed a significant decrease in perceived daily hassles after training, and the African American caregivers showed greater positive affect than the White caregivers after training.
- Positive longitudinal changes were also seen in family caregivers who participated in the FOCUSED training program: at both 6 and 12 months after training, caregivers reported a greater decrease in hassles associated with communication than did members of a control group of caregivers, and the FOCUSED caregivers also had more knowledge of AD and communication strategies than control caregivers (Ripich, Ziol, Fritsch, & Durand, 1999).
- One study examined the ability of family caregivers to *implement* one of the FOCUSED strategies (structuring of questions) and the response of the individuals with AD to that strategy (Ripich et al., 1999). At 6 and 12 months after FOCUSED training, caregivers asked significantly fewer open-ended questions (and more yes/no or multiple-choice questions), which led to more successful communication on the part of the individuals with AD.
  - Yes/no and multiple-choice questions rely on recognition memory, whereas open-ended questions (e.g., What would you like for dinner?) rely on recall memory. Reliance on recognition memory lessens the memory load of communication demands.

Memory Wallets

- These external memory aids compensate for deficits in episodic memory (Bourgeois, 1990). Picture stimuli (often photographs) are accompanied by a sentence or two. The type of wallet is not crucial; pictures may be held together with a metal ring or placed in a small photo album. Individuals with dementia use the memory aids to communicate factual information.

- Michelle Bourgeois (1992) has examined the efficacy of memory wallets on the conversational skills of persons with dementia. The following variables have been explored: severity of dementia (mild to severe), setting (private home, adult day-care center, nursing home), amount of training (none versus varying amounts), and communication partner (family members, volunteers, another person with dementia).
- The memory wallets were effective in increasing the quality of communicative exchanges on the part of the person with dementia across level of dementia severity, across communication partners, and across settings.
  - Even with no training of the communication partner or the person with dementia, improvements in communication were observed.
  - Individuals with severe dementia were less likely to make novel statements; the increased number of appropriate utterances usually consisted of statements that they read from the memory wallet.
  - There was good maintenance of the treatment effect 24–30 months posttraining under the following circumstances: subjects had mild dementia and lived in the community, partners were family members, and partners had received training in the use of the memory wallets.

Validation Therapy

- This therapy has its roots in Carl Rogers's (1961) client-centered therapy and considers the person's feelings as paramount. It is designed specifically for persons in the advanced stages of dementia. The caregiver validates what the person with dementia says, rather than correct her.
  - For example, if the person with dementia says that she has to leave the nursing home so that she can cook dinner for her husband, the caregiver might say, "I hear you were a really good cook. Your husband was a lucky man to have such a good cook for a wife. What were some of your favorite things to cook?"

■ The caregiver has validated the person's feelings and has also tried to redirect the person's behavior; the caregiver's response is an attempt to calm the person with dementia and prevent an episode of agitation.

■ Generally, reports of treatment effectiveness are anecdotal, but several data-based studies do exist. Morton and Bleathman (1991) found Validation Therapy to be effective in increasing the number of interactions and length of interactions for two of three individuals with dementia.

Reality Orientation

■ The goal is to improve orientation (Zanetti et al., 1995).
  ■ Nursing home residents are repeatedly exposed to oral and written presentations of orientation information. Confused speech and behavior are corrected. Correcting the behavior of someone who is confused may lead that person to become agitated.
  ■ Improvements have been seen on measures such as the Mini-Mental State Exam, but there has been no carryover to every day life. Questions about the functionality of Reality Orientation have been raised: does learning the date, day, and location of residence improve a person's functioning?

There are some other simple techniques that can help communication with a person with dementia.

Shorten Messages

■ Speak in short phrases or sentences. This will lessen the memory load of communication demands. It is a strategy that caregivers can use to compensate for deficits in the person's episodic memory. Evidence shows that for individuals with dementia, shortening the length of utterances led to greater improvements in auditory comprehension than simplifying the syntactic complexity of utterances (Waters, Rochon, & Caplan, 1998).

Consider the Furniture Arrangement

■ Arrange the furniture so that it is conducive to interaction among people (e.g., a semicircle arrangement). This strategy addresses the barrier of "reduced opportunity to communicate." People are more likely to talk to one another if they can see one another than if they are lined up in their wheelchairs along a wall of a nursing home.

Provide Conversational Partners

■ This strategy also addresses the barrier of "reduced opportunity to communicate."

Offer Group Activities

■ This strategy addresses the barrier of "nothing to communicate about."
■ The Breakfast Club is an example of a group activity. Residents and staff of a nursing home cook and eat breakfast together. The quantity and quality of communications are reported to improve while residents are engaging in Breakfast Club activities.

Identify Cupboard/Drawer Contents

■ Identify the contents of cupboards and drawers using written words or pictures.
  ■ For example, write the word "socks" on a 4 × 6-inch index card and tape it to the drawer containing socks. If the person with dementia can no longer understand single written words, tape a picture of socks to the sock drawer. This strategy compensates for memory deficits and may serve to decrease negative communication behaviors such as emptying the entire contents of a chest of drawers.

Provide Room Identifiers

■ Identify rooms in the house or nursing home, using written words or pictures.
  ■ For example, you might tape a picture of each nursing home resident to the door of his or her room to decrease the negative communication behavior of entering others' rooms and ransacking them. You might also write the word "bathroom" on a 5 × 7-inch index card and tape the card to the bathroom door or tape a picture of a toilet to the bathroom door to decrease the negative communication behavior of urinating on the floor. Again, this strategy compensates for memory deficits.

Provide Written Cues to Decrease Repetitious Verbalizations

■ Write the answers to questions that are asked repeatedly on a sticky note, index card, dry erase board, or any other surface that you think is appropriate. This strategy is designed to decrease repeated asking of the same question (Bourgeois, Burgio, Schulz, & Beach, 1997). Examples might include a sticky note attached to the dashboard of the car to remind the person with dementia of the destination or an index card carried in the pocket of the person with dementia that reads, "My son always visits me on Saturday afternoon."

Provide Calendars

■ Provide a daily or weekly calendar that communicates a daily schedule or weekly activities/events. The calendar can be portable, to be carried by the person with dementia, or placed in a fixed location. The activities can be communicated in written form or through the use of pictures. These strategies compensate for memory deficits.

Offer Reminiscence Therapy

■ This strategy capitalizes on one of the communication strengths in dementia: remote memory. Persons with dementia get together in a group and reminisce. Picture stimuli are often used to elicit reminiscences.

Utilize Spaced Retrieval

■ This strategy is unique in the dementia literature in that its goal is to improve the memory ability of individuals with dementia rather than to compensate for poor memory. Camp and his colleagues (1996) have explored this strategy as a means of improving the recall memory of individuals with dementia for approximately 10 years.

■ Spaced retrieval is a method of learning and retaining information by recalling information over increasingly longer periods of time.

   ■ If the subject is unable to recall the information at a particular interval of time, the correct answer is supplied by the examiner and then the subject is asked the question at half of the time interval at which recall failure occurred (e.g., if the subject cannot remember the information after 2 minutes has elapsed, the information is supplied by the examiner and then the subject is asked to recall the information 1 minute later. If failure occurs again, the answer is supplied and then the question asked 30 seconds later. The subject then works back up to recalling the information at increasing intervals of time.).

■ Frequency of training sessions has ranged from once a week to several times a week. Most sessions were 30 minutes in length. Number of sessions has ranged from 2 to 20. Severity of dementia ranged from mild to severe.

■ Camp and his colleagues have shown that the following associations can be learned: names of faces, locations of objects, names of objects, object selection, actions to be performed, pieces of information important to the subject (e.g., room number), compensatory techniques (e.g., use of a date book, use of a voice amplifier). Retention intervals have ranged from 1 week to 8 weeks, and there has been some generalization from the training sessions to real-life situations.

Supply Hearing Aids

■ This strategy addresses the barrier of hearing loss on the part of the person with dementia; it compensates for hearing loss (Palmer, Adams, Bourgeois, Durrant, & Rossi, 1999).

   ■ In a recent study using a single-subject experimental design, provided amplification for eight community-dwelling individuals with mild to moderate dementia (with one exception). Persons with dementia wore the hearing aids for an average of 4–13 hours per day. Family caregivers reported a decrease in one to four problem behaviors (out of two to four problem behaviors identified) with hearing aid use. Caregivers collected baseline data for 1.5 to 2.5 months and treatment data for approximately 2 months after hearing aid fitting. The two subjects to derive the least benefit in terms of reduction of problem behaviors were both functioning in the severe range of dementia severity: one was severely demented at the beginning of the study, and one declined into the severe range over the course of the study.

Use Audio-Assisted Memory Training

■ Individuals with dementia listen to an audiotape recorded narrative containing personally relevant information, with interactive quizzes interspersed within the narrative; the answers to the quizzes are provided on the tape after a delay of a few seconds. There are also review questions at the end of the narrative.

- Frequency and intensity of the treatment varied (e.g., one time a week for 10 weeks, two to four times a day for 3 days). Retention of information has been reported as follows: 49% to more than 75% at 1 and 2 week follow-up (Arkin, 1998), 69%–93% at 1 and 2 week follow-up (Arkin, 1992).

The Speech-Language Pathologist and the Interdisciplinary Team

- The SLP assesses and treats communicative disorders of dementia.
- Only services provided directly to clients are reimbursable at this time; although training family members and nursing home staff in the use of management strategies may be very beneficial in terms of helping the person with dementia to communicate better, such training is not reimbursable.
- As a member of an interdisciplinary care team, an SLP may devise a treatment plan (functional maintenance plan) for individuals in a nursing home but provide very little in the way of direct treatment services to persons with dementia.
- The SLP provides information to all team members about the communication strengths and weaknesses of individuals with dementia and may observe the person and/or event-specific factors that have led to behavioral disturbances.
- The SLP also solicits this information from other team members, as they may see the person with dementia in different contexts.
- The SLP may work with the physician to balance the amount of medication, positive communication behaviors, and negative communication behaviors.
- The SLP may work with other staff (nurses, nurses' aids, recreation therapists) to implement the strategies designed to improve communication.

11

End-of-Life Care for Persons With Alzheimer's Disease

More than 5 million Americans now have Alzheimer's disease and it is the seventh-leading cause of death in the United States.

Alzheimer's Association

Persons with early-stage Alzheimer's are generally cared for at home with or without regular nonprofessional caregivers. As the disease progresses to its severe stages, the requirement for long-term care assisted-living facilities or nursing homes increases dramatically. Figure 11.1 provides the natural history of AD and its progression. The changes shown in the figure represent the general range of symptoms for AD. The specific problems, along with the rate and severity of decline, can vary considerably in different individuals.

As mentioned previously, persons with end-stage AD forget to eat, essentially starving themselves. Some demonstrate morbid hunger, eating everything in sight but still losing weight. Many forget other basic activities of daily living like toileting (e.g., losing control of their bowels or bladders) and dressing. Some compulsively touch everything; some have seizures; and others pick up repetitive motor habits, like constant chewing or lip smacking. End-stage Alzheimer's persons cannot recognize their loved ones or communicate verbally. They may have difficulty walking and eventually become bedridden, responding only to tactile stimuli. Ultimately, they lose response to pain stimuli and finally lose consciousness.

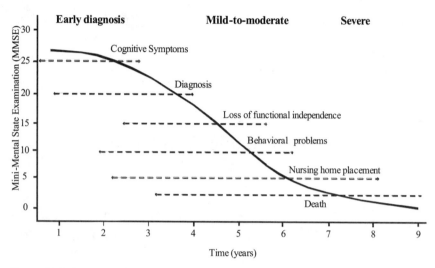

Figure 11.1 Natural history of Alzheimer's disease and its progression.
Source: "Alzheimer's Disease: Symptomatic Drugs Under Development," by H. Feldman and S. Gracon, 1996, in S. Gauthier (Ed.), *Clinical Diagnosis and Management of Alzheimer's Disease*. London: Martin Dunitz, p. 241. Copyright © 1996 Elsevier.

END-STAGE ALZHEIMER'S DISEASE CARE

As AD progresses to its later stages, individuals with the disease have no way to communicate how they feel. They will likely have lost the ability to respond to sensory stimuli, which will make it difficult to discern whether they are comfortable or uncomfortable. Caregivers attending to a person unable to respond or speak must trust their own instincts and their basic understanding of their loved one's likes and dislikes. Caregivers should also seek advice from health care professionals, Alzheimer's support organizations, and other caregivers.

There are many ways to express reassurance and love to people under care who cannot recognize their caregivers or communicate verbally. Though they might not be able to respond, people with late-stage Alzheimer's experience the world through their senses. According to the Mayo Clinic (Mayo Clinic.com, 2007e), family and friends can use senses such as touch, smell, sight, and hearing to maintain a connection with their loved one. Touching through hand-holding, kissing, combing the hair—even a gentle massage—may be reassuring to a person with Alzheimer's. Smells of favorite perfumes, flowers, and foods can be helpful. Hearing music, a tone, rhythm, or laughter can bring comfort. The sight of familiar faces or videos with scenes of nature can be relaxing. If a person is mobile or in a wheelchair, it can be stimulating to take him outside for a walk.

END-OF-LIFE CARE

The time always comes when a person with AD appears to have a very poor quality of life, and, to make matters worse, such people are unable to verbalize to others what they need and how they would like to be treated. End-of-life (EOL) care has been a common option for patients with terminal cancer, but for persons with AD, it has only recently become available.

The common issues that arise in AD's end stages are pain, difficulty breathing and swallowing, infection, lack of interest in eating food, and pressure sores (Alzheimer's Association, New York City Chapter, 2007b). People with advanced AD suffer not only from cognitive impairment but also from physical impairment. As the disease progresses, it becomes very difficult to coordinate breathing and swallowing. This problem may lead to aspiration of food and fluids into the lungs, which then become a good medium for bacterial growth, resulting in aspiration pneumonia— the most common cause of death in persons with Alzheimer's dementia. A person with advanced AD can live up to a year coordinating breathing and swallowing but might struggle with many bouts of aspiration pneumonia. Usually the person can be successfully treated with antibiotics, but the underlying problem is never corrected and the patient will redevelop the infection. If antibiotics fail to improve the pneumonia symptoms, it may be logical to withdraw them to alleviate any discomfort. Individuals experiencing difficulty breathing can be offered oxygen for labored breathing and comfort. Some people do not want oxygen, because the face mask or nasal cannula can be uncomfortable to them. People at the EOL can become congested and produce secretions in their mouth, leading to trouble with breathing. In the dying person, suctioning will only increase the amount of secretions and cause more pain. Sometimes turning a person's head to the side can be beneficial as it will help drain the mouth from the side.

A dying person almost always loses interest in eating and drinking. Caregivers at this point should not worry about nutrition and hydration. If the person is not eating due to constipation, pain, nausea, or stomach inflammation, or if the person is not near death, other modes of nutrition may be attempted. As an alternative to oral feedings, persons who have asked to have intravenous fluids and/or feeding tubes in the stomach can obtain nutrition in this manner, which will prolong life. If the person opted not to have artificial nutrition and hydration, he may die in 1 to 2 weeks without any discomfort. It has been shown that adequate hydration and nutrition are not comfort measures, that is, patients can be perfectly comfortable (if oral care is maintained), even if they are undernourished and underhydrated (Ham, 1997). An individual and family members should understand that artificial hydration in a dying person can actually worsen swelling and increase pain if the pain is caused by inflammation. The only discomfort associated with not drinking fluids is dry mouth, which can easily be managed by swabbing a person's mouth with a wet swab, placing a few ice chips in the patient's mouth, and applying lip balms and glycerin.

Some people in the EOL become bed-bound due to muscle contraction and loss of the ability to walk. If they are bed-bound and not turned regularly into different positions, people can develop pressure ulcers. This skin breakdown can become infected and very painful. Bedsores can be prevented by frequently turning and exercising the extremities every 2 hours. Special pressure-reducing mattresses or beds can help relieve pressure and pain in those who experience too much pain when their body is moved.

Up until the EOL, people with Alzheimer's and other dementias deserve respect, compassion, and access to treatment that can manage their symptoms and maintain comfort. Treatment of persons with end-stage AD should focus on managing comfort and pain until the EOL. It is important for a patient to know that care will continue right up until the EOL and that everything possible will be done to ensure that their death will be peaceful and dignified.

End-of-Life Planning

As the aging population increases and our advances in medicine allow for an increased quantity of life—but no guarantee of quality of life—individuals with Alzheimer's and caregivers must make decisions to anticipate the future. As mentioned previously, AD is a terminal disease, and currently there are no absolute cures or preventive measures available. AD progression can be slowed for a few years, but eventually there is a point where current methods need to be withdrawn because they will not make a difference in the person's quality of life.

When death becomes a real possibility, EOL decisions must be given attention. EOL decisions regarding AD almost always fall into the laps of the family and can provoke a range of strong and difficult emotions, such as anxiety, uncertainty, and sadness.

Persons at the end stage of Alzheimer's typically die within a year or two. There are some difficult questions that need to be addressed by persons with Alzheimer's and their caregivers when the final stages of AD arrive.

1   Where is the dividing line, if there is one, between living and dying?
2   When is it time to choose comfort care over lifesaving care?
3   When does medical care merely prolong a person's dying time?
4   What can caregivers do to be involved?

Preplanning for AD's end stages is also an important step. By taking the initiative early to plan for future financial and medical needs, individuals with AD and their families can be well prepared for the EOL decision-making process. This chapter focuses on the types of decisions to be made and the questions to take under consideration when dealing with the EOL of an AD-inflicted individual.

Coping With EOL

It is always difficult to accept the death of a loved one, but accepting the impending death of a loved one, which families living with AD must do, can be even more difficult. The acceptance of a looming death may be only intellectual at first, but it turns more emotional once the death actually occurs (Helpguide.com, 2007b). One way to cope with death is by learning more about the disease and its course, as described in this book and in other resources provided. It is important for caregivers to take care of their own well-being, and they should communicate with friends and relatives about their grief. Support groups are available for caregivers dealing with the impending death of a loved one with AD. Spiritual guidance, even if one is not religious, can also be helpful. Spiritual guidance can be provided by a member of the clergy, a mental health professional, or even a close friend. Among things to discuss, caregivers can talk about how they will remember the person after he is gone and how he has contributed to the caregiver's life.

In the early stages of AD, the persons may be able to discuss the progression of and the prognosis for the disease from which they are suffering. Generally, if persons with terminal illness say they are ready to die, it should be considered as a good sign, as the individual may have reached a calm acceptance of reality. In the last stage of Alzheimer's, the person will be unable to communicate at all. During the last weeks or days of the disease, caregivers and the family may notice a nonverbal indication of a willingness to let go of life. The person is communicating a readiness to die. This is a positive way of drifting into an inevitable death.

PREPARING FOR THE FUTURE

Alzheimer's disease eventually robs people of the intellectual capacity to make decisions about their own medical care. This is one of the reasons it is so important to talk about these types of choices early on in the course of the disease. Living wills should be prepared and health care proxies should be appointed as soon as the diagnosis of Alzheimer is made, but this is recommended only if the person with AD is of sound mind. Whether with AD or any other terminal disease, it is important to have legal and financial affairs in place and to assign loved ones certain responsibilities to ensure that a patient's best interests will be upheld when the end is near.

Difficult decisions about EOL include deciding what type of health care an individual will want, which is a personal decision that can vary from one person to the other. Most people will agree that quality of life supersedes quantity of life. Most physicians advise their patients to consult with family members, spiritual leaders, and others about their EOL decisions. Usually, the physician's role is to act as an advocate for their patients, but patients should always know it is their decision to make in the end.

Financial Planning

Alzheimer's disease tends to be one of the most costly chronic illnesses in America, with a far-reaching impact on such things as the ill person's estate, the well-being of the family, and their influence in the community. It is important to begin long-term financial planning before the person diagnosed with AD loses the capacity to make important decisions. Advanced planning may relieve some of the burden on caregivers and other family members when important issues arise.

Long-term care in a community setting or in an institution is expensive and can be supported only with careful and organized planning. Professional financial managers are available who specialize in financial planning for people with long-term or progressive illnesses. The family may want to assess which other financial resources may be available through community, state, or government programs. The Alzheimer's Disease Association of the Philippines (2007) lists a few financial mechanisms to consider when beginning financial planning for people diagnosed with AD:

- Potential care expenses, such as follow-up physician visits, prescription medications, care services, and housing
- Current sources of income, such as insurance, personal savings, investments, and employee or retirement benefits
- Other financial resources available through government assistance or community-based organizations

Certain documents and relationships must be put into place to ensure that the future desires of the individual with Alzheimer's will be fulfilled. Clearly written legal documents that outline wishes and decisions of the individual with Alzheimer's are essential, and these documents can authorize another person to make financial decisions on behalf of the person with AD. If the person with AD has the legal capacity, meaning the required level of mental functioning necessary to sign official documents, she should actively participate in financial planning.

Another professional to turn to is an attorney, who can be very helpful in obtaining legal advice on financial and property-related issues. Legal and financial issues of caring for someone with Alzheimer's are discussed in the following sections.

Will

A will is a document created by an individual that names an *executor* (the person who will manage the estate) and *beneficiaries* (those who will receive the estate at the time of the person's death). In other words, a will indicates how a person's assets and estate will be distributed. It also can specify arrangements for care of minors, gifts, trusts to manage the estate and funeral, and/or burial arrangements. Legal experts suggest that a newly diagnosed person with AD and family members move quickly to make or update a will and secure the estate (National Institute on Aging, 2007c).

Durable Power of Attorney for Finances

A financial power of attorney can be either durable or nondurable. A durable power of attorney for finances gives a person with AD an opportunity to authorize an agent—usually a trusted family member or friend—to make legal decisions when she is no longer competent. A durable power of attorney can help people with AD and their families avoid court actions that may take away control of financial affairs. Most people consider durable powers of attorney when there is a chronic illness involved or a date in the future when it might be foreseeable that illness can be disruptive to someone's judgment. A nondurable power of attorney, on the other hand, is generally used for limited, specific transactions, like the closing on the sale of residence or the handling of the principal's financial affairs while the principal is traveling outside of the country.

Living Trust

A living trust provides instructions about the Alzheimer's person's estate and appoints someone, often referred to as the trustee, to hold title to property and funds for the beneficiaries. The trustee follows these instructions after the person with AD can no longer manage these affairs.

Health Planning

Like financial planning, health planning should also begin soon after a diagnosis of AD has been made. Legal and medical experts encourage people recently diagnosed with a serious illness—particularly one that is expected to cause declining mental and physical health—to examine and update their health care arrangements as soon as possible (National Institute on Aging, 2007c). People with Alzheimer's may have the capacity to manage their own legal affairs during the early stage of the disease, and transitioning that power to someone else might be very difficult. Legal documents related to health care must be put into place early on or providing care can become much more legally complicated and expensive than is necessary. Medical lawyers are available who deal with health planning for people with long-term or progressive illnesses.

When discussing medical options, all parties should be aware of the risks and benefits, the probable outcome of continuing or refusing to follow a medical treatment plan, and any alternatives to the diagnostic test or procedure. The individual's decision-making capacity should be routinely assessed, since many are able to voice their desires in the mild and moderate stages of AD. Determining the decision-making capacity of a person with AD should involve an assessment of the ability to communicate choices, understand and retain relevant information, appreciate a situation and its consequences, and manipulate information rationally (Miller & Marin, 2000). Attempts to solve differences of opinion should be made via family conferences so that all members of the treatment team and concerned family members are involved.

When families begin the legal planning process, there are a number of legal documents they will need to discuss that concern the health care of the individual diagnosed with AD. Table 11.1 summarizes legal documents required for financial and health planning. Quite frequently, the term *advance directives* is used to describe these documents. There are five advance directives: a power of attorney, a health care proxy, a will, a living will, and a Do Not Resuscitate (DNR) order.

If a person with AD is under long-term care, it is the long-term institution's responsibility to ascertain the individual's wishes on admission. The following topics should be addressed in the document: DNR orders, transport to hospital, use of mechanical ventilator, use of artificial

Table 11.1

OVERVIEW OF LEGAL, MEDICAL, AND FINANCIAL PLANNING DOCUMENTS

Medical document	How it is used
Durable power of attorney for health care	Gives a designated person the authority to make health care decisions on behalf of someone else.
Living will	Describes and instructs how the person wants end-of-life health care managed.
Do not resuscitate form	Instructs health care staff not to perform specified lifesaving or other heroic measures.

Legal/financial document	
Will	Indicates how a person's assets and estate will be distributed among beneficiaries after his or her death.
Durable power of attorney for finances	Gives a designated person the authority to make legal and financial decisions on behalf of the person.
Living trust	Describes how the person wants to allocate funds and settlements.

nutrition and hydration, use of antibiotics in various forms, and renal dialysis. If there is no advance directive on record and the person with AD is not competent, it is still essential to make every effort to determine the person's wishes. Staff may consider asking nontraditional surrogates, such as a close friend or a neighbor who has cared for the person for years. At times, it may be necessary to have a surrogate appointed by the court. In an emergent situation, the physician plus a consultant may make a decision.

Durable Power of Attorney for Health Care

A durable power of attorney regarding health care is also known as a health care proxy or a medical power of attorney. A durable power of attorney for health care appoints an agent to make all decisions regarding health care, including choices regarding health care providers, medical treatment, appropriate places to live, and end-of-life decisions. It can be helpful when a person is unable to make medical decisions for herself.

Living Will

This document allows the person with AD to express his decision on the use of artificial life-support systems. There are many things that a living can resolve for people with AD if their death is impending. A person with AD must consider if he would want:

- To be hospitalized
- To be put on a respirator
- To have CPR performed
- To have surgery
- To have blood transfusions
- To have a feeding tube
- To have medicine administered
- To be resuscitated

The main difference between a living will and a durable power of attorney is simple: a living will goes into effect if a person is facing an illness, such as AD, where death is certain. The durable power of attorney for health care is a document that allows the assignee to make medical decisions for a person even if he is not facing death.

Do Not Resuscitate (DNR)

A DNR order tells the health care facility or doctor not to revive a patient whose heart or breathing has stopped. A DNR order requires the signatures of the person or a substitute and attending physician.

ETHICAL ISSUES IN ALZHEIMER'S END-OF-LIFE

According to the Alzheimer Society of Canada (2007), an ethical dilemma is a situation in which:

- One is unsure of what to do
- Two or more values may be in conflict
- Some harm may be caused, no matter what one does

When making an ethical decision, there are additional considerations, which include:

- The obligation to act
- The available options
- The best option, taking into consideration one's authority to act, one's values, the consequences, and concern for others

The Alzheimer Association's Ethics Advisory Panel proposes that efforts to prolong life in the advanced stage of Alzheimer's result in unnecessary suffering for people who could otherwise reach the end of life in relative comfort and peace (Mayo Clinic.com, 2007e). Life-sustaining treatment is any treatment that serves to prolong life without reversing the underlying medical condition. Unfortunately, advanced dementia due to AD is often not perceived by many as a terminal illness, and the prognosis is vastly overestimated. According to a study of nursing home admission, only 1% of residents with advanced dementia were perceived to have a life expectancy of less than 6 months, although 71% died during that period (Mitchell et al., 2004). A palliative approach is optimal for residents with AD, but unfortunately, studies show that nonpalliative interventions are more common—tube feeding in 25%, laboratory tests in 49%, restraints in 11%, and intravenous therapy in 10% of residents with advanced dementia (Mitchell, Kiely, & Hamel, 2004). Use of life-sustaining intensive care (e.g., mechanical ventilation, renal dialysis, antibiotics, cardiopulmonary resuscitation, and artificial nutrition and hydration) near the EOL and during the advanced stage of AD raises ethical issues.

While progress has been made in clinical and ethical decision making related to the use of life-sustaining treatment for people with advanced stage of AD, this area still remains on the margins of mainstream bioethics. Wanzer and associates (2004) defined four levels of care: (1) emergency resuscitation, (2) intensive care and advanced life support, (3) general medical care (e.g., antibiotics, surgery), and (4) comfort care. They suggest that the physician, patient, family, and other health care personnel together should make the decision regarding what level of care to assign to a person. They hold that those who receive comfort care should be clearly in the terminal phase of an irreversible illness, including dementia. The American Academy of Neurology, Ethics and Humanities Subcommittee (1996) concluded that appropriate care in advanced AD includes use of morphine for pain, mouth care, hygienic measures, grooming, skin care, bowel and bladder care, and positioning; it does not include attempts at resuscitation, hospitalization, or surgery unless imperative for comfort. Withdrawing and withholding treatment are equally justifiable, ethically and legally.

Decisions to withhold or withdraw treatment at the advanced stage of AD are increasingly important because they have to be made more frequently and more explicitly. The person with AD and the family should be involved whenever possible. Unfortunately, some health care workers and family members may be reluctant to withdraw treatments even when they believe that the patient would not have wanted them continued. The physician should prevent or resolve these situations by addressing with families feelings of guilt, fears, and concerns about withdrawing life support (American Academy of Neurology, Ethics and Humanities Subcommittee, 1996).

While many agree that patients have a clear right to refuse unwanted life-sustaining treatments, there is less consensus about patients' rights to demand those same life-sustaining treatments once a dismal prognosis has been made (Schneiderman, Jecker, & Jonsen, 1990). Many physicians, conflicted about providing this care, are looking for guidance on the question of futility. To clarify the discussion, some have defined futility in qualitative, quantitative, and physiological terms (Truog, Brett, & Frader, 1992). Qualitative futility means that applying the treatment will not improve the patient's quality of life, which is already unacceptably poor. The obvious problem with a qualitative definition of futility is that patients (or their surrogates) and physicians may disagree on exactly what constitutes a poor quality of life (Youngner, 1988). The concept of quantitative futility, on the other hand, does not consider quality-of-life issues. Under this definition, a numeric probability of survival is used to decide which treatments can be considered futile and, therefore, not offered, because the patient is unlikely to survive even with the intervention (Schneiderman, Jecker, & Jonsen, 1990). This view accords physicians much discretion, including the authority to make unilateral treatment decisions. Finally, physiological futility has been suggested to define situations in which it is impossible for the intervention to benefit the patient at all (Truog, Brett, & Frader, 1992). Under this type of definition, prolonged artificial nutrition and hydration for a patient confirmed to be in a persistent vegetative state would not be futile because the patient would physically benefit from such treatment, but performing a lung transplant for someone with widely metastatic lung cancer would be futile. While nearly everyone agrees that in cases of physiological futility physicians are not obligated to provide treatment, there is less consensus about what to do in cases of qualitative or quantitative futility, when the patient or surrogate chooses continued treatment.

Antibiotics

Most of the literature regarding the ethics of EOL care and the treatment of persons with severe dementia focuses on issues of resuscitation and the use of advanced technology. The ethical issues concerning the use of antibiotics are discussed much less frequently (Marcus, Clarfield, & Allon, 2001). People in the advanced stage of AD continue to receive antibiotics, which is consistent with the view that physicians may find the administration of these drugs to be routine and less subject to either withdrawal or withholding. Most physicians may feel more comfortable in continuing to try to correct a theoretically reversible condition by the use of antibiotics even in the face of an irreversible dying process. During the past decade, professional organizations and the medical community have raised questions based on ethical issues and on clinical studies of treatment decisions for persons with advanced stage of AD. In a study conducted by Volicer and associates (1986) in patients with advanced dementia of the Alzheimer type with symptoms of pneumonia or urinary tract infections, it was found that 62% of those patients not treated with antibiotics did not present with a significant increase in mortality during the first year. On the other hand, Loewy (1996) claims that treating a person with severe dementia for pneumonia may be justified, because such an infection poses an immediate threat at a time when a person still has a reasonable short-term ability to "profit from life." Loewy further claims that such treatment entails the relief of suffering, involves little addition of discomfort, and does not require enlisting the person's sustained cooperation to accomplish therapeutic goals. Likewise, others feel that, for persons with a terminal illness, antibiotics can be a part of comfort care (Finlay, 1996). One could also argue that, in cases in which quality of life is so poor that life itself is not worth living, any treatment that extends life, no matter how simple the treatment is, offers more burden than benefit (Brody, Campbell, Faber-Langendoen, & Ogle, 1997). Ahronheim and associates (1996) argue that antibiotics might even prolong suffering in some situations and that comfort measures, such as sedation, may be used as palliation. The debate on the use of antibiotics in advanced stage of dementia continues. The Council of Ethical and Judicial Affairs of the American Medical Association (1998) stated, "The social commitment of the physician is to sustain life and relieve suffering. Where the performance of one conflict with the other, the preferences of the patient should prevail. The principle of patient autonomy requires that physicians respect the decision to forgo life-sustaining treatment of a patient who possesses a decision-making capacity."

Nutrition and Hydration

Losing the ability to self-feed, hold food in the mouth, chew and swallow, spit, and aspire (breath) is very common in people at the late stage of AD. Gradual weight loss is also quite common in advanced stage of AD. People in advanced-stage AD may lose all interest in eating and drinking and be unable to complete sufficient oral feedings that would prevent weight loss. Eventually, the ability to swallow is also lost. At this stage, a decision on whether to have artificial nutrition and hydration (ANH) through tube feeding and intravenous hydration is inevitable, and the clinicians need to weigh the potential benefits and burdens of ANH.

There are divergent views regarding the appropriateness of ANH in individuals with advanced-stage AD. There is a frequently held belief that feeding tubes will significantly promote comfort for the individual with Alzheimer's and prevent suffering, reduce the risk of aspiration pneumonia and infections, maintain skin integrity, and prevent the person from starving to death (McCarron & McCallion, 2007). Though ANH can provide calories and prevent dehydration, there is lack of sufficient data to indicate that tube feeding in advanced dementia will prevent pneumonia, prevent or improve pressure sores, or delay mortality (Finucane, Christmas, & Travis, 1999). The lack of data to support tube feedings has led some authorities to conclude that long-term-care facilities should not offer this option in advanced AD (Gillick, 2000). Obviously, the decision to implement or withdraw tube feedings will be dependent on many factors, including institutional and state-specific policies (Teno et al., 2002). Data suggest that tube feeding is beneficial to a person with a reversible illness—which is usually not the case in persons who have advanced dementia. If a person is actively dying, his body no longer absorbs or uses nutrients. Therefore, tube feeding at the end stages of AD may not be beneficial in prolonging a person's life. Research also suggests that those persons who forgo ANH do not seem to feel thirsty or hungry. In fact, research has shown that in the absence of ANH, the body draws on endorphin, a morphine-like substance in the body that blunts nerve endings, making the person more comfortable and less likely to experience pain (Lynn & Harrold, 1999).

The Ethics Advisory Panel of the Alzheimer's Association (2000) recommends assisted oral feeding coupled with hospice care, when needed, as the compassionate alternative to tube feeding. This recommendation is based on several studies that point out that tube feeding:

- Is associated with increased diarrhea and related discomforts
- Results in increased use of physical restraints to prevent patients from pulling tubes out of their abdomens
- Does not usually improve nutritional status
- Does not lower the incidence of aspiration pneumonia or skin breakdown
- Does not improve longevity
- Denies the patient the gratification of tasting preferred foods

The Alzheimer's Association (1997) also emphasizes that "assisted oral feeding should be available to all persons with advanced Alzheimer's as needed. Neglect in this area should not be tolerated, and concerted efforts are called for to educate and support professional and family caregivers in techniques of assisted oral feeding." The only side effect of dehydration at the end of life is dry mouth, which can be relieved by good mouth care, ice chips, or moistened sponge swabs.

As with all therapies, this decision should be based primarily on the resident's wishes. If the patient's advance directive indicates that he or she does not want ANH, caregivers must respect that decision. However, if the decision was not made earlier, this is the time when the person's surrogate decision maker, together with the physician and other members of the health team, must decide whether to initiate tube feedings. The physician and health care professionals need to help families understand that forgoing ANH is not killing or starving the individual with advanced AD.

Cardiopulmonary Resuscitation

The most difficult decisions of a person's lifetime are the ones that occur when a loved one is dying. The decision to let go is extremely difficult for a family. Families occasionally choose a more aggressive course of treatment, which is really alleviating their uncomfortable emotions, rather than doing what is in the best interest of the patient. It is believed that during the advanced stage of AD, the withholding of cardiopulmonary resuscitation (CPR) in a life-or-death situation, through a document known as a No CPR order, is the only reasonable medical course. Families often have a hard time with this idea and refuse to consent to a No CPR order. Medical ethics offers three useful principles on whether or not CPR should be administered. All three are based on the patient's wishes. First, a victim of cardiopulmonary arrest should receive CPR unless compelling reasons indicate he would not want it. Second, a patient has the right to refuse CPR. Finally, if CPR will serve no therapeutic goals as defined by the patient's wishes, it should not be given (Perkins, 1986).

According to Volicer (2005), CPR is three times less likely to be successful in a person with dementia than in one who is cognitively intact. Those who do survive are taken to an intensive-care unit, where most die within 24 hours. The American Medical Association (1998) Council on Ethical and Judicial Affairs states that "Physicians are not ethically obligated to deliver care that, in their best professional judgment, will not have a reasonable chance of benefiting their patients." A judgment that CPR would not be beneficial warrants an order in the patient's record that physicians should refrain from doing it: "If, in the judgment of the attending physician, it would be inappropriate to pursue CPR, the attending physician may enter a DNR order in the patient's record." Resuscitative efforts should be considered inappropriate "only if they cannot be expected either to restore cardiac or respiratory function to the patient or to meet established ethical criteria." Some people, for personal or religious reasons, may be opposed to a DNR order. It is a physician's responsibility to let a family know that success of CPR in persons with significant cognitional impairment is very poor.

Renal Dialysis

At the end of life, even life-sustaining procedures, such as renal dialysis, may not be medically appropriate. Many people believe that dialysis is not appropriate for a person with end-stage dementia. Many physicians believe it should not be used if the person will die very soon with or without dialysis. Even if a person can survive, the choice of whether dialysis makes sense depends on the person's basic health, chances of recovery, and will to live and on the burdens and benefits of further treatment. In the view of the Alzheimer's Association's Ethics Advisory Panel (2000), use of renal dialysis in advance AD is considered a life-extension effort.

Renal dialysis is expensive, and each dialysis session is long, lasting for approximately 4 hours. Each trip to dialysis may become an ordeal. People with advanced AD may not cooperate during the dialysis. Most physicians believe that dialysis is more of a burden than a benefit for people with advanced Alzheimer's dementia. Furthermore, they feel that dialysis may be a waste of resources for someone with such a poor quality of life. Again, the decision to have a terminal patient with AD undergo renal dialysis is one that a family and a team of health care providers should make together.

Mechanical Ventilator

Quality-of-life considerations have increased the pressure on health care professionals and caregivers to assess the use of life-sustaining treatments when it comes to advanced AD. Where is the balance between a commitment to life and a commonsense willingness to "let go" when the time comes (Sullivan, 2005)? Most physicians believe that life-sustaining treatments in advanced Alzheimer's dementia can become extraordinary under one or two conditions. If they create burdens for the person to such an extent that these burdens outweigh the benefits, then the life-support treatment is considered an extraordinary means and may be withheld or withdrawn upon the request of the individual with Alzheimer's or a surrogate. The same holds true if a particular life-support treatment would benefit an individual for only a short period of time (e.g., a ventilator that extends a person's life for 2 or 3 months). Ethically, even though a benefit is offered, the use of the ventilator is considered "futile" and, therefore, optional. According to the Alzheimer's Association of the Great Plains (2007), people with Alzheimer's have the legal right to limit or forgo medical or life-sustaining treatment, including the use of mechanical ventilators.

CARE AT THE END OF LIFE

As a person progresses to the end stages of AD, it is to be hoped that he has prepared a living will and designated an appropriate health care proxy. An individual with AD has certain options to choose from in the late stages of life. They can go for exceptional medical care whose goal is to prolong life by any means necessary or may opt for a more conservative approach to care with the goal of maintaining health. An individual may also elect to continue treatment for their comorbid conditions, such as hypertension and diabetes. Finally, a person with AD may choose comfort or palliative care at the end of life, where the main objective is pain control and maintenance of quality of life through non-life-sustaining support and/or emotional and spiritual support. It should be understood that palliative care is provided when no cure exists and death is imminent. In the last stage, care may be given at home or in a hospital or nursing home, as was discussed in the preceding chapters of this book. An individual may also choose to receive care through hospice—a form of palliative care and emotional and spiritual support in the late stages of a terminal illness. The physician can continue to direct care and to guide the patient and the family to other resources as needed.

Dying With Dignity: Comfort, Not Life Extension

Helping someone with Alzheimer's through the last years of their life is one of the most difficult parts of caring for the disease. As the disease progresses, caregivers end up making more and more decisions based on the individual's advance directives or their simple wishes. Among the most profound of these responsibilities is ensuring that the person's most basic needs for respect, dignity, and physical comfort are sustained until the end of life (Mayo Clinic.com, 2007e). Health care providers, caregivers, family, and friends need to ensure that dying people are treated with dignity and respect.

Hospice

Alzheimer's disease is considered incurable and terminal, so pain management, comfort care, and a focus on quality of life are priorities (Haak & Peters, 2004). Hospice provides a special way of caring for a person who is terminally ill and for the person's family. Hospice is a philosophy of care where death is recognized as a natural stage of life. People with AD can benefit from hospice in many ways. Symptoms are controlled, so days are filled with dignity and quality, while being shared with loved ones. Hospice care is typically reserved for people who have 6 months or less to live. Delivered by highly skilled professionals with expertise and compassion, hospice offers care to the patient and support for the family unit as a whole.

A hospice is a program designed to care for the dying and their special needs (ALS Society of Alberta, 2006). Among these services, all hospice programs should include:

- Control of pain and other symptoms through medication, environmental adjustment, and education
- Psychosocial support for both the patient and family, from diagnosis through bereavement
- Medical services commensurate with the needs of the patient
- Interdisciplinary team approach to patient care, patient and family support, and education with physician leadership
- Integration into existing facilities where possible
- Specially trained personnel with expertise in the care of the dying and their families

Unfortunately, hospice services are not as commonly used for persons with AD as they are for cancer patients. In fact, fewer than 3% of the nation's hospice census comprises patients with AD (Hoyert & Rosenberg, 1999), whereas 80% of Medicare cancer patients are enrolled in hospice (Matzo, 2004). This is partly because it is difficult to predict how long a person with end-stage Alzheimer's will live. The National Hospice and Palliative Care Organization (NHPCO) has published guidelines to help determine which individuals with dementia are likely to have a prognosis of 6 months or less, which may help physicians determine when hospice is appropriate for people with AD. In general, the guidelines require a severity of dementia in which the person has lost the ability to communicate in any meaningful way and can no longer walk without assistance. In addition, the guidelines require that at least one dementia-related medical complication be present, such as aspiration pneumonia, upper urinary tract infection, sepsis or other overwhelming infection, worsening bedsores, or weight loss greater than 10% over the past 6 months.

If persons with AD qualify for hospice care, they can get medical and support services, including nursing care, social services, physician services, counseling, homemaker services, and other types of services. Depending on the person's medical condition, hospice care can be provided in the home, a hospice facility, an assisted living facility, or a nursing home. A team of physicians, nurses, home health aides, social workers, counselors, and trained volunteers is available to help the dying person and the family to cope with the illness. Hospice services are provided by a multidisciplinary team of professionals who work to maximize comfort for the terminally ill person and to help support the family members and loved ones.

A hospice care team consists of:

Physicians. Both a primary-care physician and the hospice's medical director oversee the care. The primary-care physician remains the main physician in charge, but the hospice medical director often has added expertise in symptoms management and end-of-life care that can supplement the care provided by the primary physician.

Nurses. Nurses come to the home or other care setting for regular evaluations and report back to the physician. Nurses also provide help and support for family members and friends. They can address any concerns the caregivers may have about EOL issues and symptoms management. The frequency of nursing visits depends upon the amount of care needed. Nurses are available at all times for emergency visits in case a change or crisis develops. They can also offer support and guidance at the time of death.

Home Health Aides. Home health aides and homemaker services can assist the caregiver in caring for individual with AD. Home health aides provide extra support for routine care, such as helping the person with dressing, bathing, and eating.

Spiritual Counselors. Chaplains, priests, lay ministers, or other spiritual counselors are available to the person with AD and his family. Many people in hospice care have connections to some spiritual services in their community, but the hospice can provide additional services, if desired.

Social Workers. Social workers provide counseling and support. They can also help you sort out insurance and other financial concerns.

Volunteers. Trained hospice volunteers provide a variety of services, such as staying with the individual with AD while the caregiver runs errands, providing transportation assistance, or just being a companion by playing cards or reading to her.

Bereavement Counselors. Trained bereavement counselors offer support and guidance for the family during and after the death of the person with Alzheimer's. Bereavement counselors continue to provide support for up to a year after death.

Medicare Hospice Benefit (Center to Advance Palliative Care, 2002) limits care to patients who:

■ Agree to therapy with a palliative intent
■ Have a life expectancy of less than 6 months if the disease runs its usual course in the judgment of the patient's attending physician and the hospice medical director
■ Elect the Medicare Hospice Benefit for coverage of all services related to their terminal illness

Palliative Care

The field of palliative care is one response to the changing profile of death in the twenty-first century. To *palliate* means to make comfortable by treating a person's symptoms from an illness or a disease. Various groups have defined palliative care in diverse ways, but each of the proposed definitions shares the same goals: relieving suffering and improving quality of life. The Institute of Medicine (1997) defines palliative care as follows: "Palliative care seeks to prevent, relieve, reduce or soothe the symptoms of disease or disorder without effecting a cure....Palliative care in this broad sense is not restricted to those who are dying or those enrolled in hospice programs....It attends closely to the emotional, spiritual, and practical needs and goals of patients and those close to them."

The World Health Organization (WHO) (1990) defines palliative care as "The active total care of patients whose disease is not responsive to curative treatment. Control of pain, of other symptoms, and of psychological, social and spiritual problems, is paramount. The goal of palliative care is achievement of the best quality of life for patients and their families. Many aspects of palliative care are also applicable earlier in the course of the illness in conjunction with anti-cancer treatment." Further elaborating this definition, the WHO notes that palliative care:

- Affirms life and regards dying as a normal process
- Neither hastens nor postpones death
- Provides relief from pain and other distressing symptoms
- Integrates the psychological and spiritual aspects of care, fostering opportunities to grow
- Offers an interdisciplinary team to help patients live as actively as possible until death
- Offers a support system for the family during the patient's illness and their own bereavement

Palliative care is not just limited to cancer (as it was in the past). It now encompasses any illness or disease that cannot be cured. It is a type of care designed for people who have illnesses that do not go away and often get worse with time.

The goal of palliative care for a person with AD is to improve quality of life in a physical, emotional, spiritual, and psychosocial sense. It can help people cope with their feelings about living with a chronic illness, and it can also help manage symptoms, pain, or side effects from treatment. Hospice may be the standard method for providing quality EOL care in the United States, but studies reveal that persons with AD are infrequently referred to hospice. According to these studies, barriers to hospice exist in this population, even though patients with AD would benefit from hospice or hospice-like services earlier in the course of the disease. To respond to these discrepancies, the Palliative Excellence in Alzheimer Care Efforts (PEACE) program was implemented by the University of Chicago Medical Center. The PEACE program is a disease-management model for dementia that incorporates advance planning, patient-centered care, family support, and a palliative-care focus from the diagnosis of dementia through its terminal stages (Shega et al., 2003).

Pain Management

Research reports that a direct relationship exists between cognitive impairment and pain. People suffering from AD with impaired cognition suffer a great deal of untreated pain (Haley et al., 1995). As many as 45%–80% of nursing home residents have pain that contributes materially to functional impairment and decreased quality of life (Farrell, 1995). Pain control in a person with end-stage Alzheimer's dementia may be inadequate. One of the causes for inadequate pain control among patients with advanced AD is the difficulty in detecting and assessing intensity of pain (Kim, Yeaman, & Keene, 2005). Patients in AD's late stages cannot express pain level on the 0–10 pain measurement scale, because they can't communicate in general. Another reason pain control is tricky is because elderly people with AD may have different, less obvious ways of expressing pain. A sudden increase in disruptive behavior, such as shouting and striking out at caregivers, may be a sign of inadequate pain control (Mayo Clinic.com, 2007e).

Effective pain management may have important implications for improving quality of life among individuals with end-stage AD (Kim, Yeaman, & Keene, 2005). Pain can be alleviated in end-stage Alzheimer's through the careful use of analgesic drugs combined with nonpharmacologic strategies, including exercise programs and other physical therapy modalities. Elderly people are more sensitive to the side effects associated with many pain medications, but this does not justify a failure to treat pain, especially in those who are terminally ill or near the end of life (Farrell, 1995). If a person with end-stage AD is observed to be in any type of discomfort, it is advised that they will benefit from a standing order for pain medication. This means a person gets Tylenol or morphine every 4 hours around the clock. Pain medications can be over-the-counter, like Advil and Tylenol, or strong narcotics, like morphine. Sometimes a combination of such medications is best. There are times during the dying process where breathing may become somewhat noisy. Morphine may ease breathing and suppress gurgling. Morphine or other pain medication may be administered by injection, via a patch, or, most often, in a form that can be dissolved under the tongue. However, clinicians should be aware that morphine and other opiate drugs can increase confusion among persons with end-stage AD (Kim, Yeaman, & Keene, 2005). In addition to medications, alternative means can provide pain control for patients who can hear and respond. These include guided mental imagery, hypnosis, and relaxation, counseling for stress and anxiety, and spiritual support. Pain control is clearly an area to target at the EOL. But one study revealed that despite the effectiveness of pain controls, one out of five persons does not get relief from pain and uncomfortable symptoms as death approaches (Massachusetts Compassionate Care Coalition, 2007). According to the study, all the modalities are available that are required to ensure that no one dies in pain.

Grief and Bereavement

Grief is a normal and healthy reaction to loss. In the case of AD, it is normal for caregivers to experience loss as the disease progresses. *Anticipatory grief* is the term sometimes used to describe the mixed emotions of a caregiver while a person with Alzheimer's is still alive. Some studies

Table 11.2

FINDING SUPPORT AFTER A LOSS

Friends	Let people who care about you take care of you, even if you take pride in being strong and self-sufficient. Especially when you live away from family, true friends can offer shoulders for you to cry on until you begin to recover.
Family	The death of a relative can create a path for reunion, and even reconciliation, among surviving relatives. (It can also tear families apart, especially in the case of a sudden or violent death, so it's important to be sensitive to one another's approaches to grief and to refrain from accusation.) Sharing your loss can make the burden of grief easier to carry. Reminiscing about the person all of you lost may help everyone recover. If you've lost a friend or spouse, family members can form a caring community.
Your faith community	If you follow a religious tradition, embrace the comfort its mourning rituals can provide. Allow people within your religious community to give you emotional support. If you're estranged from your faith community or have none, this may be a good time to reconnect or to explore alternatives.
Support groups	There are many support groups for people who are grieving, including specialized groups (such as, people who have lost children, survivors of suicides).
Therapists and other professionals	Talking with a psychotherapist or grief counselor may be a good idea if the intensity of your grief doesn't diminish over time, that is, months go by and you still have physical symptoms, such as trouble with eating or sleeping; or your emotional state impairs your ability to go about your daily routine.

Source: "Coping With Grief and Loss: Guide to Grieving and Bereavement," by E. Jaffe-Gill, M. Smith, and J. Segal, 2007, Helpguide.org. Retrieved December 2007, from http://www.helpguide.org/mental/grief_loss.htm. Reprinted with permission from http://www.helpguide.org/. Copyright © 2008 Helpguide.org. All rights reserved.

(Brown & Stoudemire, 1983) suggest that anticipatory grief helps to prepare one for the loss of a loved one, while other studies point out that it makes very little difference (Hill, Thompson, & Gallagher, 1988). Even though the caregiver has experienced anticipatory grief and knows the death will occur, the actual event triggers a new kind of grief. There may be some sense of relief mixed in with the sense of loss (helpguide.com, 2007c). The feelings of guilt, anger, anxiety, depression, and helplessness that are usually associated with the burden of caregiving also add to the grief. In her book *On Death and Dying*, Elisabeth Kübler-Ross (1997) introduced the Five Stages of Grief. These are five stages that a dying person experiences when informed of his terminal prognosis:

1 Denial (*this isn't happening to me*)
2 Anger (*why is this happening to me?*)
3 Bargaining (*I promise I'll be a better person if…*)
4 Depression (*I don't care anymore*)
5 Acceptance (*I'm ready for whatever comes*)

Many people believe that these stages of grief are also experienced by those who are coping with the loss of a loved one. The single most important factor in healing from loss is having the support of friends, family, and professionals. Table 11.2 presents various sources of support.

It is important for caregivers to share their feelings when grieving. Knowing that others know and understand their grieving will make them feel less alone and will ultimately help them heal.

References

About.com. (2007). *Diagnosis of Alzheimer's disease.* Retrieved August 2007, from http://alzheimers.about.com/od/diagnosisissues/Diagnosis_of_Alzheimers_Disease.htm

Abreu, B. C. (1990). *The quadraphonic approach: Evaluation and treatment of the brain injured patient.* New York: Therapeutic Service Systems.

Abreu, B. C. (2000). Self-care management for persons with cognitive deficits after Alzheimer's disease and traumatic brain injury. In C. Christiansen (Ed.), *Ways of living: Self-care strategies for special needs* (pp. 85–121). (2nd ed.). Bethesda, MD: American Occupational Therapy Association.

A.D.A.M. Healthcare Center. (2004a). *Alzheimer's disease.* Retrieved June 2007, from http://adam.about.com/reports/000002_1.htm

A.D.A.M. Healthcare Center. (2004b). *Alzheimer's disease.* Retrieved June 2007, from http://adam.about.com/reports/000002_3.htm

Adelman, A. M., & Daly, M. P. (2005). Initial evaluation of the patient with suspected dementia. *American Family Physician, 71,* 1745–1750.

Administration on Aging, U.S. Department of Health and Human Services. (2007). *AOA fact sheet on Alzheimer's disease.* Retrieved June 2007, from http://www.aoa.gov/alz/public/alzcarefam/disease_info/facts_alz/aoa_factsheet.asp

Administration on Aging Fact Sheet, U.S. Department of Health and Human Services. (2007, September). *Assisted living.* Retrieved October 2007, from http://www.aoa.gov/PRESS/fact/pdf/fs_Assistedliving.doc

Agarwal, K. (2002). Assessment of pain in patients with dementia. *Pain Relief Connection, 1,* 3–6.

Aguero-Torres, H., Fratiglioni, L., Guo, Z., Viitanen, M., Strauss, E. V., & Vinblad, B. (1998). Dementia is the major cause of functional dependence in the elderly: 3-year follow-up data from a population-based study. *American Journal of Public Health, 88,* 1452–1456.

Ahronheim, J. C., Morrison, R. S., Baskin, S. A., Morris, J., & Meier, D. E. (1996). Treatment of the dying in the acute care hospital: Advanced dementia and metastatic disease. *Archives of Internal Medicine, 156,* 2094–2100.

Alexander, M. (2001). The charms of music: Step by step prescription for patients. *North Carolina Medical Journal, 62,* 91–94.

Alexandrov, P. N., Zhao, Y., Pogue, A. I., Tarr, M. A., Kruck, T.P., & Percy, M. E., et al. (2005). Synergistic effects of iron and aluminum on stress-related gene expression in primary human neural cells. *Journal of Alzheimer's Disease, 8,* 117–127.

Allen, C. K. (1982). Independence through activity: The practice of occupational therapy (Psychiatry). *American Journal of Occupational Therapy, 36,* 731–739.

309

Allen, C. K., Earhart, C. A., & Blue, T. (1992). *Occupational therapy treatment goals for the physically and cognitively disabled.* Rockville, MD: American Occupational Therapy Association.

Almor, A., Kempler, D., MacDonald, M. C., Andersen, E. S., & Tyler, L. K. (1999). Why do Alzheimer patients have difficulty with pronouns? Working memory, semantics, and reference in comprehension and production in Alzheimer's disease. *Brain and Language, 67,* 202–227.

Alzheimer Research Forum. (2007, October). *Tests.* Retrieved November 2007, from http://www.alzforum.org/dis/dia/tes/default.asp

Alzheimer's Association. (1997). *Ethical considerations: Issues in death and dying.* Retrieved November 2007, from http://www.alz.org

Alzheimer's Association. (2003a). *Facts: About depression and Alzheimer's disease.* (Prepared by the Clinical Issues and Interventions Work Group of the Alzheimer's Association). Retrieved September 2007, from http://www.alz.org.

Alzheimer's Association. (2003b). *Sleep changes in Alzheimer's disease.* Prepared in consultation with the Clinical Issues and Interventions Work Group of the Alzheimer's Association. Retrieved September 2007, from http://www.alzdsw.org/pdf_documents/factsheets/sleep.pdf

Alzheimer's Association. (2004). *Annual Report; Fiscal Year 2004.* Retrieved July 2007, from http://www.alz-nca.org/annualreport/fy04.pdf

Alzheimer's Association. (2005a). *Living with Alzheimer's: Personal care.* Retrieved August 2007, from http://www.alz.org/living_with_alzheimers_personal_care.asp

Alzheimer's Association. (2005b). *Personal care: Assisting the person with dementia with changing daily needs.* Retrieved September 2007, from http://www.alznyc.org/store/index.php?main_page=popup_image&pID=244

Alzheimer's Association. (2005c). *10 warning signs of Alzheimer's disease.* Retrieved August 2007, from http://www.tnalz.org/10-Warning-Signs.pdf

Alzheimer's Association. (2007a). *Caregivers Forum.* Retrieved September 2007, from http://alzheimers.infopop.cc/eve/forums/a/tpc/f/214102241/m/5731072852

Alzheimer's Association. (2007b). *Steps to diagnosis.* Retrieved November 2007, from http://www.alz.org/alzheimers_disease_steps_to_diagnosis.asp

Alzheimer's Association (2007c). *Alzheimer's Stages.* Retrieved September 2007, from http://www.alz.org/alzheimers_disease_stages_of_alzheimers.asp

Alzheimer's Association. (2007d). *Alzheimer's disease.* Retrieved December 2007, from http://www.alz.org/alheimers_disease.asp

Alzheimer's Association. (2008). *About Alzheimer's.* Retrieved January 2008, from http://www.centralcoastalz.org/about_ad/about_alz.html

Alzheimer's Association, Ethics Advisory Panel. (2000). *Assisted oral feeding and tube feeding.* Retrieved December 2007, from http://www.alz.org/documents/national/FSOralfeeding.pdf

Alzheimer's Association, New York City Chapter. (2007a). *Incontinence and toileting.* Retrieved September 2007, from http://www.alznyc.org/caregivers/incontinence.asp

Alzheimer's Association, New York City Chapter. (2007b). *Late stage care.* Retrieved November 2007, from http://www.alznyc.org/caregivers/latestage.asp

Alzheimer's Association of the Great Plains. (2007). *Late-stage care.* Retrieved November 2007, from http://www.alzgreatplains.org/alzheimers/day_to_day.html?day_to_day_item=1090&db_item=listitem

Alzheimer's Disease Association of the Philippines. (2007). *About Alzheimer's.* Retrieved November 2007, from http://www.alzphilippines.com/faqs.html

Alzheimer's Disease Education & Referral Center. (2002, July). Frontotemporal dementia: Growing interest in a rare dementia. *Connections, 9,* 4. Retrieved August 2007, from http://www.nia.nih.gov/NR/rdonlyres/88A32A1B-860B-4C47-9701-4FC0CD54 C144/3958/FTDReprint.pdf

Alzheimer's Disease International. (1999, April). *Factsheet 3: The prevalence of dementia.* Retrieved July 2007, from http://www.alz.co.uk/adi/pdf/3preval.pdf

Alzheimer's Disease International. (2004). *Tips to meet daily challenges.* Retrieved July 2007, from http://www.alz.co.uk/carers/tips.html

Alzheimer's Foundation of America. (2007). *Alzheimer's symptoms.* Retrieved August 2007, from http://www.alzfdn.org/alzheimers/symptoms.shtml

AlzheimersOnline. (2007). *Stages of Alzheimer's disease.* Retrieved September 2007, from http://www.alzheimersonline.com/understand/stages.aspx

Alzheimer's Outreach. (1996). *Memory-related communication problems.* Retrieved September 2007, from http://www.zarcrom.com/users/alzheimers/t-03.html

Alzheimer's Outreach. (2007). *Challenging behaviors for the caregiver.* Retrieved September 2007, from http://www.zarcrom.com/users/alzheimers/c-08a.html

Alzheimer's Society. (2007a). *Alzheimer's disease: What is Alzheimer's disease?* Retrieved September 2007, from http://www.alzheimer.ca/english/disease/whatisit-effects.htm

Alzheimer's Society. (2007b). *Am I at risk of developing dementia?* Retrieved June 2007, from http://www.alzheimers.org.uk/site/scripts/documents_info.php?document ID=102

Alzheimer's Society. (2007c). *Genetics and dementia.* Retrieved June 2007, from http://www.alzheimers.org.uk/site/scripts/documents_info.php?documentID=168

Alzheimer's Society. (2007d). *Food for thought: Eating and nutrition.* Retrieved September 2007, from http://www.alzheimers.org.uk/site/scripts/documents_info.php? documentID=364

Alzheimer's Society of Canada. (2007). *Caring for someone with Alzheimer's disease? Take care of yourself too!* Retrieved July 2007, from http://www.alzheimer.ca/english/ care/caregivers-selfcare.htm

Alzheimersinfo101.org. (2007). *Alzheimer's signs and early stages.* Retrieved August 2007, from http://www.alzheimersinfo101.org/alzheimers-signs.html

American Academy of Family Physicians. (2007). *Sleep apnea.* Retrieved July 2007, from http://familydoctor.org/online/famdocen/home/articles/212.html

American Academy of Neurology, Ethics and Humanities Subcommittee. (1996). Ethical issues in the management of the demented patient. *Neurology, 48,* 1180–1183.

American Association for Geriatric Psychiatry. (2003). *Designing brief Alzheimer's screening tests for use in general medical practice.* Retrieved August 2007, from http://www. cmecorner.com/macmcm/AAGP/aagp2003_07.htm

American Health Assistance Foundation. (2006). *About Alzheimer's: The facts on Alzheimer's disease.* Retrieved March 2007, from http://www.ahaf.org/SubIndex/AD_ PDF_FactSheets/AD_stats.pdf

American Medical Association. (1997). American Medical Association Council on Ethical and Judicial Affairs Code of Medical Ethics. Chicago, IL.

American Medical Association. (1998). Council on Ethical and Judicial Affairs. Code of Medical Ethics: Current Opinions with Annotations. Chicago, IL.

American Occupational Therapy Association. (1994). Statement: Occupational therapy services for persons with Alzheimer's disease and other dementias. *American Journal of Occupational Therapy, 48,* 1029–1031.

American Psychiatric Association. (1994). *Diagnostic and statistical manual of mental disorders* (4th ed.). Washington, DC: Author.

American Psychiatric Association. (2006). American Psychiatric Association practice guidelines for the treatment of psychiatric disorders: Compendium 2006. Arlington, VA: American Psychiatric Publishing.

Angevaren, M., Vanhees, L., Wendel-Vos, W., Verhaar, H. J., Aufdemkampe, G., & Aleman, A., et al. (2007). Intensity, but not duration, of physical activities is related to cognitive function. *European Journal of Cardiovascular and Preventive Rehabilitation, 14,* 825–830.

APA Practice Guidelines (4th ed.). (2007). *Practice guideline for the treatment of patients with Alzheimer's disease and other dementias.* Retrieved from http://ajp.psychiatryonline.org/cgi/data/164/12/A48/DC2/1

Arkin, S. (1998). *Alzheimer memory training: Long term retention achieved.* Unpublished manuscript.

Arkin, S. (2006). *Introduction to Alzheimer's disease and exercise.* National Center on Physical Activity and Disability. Retrieved September 2007, from http://www.ncpad.org/disability/fact_sheet.php?sheet=138

Arkin, S. M. (1992). Audio-assisted memory training with early Alzheimer's patients: Two single subject experiments. *Clinical Gerontologist, 12,* 77–96.

Arkin, S. M. (2001). Alzheimer rehabilitation by students: Interventions and outcomes. *Neuropsychological Rehabilitation, 11,* 273–317.

Armstrong, R. A., Anderson, J., Cowburn, J. D., Cox, J., & Blair, J. A. (1992). Aluminum administered in drinking water but not in the diet influences biopterin metabolism in the rodent. *Biolological Chemistry, 373,* 1075–1078.

Arvanitakis, Z., Wilson, R. S., Bienias, J. L., Evans, D. A., & Bennett, D. A. (2004). Diabetes mellitus and risk of Alzheimer disease and decline in cognitive function. *Archives of Neurology, 61,* 661–666.

Austen, B. M., Sidera, C., Liu, C., & Frears, E. (2003). The role of intracellular cholesterol on the processing of the beta-amyloid precursor protein. *Journal of Nutrition, Health & Aging, 7,* 31–36.

Bach, D., Bach, M., Bohmer, F., Fruhwald, T., & Grilc, B. (1995). Reactivating occupational therapy: A method to improve cognitive performance in geriatric patients. *Age and Ageing, 24,* 222–226.

Ballard, C., Fossey, J., Chithramohan, R., Howard, R., Burns, A., & Thompson, P., et al. (2001). Quality of care in private sector and NHS facilities for people with dementia: cross sectional survey. *British Medical Journal, 323,* 426–427.

Barnes, L. L., Wilson, R. S., Li, Y., Aggarwal, N. T., Gilley, D. W., & McCann, J., et al. (2005). Racial differences in the progression of cognitive decline in Alzheimer disease. *American Journal of Geriatric Psychiatry, 13,* 959–967.

Barone, P., Amboni, M., Vitale, C., & Bonavita, V. (2004). Treatment of nocturnal disturbances and excessive daytime sleepiness in Parkinson's disease. *Neurology, 63,* S35–S38.

Beatty, W. W., Brumback, R. A., & Vonsatte, J. P. (1997). Autopsy-proven Alzheimer disease in a patient with dementia who retained musical skill in life. *Archives of Neurology, 54,* 1448.

Bejjani, G. K., & Hammer, M. D. (2005). Normal-pressure hydrocephalus: Another treatable "dementia": Part I. *Contemporary Neurosurgery, 27,* 1–4.

Bennett, D. A. (1999). Foreword. In D. Kuhn, *Alzheimer's early stages.* Berkeley, CA: Hunter House.

Bickel, H. (1996). The hierarchic dementia scale: Usage. *International Psychogeriatrics, 8,* 213–224.

Billings, L. M., Green, K. N., McGaugh, J. L., & LaFerla, F. M. (2007). Learning decreases A beta°56 and tau pathology and ameliorates behavioral decline in 3xTg-AD mice. *Journal of Neuroscience, 27,* 751–761.

Birks, J., Grimley, E. V., & Van Dongen, M. (2002). Ginkgo biloba for cognitive impairment and dementia. *Cochrane Database Systematic Review, 4,* CD003120.

Blessed, G., Tomlinson, B. E., & Roth, M. (1968). The association between quantitative measures of dementia and of senile change in the cerebral grey matter of elderly subjects. *British Journal of Psychiatry, 114,* 797–811.

Bonner, A. P., & Cousins, S. O. (1996). Exercise and Alzheimer's disease benefits and barriers. *Activities, Adaptation & Aging, 20,* 21–34.

Bourgeois, M. S. (1990). Enhancing conversations in Alzheimer's disease using a prosthetic memory aid. *Journal of Applied Behavior Analysis, 23,* 29–42.

Bourgeois, M. S. (1992). Evaluating memory wallets in conversations with persons with dementia. *Journal of Speech and Hearing Research, 35,* 1344–1357.

Bourgeois, M. S., Burgio, L. D., Schulz, R., & Beach, S. (1997). Modifying repetitive verbalizations of community-dwelling patients with AD. *Gerontologist, 37,* 30–39.

Breitner, J. C. S., Gau, B. A., Welsh, K. A., Plassman, B. L., McDonald, W. M., & Helms, M. J., et al. (1994). Inverse association of anti-inflammatory treatments and Alzheimer's disease: Initial results of a co-twin control study. *Neurology, 44,* 227–232.

Brody, H., Campbell, M. L., Faber-Langendoen, K., & Ogle, K. S. (1997). Withdrawing intensive life-sustaining treatment—Recommendations for compassionate clinical management. *New England Journal of Medicine, 336,* 652–657.

Brookmeyer, R., Gray, S., & Kawas, C. (1998). Projections of Alzheimer's disease in the United States and the public health impact of delaying disease onset. *American Journal of Public Health, 88,* 1337–1342.

Brotons, M., & Koger, S. M. (2000). The impact of music therapy on language. *Journal of Music Therapy 37,* 183–195.

Brown, J. T., & Stoudemire, A. (1983). Normal and pathological grief. *Journal of the American Medical Association, 250,* 378–382.

Bryce, N. (2000). *Maintaining selfhood and dignity in patients with Alzheimer's disease.* ElderCare Online. Retrieved June 2000, from http://www.ec-online.net/Knowledge/Articles/selfhood.html

Brynes, G. (2007). *Dealing with dementia.* Northern County Psychiatric Associates. Retrieved May 2007, from http://www.ncpamd.com/dementia.htm

Buchner, D., & Larson, E. (1987). Falls and fractures in patients with Alzheimer-type dementia. *Journal of the American Medical Association, 257,* 1492–1495.

Buckwalter, J. G., Sobel, E., Dunn, M. E., Diz, M. M., & Henderson, V. W. (1993). Gender differences on a brief measure of cognitive functioning in Alzheimer's disease. *Archives of Neurology, 50,* 757–760.

Burns, T., Mortimer, J. A., & Merchak, P. (1994). The Cognitive Performance Test: A new approach to functional assessment in Alzheimer's disease. *Journal of Geriatric Psychiatry and Neurology, 7,* 46–54.

California Long Term Care Ombudsman. (2007). *The Long Term Care Ombudsman Program*. Retrieved October 2007, from http://teampublish.allsoldout.net/teampubv3/includes/CALTCOBrochure.pdf

Camp, C. J., Foss, J. W., O'Hanlon, A. M., & Stevens, A. B. (1996). Memory interventions for persons with dementia. *Applied Cognitive Psychology, 10,* 193–210.

Canadian Study of Health and Aging Working Group. (1994). The Canadian Study of Health and Aging: Risk factors for Alzheimer's disease in Canada. *Neurology, 44,* 2073–2080.

Cannuscio, C. C., Jones, C., Kawachi, I., Colditz, G. A., Berkman, L., & Rimm, E. (2002) Reverberation of family illness: A longitudinal assessment of informal caregiver and mental health status in the nurses' health study. *American Journal of Public Health, 92,* 305–1311.

Capezuti, E. (1996). Falls. In R. J. Lavizzo-Mourey & M. A. Forciea (Eds.), *Geriatric secrets* (pp. 110–115). Philadelphia: Hanley & Belfus.

Carlsson, C. M., Gleason, C. E., & Asthana, S. (2005, May). Update on diagnosis and treatment of Alzheimer disease. *Applied Neurology.* Retrieved August 2007, from http://appneurology.com/showArticle.jhtml?articleId=163105707

Case Western Reserve University. (2000, July). *Findings presented on Alzheimer's disease, brain gymnastics, and lead.* Retrieved March 2007, from http://www.case.edu/pubaff/univcomm/reports.htm

Casserly, I., & Topol, E. (2004). Convergence of atherosclerosis and Alzheimer's disease: Inflammation, cholesterol, and misfolded proteins. *Lancet, 363,* 1139–1146.

Center to Advance Palliative Care. (2002). *Differences between hospice and palliative care programs.* Retrieved December 2007, from http://64.85.16.230/educate/content/elements/differencebetweenhpc.html

Chiu, N., Lee, B., Hsiao, S., & Pai, M. (2004). Educational level influences regional cerebral blood flow in patients with Alzheimer's disease. *Journal of Nuclear Medicine, 45,* 1860–1863.

Civic Ventures. (2006). *Get the facts: Experience is America's only growing natural resource.* Retrieved March 2007, from http://www.civicventures.org/the_facts.cfm

Cleveland Clinic Health System. (2004). *Types of Alzheimer's disease.* Retrieved June 2007, from http://www.cchs.net/health/health-info/docs/2300/2341.asp?index=9171

CLSC Côte-des-Neiges. (2001). *S.A.S. safety assessment scale.* Retrieved October 2007, from http://www.alzheimersupport.com/articles/1567.pdf

Cohen, D., Eisdorfer, C., Gorelick, P., Luchins, D., Freels, S., & Semla, T., et al. (1993). Sex differences in the psychiatric manifestations of Alzheimer's disease. *Journal of American Geriatric Society, 41,* 229–232.

Committee on Government Reform, U.S. House of Representatives. (2001, July). *Abuse of residents is a major problem in U.S. nursing homes.* Prepared for Rep. Henry A. Waxman. Retrieved October 2007, from http://oversight.house.gov/documents/20040830113750-34049.pdf

Commonwealth Fund. (2000, June 7). *Malnutrition and dehydration plague nursing home residents.* Retrieved October 2007, from http://www.commonwealthfund.org/newsroom/newsroom_show.htm?doc_id=223638

Coogler, C. E., & Wolf, S. L. (1999). Falls. In W. R. Hazzard, R. Andres, & E. L. Bierman (Eds.), *Principles of geriatric medicine and gerontology* (4th ed., pp. 1192–1199). New York: McGraw-Hill.

Coste, J. K. (2004). *Learning to speak Alzheimer's: A groundbreaking approach for everyone dealing with the disease.* New York: Houghton Mifflin.

Council on Ethical and Judical Affairs, American Medical Association. (1998–1999). Opinion E2.20: Withholding or withdrawing life-sustaining medical treatment. In *Code of medical ethics: Current opinions with annotations.* Chicago: American Medical Association.

Cruz, E. D. (2004). *Tips for occupational therapists working with clients who have dementia.* The University of Texas Medical Branch at Galveston. Retrieved September 2007, from http://etgec.utmb.edu/dementia/ot_therapist.html

Cullen, B., Coen, R. F., Lynch, C. A., Cunningham, C. J., Coakley, D., Robertson, I. H., et al. (2005). Repetitive behaviour in Alzheimer's disease: Description, correlates and functions. *International Journal of Geriatric Psychiatry, 20,* 686–693.

Cummings, J. L., Frank, J. C., Cherry, D., Kohatsu, N. D., Kemp, B., Hewett, L., et al. (2002). Guidelines for managing Alzheimer's disease: Part I: Assessment. *American Family Physician, 65,* 2263–2272.

Cummings, J. L., Frank, J. C., Cherry, D., Kohatsu, N. D., Kemp, B., Hewett, L. et al. (2002). Guidelines for managing Alzheimer's disease: Part II: Treatment. Assessment. *American Family Physician, 65,* 2525–2534.

Daly, M. P. (1999). Diagnosis and management of Alzheimer disease. *American Board of Family Practice, 12,* 375–384.

dbs Productions. (2007). *Alzheimer's disease and related disorders: Wandering overview.* Retrieved September 2007, from http://www.dbs-sar.com/SAR_Research/wandering.htm

DeAngelo, A., & Halliday, A. (2005, September). *Wernicke-Korsakoff Syndrome.* Retrieved June 2007, from http://www.emedicine.com/med/topic2405.htm

DeCarli, C. (2003). Mild cognitive impairment: Prevalence, prognosis, aetiology, and treatment. *Lancet Neurology, 2,* 15–21.

DeNoon, D. J. (2005, August). *Obesity and Alzheimer's: High insulin levels linked to Alzheimer's.* Retrieved August 2007, from http://www.webmd.com/alzheimers/guide/20061101/obesity-alzheimers-risk

Doraiswamy, P. M., Leon, J., Cummings, J. L., Marin, D., & Neumann, P. J. (2002). Prevalence and impact of medical comorbidity in Alzheimer's disease. *The Journals of Gerontology Series A: Biological Sciences and Medical Sciences, 57,* M173–M177.

Doskoch, P. (2000, October). *Brain injury and Alzheimer's disease: What is the link? Neuropsychiatry Reviews, 1*(5). Retrieved August 2007, from http://www.neuropsychiatryreviews.com/oct00/npr_oct00_brain.html

Duan, W., Ladenheim, B., Cutler, R. G., Kruman I. I., Cadet, J. L., & Mattson, M. P. (2002). Dietary folate deficiency and elevated homocysteine levels endanger dopaminergic neurons in models of Parkinson's disease. *Journal of Neurochemistry, 80,* 101–110.

Dubinsky, R. M., Stein, A. C., & Lyons, K. (2000). Practice parameter: Risk of driving and Alzheimer's disease (an evidence-based review): Report of the quality standards subcommittee of the American Academy of Neurology. *Neurology, 54,* 2205–2211.

Dura, J. R., Stukenberg, K. W., & Kiecolt-Glaser, J. K. (1991). Anxiety and depressive disorders in adult children caring for demented parents. *Psychology & Aging, 6,* 467–473.

Edwardson, J., & Morris, C. (1998). The genetics of Alzheimer's disease: The number of genetic risk factors associated with this disorder is increasing steadily. *British Medical Journal, 317,* 361–362.

eMedicineHealth. (2005a). *Alzheimer disease overview.* Retrieved June 2007, from http://www.emedicinehealth.com/alzheimer_disease/article_em.htm

eMedicineHealth. (2005b). *Dementia with Lewy bodies.* Retrieved June 2007, from http://www.emedicinehealth.com/dementia_with_lewy_bodies/article_em.htm

Engelhart, M. J., Geerlings, M. I., Ruitenberg, A., van Swieten, J. C., Hofman, A., Witteman, J. C., et al. (2002). Dietary intake of antioxidants and risk of Alzheimer disease. *Journal of the American Medical Association, 287,* 3223–3229.

Ernst, R. L., & Hay, J. W. (1994). The U.S. economic and social costs of Alzheimer's disease revisited. *American Journal of Public Health, 84,* 1261–1264.

Ertekin-Taner, N., Graff-Radford, N., Younkin, L. H., Eckman, C., Baker, M., Adamson, J., et al. (2000). Linkage of plasma Abeta42 to a quantitative locus on chromosome 10 in late-onset Alzheimer's disease pedigrees. *Science, 290,* 2303–2304.

Evans, D. A., Funkenstein, H. H., Albert, M. S., Scherr, P. A., Cook, N. R., Chown, M. J., et al. (1989). Prevalence of Alzheimer's disease in a community population of older persons: Higher than previously reported. *Journal of the American Medical Association, 262,* 2551–2556.

Farrell, B. (1995). Pain evaluation and management in the nursing home. *Annals of Internal Medicine, 123,* 681–687.

Feldman, H., & Gracon, S. (1996). Alzheimer's disease: Symptomatic drugs under development. In S. Gauthier (Ed.), *Clinical diagnosis and management of Alzheimer's disease* (pp. 239–253). London: Martin Dunitz.

Feldt, K. S. (2000). The Checklist of Nonverbal Pain Indicators (CNPI). *Pain Management Nursing, 1,* 13–21.

Field, M. J., & Cassel, C. K. (Eds.). (1997). *Committee on Care at the End of Life, Institute of Medicine: Approaching death: improving care at the end of life.* Washington, DC: National Academy Press.

Finlay, I. (1996). Difficult decisions in palliative care. *British Journal of Hospital Medicine, 56,* 264–267.

Finucane, T. E., Christmas, C., & Travis, K. (1999). Tube feeding in patients with advanced dementia: A review of the evidence. *Journal of the American Medical Association, 282,* 1365–1370.

Fisher Center for Alzheimer's Research Foundation. (2007). *Understanding Alzheimer's disease.* Retrieved September 2007, from http://www.alzinfo.org/Understanding-Alzheimers-Disease.asp

Folstein, M. F., Folstein, S. E., & McHugh, P. R. (1975). Mini-mental state. A practical method for grading the cognitive state of patients for the clinician. *Journal of Psychiatric Research, 12,* 189–198.

Forbes, K. E., Shanks, M. F., & Venneri, A. (2004). The evolution of dysgraphia in Alzheimer's disease. *Brain Research Bulletin, 63,* 119–124.

Fornazzari, L. R. (2005). Preserved painting creativity in an artist with Alzheimer's disease. *European Journal of Neurology, 12,* 419–424.

Friedland, R. P., Koss, E., Kumar, A., Gaine, S., Metzler, D., Haxby, J. V., et al. (1988). Motor vehicle crashes in dementia of the Alzheimer type. *Annals of Neurology, 24,* 782–786.

Fuchs-Lacelle, S., & Hadjistavropoulos, T. (2004). Development and preliminary validation of the Pain Assessment Checklist for Seniors with Limited Ability to Communicate (PACSLAC). *Pain Management Nursing, 5,* 37–49.

Fuller, G. F. (2000). Falls in the elderly. *American Family Physician, 61,* 2159–2168.

Galasko, D. (1998). An integrated approach to the management of Alzheimer's disease: Assessing cognition, function and behaviour. *European Journal of Neurology, 5,* S9–S17.

Galasko, D., Bennett, D., Sano, M., Ernesto, C., Thomas, R., Grundman, M., et al. (1997). An inventory to assess activities of daily living for clinical trials in Alzheimer's disease: The Alzheimer's Disease Cooperative Study. *Alzheimer Disease and Associated Disorders, 11*(Suppl. 2), S33–S39.

Gauthier, S. (2000). *Alzheimer's disease.* Retrieved August 2007, from http://www.agis.com/

Geldmacher, D. S., & Whitehouse, P. J. (1997). Differential diagnosis of Alzheimer's disease. *Neurology, 48*(Suppl. 6), S2–S9.

Gerdner, L., & Swanson, E. A. (2001). Effects of individualized music on confused and agitated elderly patients. *Archives of Psychiatric Nursing, 7,* 284–291.

Gillick, M. R. (2000). Rethinking the role of tube feeding in patients with advanced dementia. *New England Journal of Medicine, 342,* 206–210.

Goldberg, B. (1996, Fall). A very long goodbye: The ravages of Alzheimer's disease. *ASHA, 38,* 25–31.

Gorina, Y., Hoyert, D., Lentzner, H., & Goulding, M. (2006). Trends in causes of death among older persons in the United States. *Aging trends, 6.* Hyattsville, MD: National Center for Health Statistics.

Green, R. C., Cupples, L. A., Go, R., Benke, K. S., & Edeki, T. (2002). Risk of dementia among White and African American relatives of patients with Alzheimer disease. *Journal of the American Medical Association, 287,* 329–336.

Grossberg, G., Dharmarajan, T. S., Fillit, H., & Ringel, M. (2007). Slowing disease progression: Practical management of dementia in primary care: Part 3: Alzheimer's disease: Caring for the caregiver. *Family Practice Recertification, 29,* 1–8.

Gurwitz, J. H., Fields, T. S., Judge, J., Rochon, P., Harrold, L. R., Cadoret, C., et al. (2005). The incidence of adverse drug events in two large academic long-term care facilities. *American Journal of Medicine, 118,* 261–258.

Gustafson, D., Rothenberg, E., Blennow, K., Steen, B., & Skoog, I. (2003). An 18-year follow-up of overweight and risk of Alzheimer disease. *Archives of Internal Medicine, 163,* 1524–1528.

Gwyther, L. (1985). *Care of Alzheimer's patients: A manual for nursing home staff.* Washington, DC: American Health Care Association.

Haak, N., & Peters, M. (2004). Pilgrimages in partnering with palliative care. *Alzheimer's Care Quarterly, 5,* 300–312.

Hachinski, V. C. (1989). Effect of strokes on musical ability and performance. *Seminars in Neurology, 9,* 159–162.

Haddon, W. J. (1968). The changing approach to the epidemiology, prevention, and amelioration of trauma: The transition to approaches etiologically rather than descriptively based. *American Journal of Public Health, 58,* 1431–1438.

Haddon, W. (1980). The basic strategies for reducing damage from hazards of all kinds. *Hazard Prevention, 16,* 8–12.

Hake, A. M. (2001). Use of cholinesterase inhibitors for treatment of Alzheimer disease. *Cleveland Clinic Journal of Medicine, 68,* 608–616.

Haley, W. E., West, C. A., Wadley, V. G., Ford, G. R., White, F. A., Barrett, J. J., et al. (1995). Psychological, social, and health impact of caregiving: A comparison of black and white dementia family caregivers and noncaregivers. *Psychology and Aging, 10,* 540–552.

Hall, K. S., Gao, S., Unverzagt, F. W., & Hendrie, H. C. (2000). Low education and childhood rural residence: Risk for Alzheimer's disease in African Americans. *Neurology, 54,* 95–99.

Ham, R. J. (1997). After the diagnosis: Supporting Alzheimer's patients and their families. *Postgraduate Medicine, 101,* 6–8.

Hardy, J., & Selkoe, D. J. (2002). The amyloid hypothesis of Alzheimer's disease: Progress and problems on the road to therapeutics. *Science, 297,* 353–356.

Harvard Health Publications. (2007). *Anticipating the future: The stages of Alzheimer's.* Retrieved September 2007, from http://mercksource.com/ppdocs/us/cns/harvard-health-reports/MerckSHR-Alzheimers082906/sections/sect12.htm

Harvard Health Publications. (2007, January). *Diagnosing Alzheimer's disease.* Retrieved August 2007, from http://body.aol.com/learn-about-it/alzheimers/diagnosing-alzheimers-disease/the-evaluation-process?cc=70

Hausdorff, J. M., Rios D., & Edelberg, H. K. (2001). Gait variability and fall risk in community-living older adults: A 1-year prospective study. *Archives of Physical Medicine & Rehabilitation, 82,* 31–35.

Heath, B. (2004, November 28). Nursing home patients die from malnutrition. *The Detroit News.* Retrieved October 2007, from http://www.detnews.com/2004/special report/0411/30/A01-17436.htm

Hebert, L. E., Beckett, L. A., Scherr, P. A., & Evans, D. A. (2001). Annual incidence of Alzheimer disease in the United States projected to the years 2000 through 2050. *Alzheimer Disease and Associated Disorders, 15*(4), 169–173.

Hebert, L. E., Scherr, P. A., Bienias, J. L., Bennett, D. A., & Evans, D. A. (2003). Alzheimer's disease in the U.S. population: Prevalence estimates using the 2000 consensus. *Archives of Neurology, 60,* 1119–1122.

Hebert, L. E., Scherr, P. A., McCann, J. J., Beckett, L. A., & Evans, D. A. (2001). Is the risk of developing Alzheimer's disease greater for women than for men? *American Journal of Epidemiology, 153,* 132–136.

Hebert, L. E., Wilson, R. S., Gilley, D. W., Beckett, L. A., Scherr, P. A., Bennett, D. A., et al. (2000). Decline of language among women and men with Alzheimer's disease. *Journal of Gerontology, Psychological Sciences and Social Sciences, 55*(Series B), 354–360.

Hellen, C. R. (1998). *Alzheimer's disease: Activity focused care* (2nd ed.). Burlington, MA: Butterworth-Heinemann.

Helpguide.com. (2007a). *Alzheimer's Caregivers Guide.* Retrieved September 2007, from http://www.helpguide.org/elder/alzheimers_disease_dementias_caring_caregivers.htm

Helpguide.com. (2007b). *Final stage Alzheimer's care: Caring for a person in the final stage of Alzheimer's disease or another dementia.* Retrieved December 2007, from http://www.helpguide.org/elder/alzheimers_disease_dementia_caring_final_stage.htm

Helpguide.com. (2007c). *Late stage and end-of-life Alzheimer's care*. Retrieved November 2007, from http://www.helpguide.org/elder/alzheimers_disease_dementia_caring_final_stage.htm

Hill, C. D., Thompson, L. W., & Gallagher, D. (1988). The role of anticipatory bereavement in older women's adjustment to widowhood. *The Gerontologist, 28,* 792–796.

Hill, J. W., Futterman, R., Duttagupta, S., Mastey, V., Lloyd, J. R., & Fillit, H. (2002). Alzheimer's disease and related dementias increase costs of comorbidities in managed Medicare. *Neurology, 58,* 62–70.

Hingley, A. T. (1998). *Alzheimer's: Few clues on the mysteries of memory. U.S. Food and Drug Administration*. Retrieved April 2007, from http://www.fda.gov/Fdac/features/1998/398_alz.html

Hinman, R. M. (2004). *Dementia education: General management strategies*. The University of Texas Medical Branch at Galveston. Retrieved September 2007, from http://etgec.utmb.edu/dementia/physicaltherapist.html

Hoffman, M. T., Bankes, P. F., Javed, A., & Selhat, M. (2003). Decreasing the incidence of falls in the nursing home in a cost-conscious environment: A pilot study. *Journal of the American Medical Directors Association, 4,* 95–97.

Holland, A. J. (1999). Down's syndrome. In M. P. Janicki & A. J. Dalton (Eds.), *Dementia, aging and intellectual disabilities: A handbook* (pp. 183–197). Philadelphia: Bunner/Mazel.

Hollmann, W., Struder, H. K., Tagarakis, C. V. M., & King, G. (2007). Physical activity and the elderly: Review. *European Journal of Cardiovascular Prevention & Rehabilitation, 14,* 730–739.

Hoyert, D. L., & Rosenberg, H. M. (1999, June 30). Mortality from Alzheimer's disease: An update. *National Vital Statistics, 47*(20), 1–6.

Hugonot-Diener, L., Verny, M., Devouche, E., Saxton, J., Mecocci, P., & Boller, F. (2003). *Psychologie & NeuroPsychiatrie du vieillissement, 4,* 273–283. [Abridged version of the severe impairment battery (SIB); Article in French.]

Hurley, A. C., Volicer, B. J., Hanrahan, P. A., Houde, S., & Volicer, L. (1992). Assessment of discomfort in advanced Alzheimer patients. *Research in Nursing & Health, 15,* 369–377.

Information from your family doctor. (2003). Memory loss. *American Family Physician, 67,* 1047–1048.

Institute for Ethics at the American Medical Association. (1999). Education for Physicians on End-of-life Care: Participant's Handbook. Retrieved January, 2008, from http://www.ama-assn.org/ethic/epec/download/plenary_3.pdf

Inverarity, L., (2007). *Alzheimer's disease and exercise: Overview*. About.com: Physical therapy. Retrieved October 2007, from http://physicaltherapy.about.com/od/typesofphysicaltherapy/ss/Alzheimers.htm

Jackson, S. (2007). *The role of the speech-language pathologist in the assessment and management of behavioral disturbances in dementia*. The University of Kansas Medical Center. Retrieved September 2007, from http://coa.kumc.edu/GEC/modules/BehavDisorder/SpeechTherapy/ST_FrameOverview.htm

Jaffe-Gill, E., Smith, M., & Segal, J. (2007). *Coping with grief and loss: Guide to grieving and bereavement*. HELPGUIDE.org. Retrieved December 2007, from http://www.helpguide.org/mental/grief_loss.htm

Johnson, J. K., Cotman, C. W., Tasaki, C. S., & Shaw, G. L. (1998). Enhancement of spatial-temporal reasoning after a Mozart listening condition in Alzheimer's disease: A case study. *Neurology Research, 20,* 666–672.

The Junior League of New York City. (1988). *Alzheimer's disease: Early warning signs and diagnostic resources.* Retrieved April 2007, from http://www.searo.who.int/en/Section1174/Section1199/Section1567/Section1823_8057.htm

Kalmijn, S., Launer, L. J., Ott, A., Witteman, J. C., Hofman, A., Breteler, M., et al. (1997). Dietary fat intake and the risk of incident dementia in the Rotterdam Study. *Annals of Neurology, 42,* 776–782.

Kannus, P., Parkarri, J., Koskinen, S., Niemi, S., Palvanen, M., Jarvinen, M., et al. (1999). Fall-induced injuries and deaths among older adults. *Journal of the American Medical Association, 281,* 1895–1899.

Katz, S., Down, T. D., Cash, H. R., & Grotz, R. C. (1970). Progress in the development of the index of ADL. *Gerontologist, 10,* 20–30.

Kennard, C. (2006a). *Alzheimer's disease: Causes of fecal incontinence.* About.com. Retrieved September 2007, from http://alzheimers.about.com/od/practicalcare/a/fecal_causes.htm

Kennard, C. (2006b). *Driving with Alzheimer's disease.* Retrieved July 2007, from http://alzheimers.about.com/cs/diagnosisissues/a/Driving.htm

Kennard, C. (2006c). *How people with dementia behave when they get lost.* Retrieved September 2007, from http://alzheimers.about.com/od/whattoexpect/a/wandering.htm

Kim, K. Y., Yeaman, P. A., & Keene, R. L. (2005). Practical geriatrics: End-of-life care for persons with Alzheimer's disease. *Psychiatric Services, 56,* 139–141.

King's College London. (2005, December). *Molecule links Down syndrome to Alzheimer's. Science Daily.* Retrieved June 2007, from http://www.sciencedaily.com/releases/2005/12/051206090403.htm

Kivipelto, M., Helkala, E. L., Laakso, M. P., Hänninen, T., & Hallikainen, M. (2001). Midlife vascular risk factors and Alzheimer's disease in later life: Longitudinal, population based study. *British Medical Journal, 322,* 1447–1451.

Knopman, D. S., DeKosky, S. T., Cummings, J. L., Chui, H., Corey-Bloom, J., Relkin, N., et al. (2001). Practice parameter: Diagnosis of dementia (an evidence based review). Report of the Quality Standards Subcommittee of the American Academy of Neurology. *Neurology, 56,* 1143–1153.

Koger, S. M., Chapin, K., & Brotons, M. (1999). Is music therapy an effective intervention for dementia? A meta-analytic review of literature. *Journal of Music Therapy, 36,* 2–15.

Koppel, R. (2002). *Alzheimer's disease: The costs to U.S. businesses in 2002.* Washington, DC: Alzheimer's Association.

Kübler-Ross, E. (1997). *On death and dying.* New York: Scribner.

Kuhn, D. (1999). *Alzheimer's early stages.* Berkeley, CA: Hunter House.

Kukull, W. A., Larson, E. B., Bowen, J. D., McCormick, W. C., & Teri, L. (1995). Solvent exposure as a risk factor for Alzheimer's disease: A case-control study. *American Journal of Epidemiology, 141,* 1059–1071.

Kukull, W. A., & Martin, G. M. (1998). APOE polymorphisms and late-onset Alzheimer disease: The importance of ethnicity. *Journal of the American Medical Association, 279,* 788–789.

Kumar-Singh, S., & Broeckhoven, C. V. (2007). Frontotemporal lobar degeneration: Current concepts in the light of recent advances. *Brain Pathology, 17,* 104–114.

Lach, H. (1998, July-August). Safety and falls in long-term care settings. (Newsletter). Alzheimer's Association Omaha-Eastern Nebraska Chapter.

Larson, E. B., Wang, L., Bowen, J. D., McCormick, W. C., Teri, L., Crane, P., et al. (2006). Exercise is associated with reduced risk for incident dementia among persons 65 years of age and older. *Annals of Internal Medicine, 144,* 73–81.

Lautenschlager, N. T., Cupples, L. A., Rao, V. S., Auerbach, S. A., Becker, R., Chui, H., et al. (1996). Risk of dementia among relatives of Alzheimer disease patients in the MIRAGE study: What is in store for the Oldest Old? *Neurology, 46,* 641–650.

Lawton, M. P., & Brody, E. M. (1969). Assessment of older people: Self-maintaining and instrumental activities of daily living. *Gerontologist, 9,* 179–186.

Lazowski, D. A., Ecclestone, N. A., Myers, A. M., Peterson, D. H., Tudor-Locke, C., Fitzgerald, C., et al. (1999). A randomized outcome evaluation of group exercise programs in long-term care institutions. *Journals of Gerontology Series A: Biological Sciences and Medical Sciences, 54A,* M621–M628.

LeBlanc, E. S., Janowski, J., Chan, B. K., & Nelson, H. D. (2001). Hormone replacement therapy and cognition: Systematic review and meta-analysis. *Journal of the American Medical Association, 285,* 1489–1499.

Leon, J., Cheng, C., & Neumann, P. (1998). Alzheimer's disease care: Costs and potential savings. *Health Affairs, 17,* 206–216.

Leroi, I., & Burns, A. (2007). Behavioural and psychological symptoms of dementia associated with Parkinson's disease. *Journal of Neurology, Neurosurgery & Psychiatry, 78,* 2–3.

Letenneur, L., Gilleron, V., Commenges, D., Helmer, C., Orgogonzo, J. M., Dartigues, J. F. (1999). Are sex and educational level independent predictors of dementia and Alzheimer's disease? Incidence data from the PAQUID project. *Journal of Neurology, Neurosurgery and Psychiatry, 66,* 177–183.

Loewy, E. H. (1996). *Textbook of healthcare ethics.* New York: Plenum Press.

Logemann, J. A. (1998). *Roles of speech-language pathologists in swallowing and feeding disorders: Technical report.* American Speech-Language-Hearing Association. Retrieved September 2007, from http://www.asha.org/NR/rdonlyres/B8DE1480-C7B4-4383-A1F6-5829E9CB0CF5/0/v3TRRolesSLPSwallowingFeeding.pdf

Logemann, J. A. (2007). *Dysphagia and dementia: The challenge of dual diagnosis.* American Speech-Language-Hearing Association. Retrieved September 2007, from http://www.asha.org/about/publications/leader-online/archives/2003/q1/030218g.htm

Lucas-Blaustein, M. J., Filipp, L., Dungan, C., & Tune, L. (1988). Driving in patients with dementia. *Journal of American Geriatrics, 36,* 1087–1097.

Luchsinger, J. A., Tang, M. X., Shea, S., & Mayeux, R. (2002). Caloric intake and the risk of Alzheimer disease. *Archives of Neurology, 59,* 1258–1263.

Lynn, J., & Harrold, J. (1999). *Handbook for mortals: Guidance for people facing serious illness.* New York: Oxford University Press.

Madan, S. (2005). Music intervention for disruptive behaviors in long-term care residents with dementia. *Annals of Long-Term Care: Clinical Care and Aging, 13,* 33–36.

Mahoney, F. I., & Barthel, D. (1965). Functional evaluation: The Barthel Index. *Maryland State Medical Journal, 14,* 56–61.

Marcus, E. L., Clarfield, A. M., & Allon, E. (2001). Ethical issues relating to the use of antimicrobial therapy in older adults. *Clinical Infectious Diseases, 33,* 1697–1705.

Markesbury, W. R. (1996). Trace elements in Alzheimer's disease. In Z. S. Khachaturan & T. S. Radebaugh (Eds.), *Alzheimer's disease: Cause(s), diagnosis, treatment, and care* (pp. 233–238). Boca Raton, FL: CRC Press.

Massachusetts Compassionate Care Coalition (Newsletter). (2007). Retrieved December 2007, from http://www.massccc.com/news.html

Mattern, J. M., & Camp, C. J. (1998). Increasing the use of foreign language phrases by direct care staff in a nursing home setting. *Clinical Gerontologist, 19,* 84–86.

Mattson, M. P. (1998). Experimental models of Alzheimer's disease. *Science & Medicine, 5,* 16–25.

Matzo, M. L. (2004). Palliative care: Prognostication and the chronically ill. *American Journal of Nursing, 104,* 40–49.

Mayo Clinic. (2007). *Diagnosis of Alzheimer's disease at Mayo Clinic.* Retrieved August 2007, from http://www.mayoclinic.org/alzheimers-disease/diagnosis.htmi

MayoClinic.com. (2005). *Alzheimer's: Understand and control wandering.* Retrieved September 2007, from http://www.riversideonline.com/health_reference/Alzheimers/HQ00218.cfm?RenderForPrint=1

MayoClinic.com. (2006a). Alzheimer's stages: *How the disease progresses.* Retrieved September 2007, from http://www.mayoclinic.com/health/alzheimers-stages/AZ00041

MayoClinic.com. (2006b). *Ginkgo (Ginkgo biloba L.).* Retrieved September 2007, from http://www.mayoclinic.com/health/ginkgo-biloba/NS_patient-ginkgo

MayoClinic.com. (2007a). *Alzheimer's disease.* Retrieved September 2007, from http://www.mayoclinic.com/health/alzheimers-disease/DS00161/DSECTION=6

MayoClinic.com. (2007b). *Alzheimer's disease.* Retrieved September 2007, from http://www.mayoclinic.com/health/alzheimers-disease/DS00161/DSECTION=8

Mayo Clinic.com. (2007c). *Alzheimer's or depression: Could it be both?* Retrieved June 2007, from http://www.mayoclinic.com/health/alzheimers/HQ00212

MayoClinic.com. (2007d). *Alzheimer's: Understand and control wandering.* Retrieved September 2007, from http://www.mayoclinic.com/health/alzheimers/HQ00218

Mayo Clinic.com. (2007e). *Anticipating end-of-life needs of people with Alzheimer's disease.* Retrieved, June 2008, from http://www.mayoclinic.com/health/alzheimers/HQ00618

Mayo Clinic.com (2007f). *Early-onset Alzheimer's: When symptoms begin before 65.* Retrieved June 2007, from http://www.mayoclinic.com/health/alzheimers/AZ00009

McCarron, M., & McCallion, P. (2007). End-of-life care challenges for persons with intellectual disability and dementia: Making decisions about tube feeding. *Intellectual and Developmental Disabilities, 45,* 128–131.

McHorney, C. A., & Rosenbek, J. C. (1998). Functional outcome assessment of adults with oropharyngeal dysphagia. *Seminars in Speech and Language, 19,* 235–247.

McKeith, I., Del Ser, T., Spano, P., Emre, M., Wesnes, K., Anand, R., et al. (2000). Efficacy of rivastigmine in dementia with Lewy bodies: A randomised, double-blind, placebo-controlled international study. *Lancet, 356,* 2031–2036.

McKeith, I. G., Dickson, D., Emre, M., O'Brien, J. T., Feldman, H., Cummings, J., et al. (2005). Diagnosis and management of dementia with Lewy bodies: Third report of the DLB Consortium. *Neurology, 65,* 1863–1872.

McKhahnn, G. M., Albert, M. S., Grossman, M., Miller, B., Dickson, D., Trojanowski, J. Q., et al. (2001). Clinical and pathological diagnosis of frontotemporal dementia: Report of the work group on frontotemporal dementia and Pick's disease. *Archives of Neurology, 58*, 1803–1809.

McKhann, G., Drachman, D. D., Folstein, M., Katzman, R., Price, D., & Stadlan, E. M. (1984). Clinical diagnosis of Alzheimer's disease: Report of the NINCDS-ADRDA Work Group under the auspices of the Department of Health and Human Services Task Force on Alzheimer's Disease. *Neurology, 34*, 939–944.

Medicine Online. (2007). *Alzheimer's disease*. Retrieved September 2007, from http://www.medicineonline.com/articles/A/1/Alzheimer-Disease.html

Merck Manual of Health & Aging. (2007). *Alzheimer's disease*. Retrieved September 2007, from http://www.merck.com/pubs/mmanual_ha/sec3/ch27/ch27b.html

Merino, J. G., & Luchsinger, J. (2004). *Parkinson disease dementia*. Retrieved May 2007, from http://www.emedicine.com/Med/topic3110.htm

Metlife Mature Market Institute (MMMI). 2005. *Demographic profile: American baby boomers*. Retrieved April 2007, from http://www.metlife.com/WPSAssets/344 42486101113318029V1FBoomer%20Profile%202005.pdf

Miller, S. S., & Marin, D. B. (2000). Assessing capacity. *Emergency Medicine Clinics of North America, 18*, 233–242.

Mintzer, J., & Targum, S. (2003). Psychosis in elderly patients: Classification and pharmacotherapy. *Journal of Geriatric Psychiatry and Neurology, 16*, 199–206.

Mitchell, S. L., Kiely, D. K., & Hamel, M. B. (2004). Dying with advanced dementia in the nursing home. *Archives of Internal Medicine, 164*, 321–326.

Mitchell, S. L., Kiely, D. K., Hamel, M. B., Park, P. S., Morris, J. N., & Fries, B. E. (2004). Estimating prognosis for nursing home residents with advanced dementia. *Journal of the American Medical Association, 291*, 2734–2740.

Mittelman, M. S., Ferris, S. H., Shulman, E., Steinberg, G., & Levin, B. (1996). A family intervention to delay nursing home placement of patients with Alzheimer disease. *Journal of the American Medical Association, 276*, 1725–1731.

Mittelman, M. S., Haley, W. E., Clay, O. J., & Roth, D. L. (2006). Improving caregiver well-being delays nursing home placement of patients with Alzheimer disease. *Neurology, 67*, 1592–1599.

Mobily, P. R., Herr, K. A., Clark, M. K., & Wallace, R. B. (1994). An epidemiologic analysis of pain in the elderly: The Iowa 65+Rural Health Study. *Journal of Aging and Health, 6*, 139–154.

Mohs, R. C., Breitner, J. C., Silverman, J. M., & Davis, K. L. (1987). Alzheimer's disease. Morbid risk among first-degree relatives approximates 50% by 90 years of age. *Archives of General Psychiatry, 44*, 405–408.

Morley, J. E. (2007). *Managing cognitive dysfunction*. interMDnet Corporation. Retrieved September 2007, from http://www.thedoctorwillseeyounow.com/articles/senior_living/cogdys_6/

Morris, J. C. (2006, July 15–20). Presentation, International Conference on Alzheimer's Disease and Related Disorders, Madrid, Spain.

Morris, M. C., Evans, D. A., Bienias, J. L., Tangney, C. C., & Wilson, R. S. (2004). Dietary fat intake and 6-year cognitive change in an older biracial community population. *Neurology, 62*, 1573–1579.

Morton, I., & Bleathman, C. (1991). The effectiveness of Validation Therapy in dementia: A pilot study. *International Journal of Geriatric Psychiatry, 6*, 327–330.

Mullan, M., Bennett, C., Figueredo, C., Hughes, D., Mant, R., Owen, M., et al. (1995). Clinical features of early onset, familial Alzheimer's disease linked to chromosome 14. *American Journal of Medical Genetics, 60,* 44–52.

Munoz, D. J., & Feldman, H. (2000). Causes of Alzheimer's disease. *Canadian Medical Association Journal, 162,* 65–72.

National Academy on an Aging Society. (2000). 1993 Study of Assets and Health Dynamic Among the Oldest Old. *Caregiving, 7,* 1–5.

National Family Caregivers Association. (2000). *Caregiving across the life cycle.* Retrieved July 2007, from http://nfcacares.org/survey.html

National Hospice and Palliative Care Organization (NHPCO). (2005). *NHPCO's 2005 Facts and Figures on Hospice.* Retrieved December 2007, from http://www.nhpco.org/i4a/pages/index.cfm?pageid=3274

National Institute on Aging. (2002). *Folic acid possibly a key factor in Alzheimer's disease prevention.* Retrieved July 2007, from http://www.nih.gov/news/pr/mar2002/nia-01.htm

National Institute on Aging. (2006). *Plaques and tangles: The hallmarks of AD.* Retrieved June 2007, from http://www.nia.nih.gov/Alzheimers/Publications/Unraveling TheMystery/Part1/Hallmarks.htm

National Institute on Aging. (2007a). *Caregiver guide: Tips for caregivers of people with Alzheimer's disease.* NIH Publication No. 01–4013. U.S. Department of Health and Human Services.

National Institute on Aging. (2007b). *Home safety for people with Alzheimer's disease.* NIH Publication No. 02–6179. U.S. Department of Health and Human Services.

National Institute on Aging. (2007c). *Legal and financial planning for people with Alzheimer's disease.* Retrieved November 2007, from http://www.nia.nih.gov/Alzheimers/Publications/legaltips.htm

National Institute on Aging. (2007d). *2005–2006 Progress report on Alzheimer's disease.* NIH Publication number 06-6047. U.S. Department of Health and Human Services.

National Institute on Aging, Alzheimer's Disease Education and Referral Center (ADEAR). (2007). *What drugs are currently available to treat AD?* Retrieved April 2007, from http://www.nia.nih.gov/Alzheimers/AlzheimersInformation/Treatment/

National Institute on Health. (2003, December). *Alzheimer's disease: Unraveling the mystery.* NIH Publication Number 02-3782.

National Institute of Neurological Disorders and Stroke. (2007). *Dementia with Lewy bodies.* Retrieved June 2007, from http://www.ninds.nih.gov/disorders/dementiawith lewybodies/dementiawithlewybodies.htm

National Long-Term-Care Ombudsman Resource Center. (2007). Retrieved October 2007, from http://www.ltcombudsman.org/ombpublic/49_151_855.CFM

National Respite Coalition. (2000). *Lifespan respite.* Retrieved June 2007, from http://www.archrespite.org/NRC-Lifespan.htm

Nemetz, P. N., Leibson, C., Naessens, J. M., Beard, M., Kokmen, E., & John, F., et al. (1999). Traumatic brain injury and time to onset of Alzheimer's disease: A population-based study. *American Journal of Epidemiology, 149,* 32–40.

Neurologyreviews.com. (2003, November). *Literature monitor: Recent articles of interest in neurology.* Retrieved September 2007, from http://www.neurologyreviews.com/nov03/nr_nov03_litmon.html

New York City Department for the Aging. (2007). *Senior housing.* Retrieved October 2007, from http://www.nyc.gov/html/dfta/html/senior/housing.shtml

Nurmi, I., & Luthje, P. (2002). Incidence and cost of falls and fall injuries among elderly in institutional care. *Scandinavian Journal of Primary Health Care, 20,* 118–122.

Nursing Home Reform Act. (1987). Retrieved October 2007, from http://www.ltcom budsman.org/ombpublic/49_346_1023.cfm

O'Malley, K., Sabogal, F., Lee, J. R., Engelman, M., Larson, M., & Cadogan, M. (2006). The Pain Assessment in Advanced Dementia (PAINAD) scale. *CAHQ Journal, 3,* 42–48.

Ono, K., Hasegawa, K., Naiki, H., & Yamada, M. (2004). Curcumin has potent anti-amyloidogenic effects for Alzheimer's beta-amyloid fibrils in vitro. *Journal of Neuroscience Research, 75,* 742–750.

Paganini-Hill, A., & Henderson, V. W. (1994). Estrogen deficiency and risk of Alzheimer's disease in women. *American Journal of Epidemiology, 140,* 256–261.

Palmer, C. V., Adams, S. W., Bourgeois, M. S., Durrant, J., & Rossi, M. (1999). Reduction in caregiver-identified problem behaviors in patients with Alzheimer's disease post-hearing-aid fitting. *Journal of Speech, Language, and Hearing Research, 42,* 312–328.

Perkins, H. S. (1986). Ethics at the end of life: Practical principles for making resuscitation decisions. *Journal of General Internal Medicine, 1,* 170–176.

Peskind, E. R. (1996). Neurobiology of Alzheimer's disease. *Journal of Clinical Psychiatry, 57,* 5–8.

Petersen, R. C. (2004). Mild cognitive impairment as a diagnostic entity. *Journal of Internal Medicine, 256,* 183–194.

Petersen, R. C., Doody, R., Kurz, A., Mohs, R. C., Morris, J. C., Robins, P. V., et al. (2001). Current concepts in mild cognitive impairment. *Archives of Neurology, 58,* 1985–1992.

Petersen, R. C., Stevens, J. C., Ganguli, M., Tangalos, E. G., Cummings, J. L., DeKosky, S. T., et al. (2001). Practice parameter: Early detection of dementia: Mild cognitive impairment (An evidence-based review). Report of the Quality Standards Subcommittee of the American Academy of Neurology. *Neurology, 56,* 1133–1142.

Pfeifer, E., & Davis, G. C. (1971). Measurement of functional activities in older adults in the community. *Journal of Gerontology, 37,* 323–329.

Phillips, C. D., Hawes, C., Spry, K., & Rose, M. (2000, June). *Residents leaving assisted living: Descriptive and analytic results from a national survey.* U.S. Department of Health and Human Services. Retrieved June, 2008, from http://aspe.hhs.gov/daltcp/reports/alresid.htm

Pillemer, K., & Suitor, J. J. (1992). Violence and violent feelings: What causes them among family caregivers? *Journal of Gerontology, 47*(Suppl.), 165–172.

Press, D., & Alexander, M. (2007a). *Cholinesterase inhibitors in dementia.* UpToDate.com. Retrieved September 2007, from http://www.utdol.com/utd/content/topic.do?topic Key=nuroegen/2069&selectedTitle=3~150&source=search_result

Press, D., & Alexander, M. (2007b). *Prevention of dementia.* UpToDate.com. Retrieved September 2007, from http://www.utdol.com/utd/content/topic.do?topicKey=nuro egen/1445&selectedTitle=6~150&source=search_result

Qiu, C., Bäckman, L., Winblad, B., Agüero-Torres, H., & Fratiglioni, L. (2001). The influence of education on clinically diagnosed dementia incidence and mortality: Data from the Kungsholmen project. *Archives of Neurology, 58,* 2034–2039.

Ramakrishnan, K., & Scheid, D. C. (2007). Treatment options for insomnia. *American Family Physician, 76,* 517–526.

Rapp, M. A., Schnaider-Beeri, M., Grossman, H. T., Sano, M., Perl, D. P., Purohit, D. P., et al. (2006). Increased hippocampal plaques and tangles in patients with Alzheimer disease with a lifetime history of major depression. *Archives of General Psychiatry, 63,* 161–167.

Reagan, R. (1994). *Ronald Reagan's announcement of Alzheimer's disease.* Retrieved March 2007, from http: //www.medaloffreedom.com/RonaldReaganAlzheimersAnnouncement.htm

Reisberg, B. (1988). Functional Assessment Staging (FAST). *Psychopharmacology Bulletin, 24,* 653–659.

Reisberg, B., Ferris, S. H., De Leon, M. J., & Crook, T. (1982). The Global Deterioration Scale for assessment of primary degenerative dementia. *American Journal of Psychiatry, 139,* 1136–1139.

Reisberg, B., Schneck, M. K., Ferris, S. H., Schwartz, G. E., & deLeon, M. J. (1983). The brief cognitive rating scale (BCRS): Findings in primary degenerative dementia (PDD). *Psychopharmacology Bulletin, 19,* 47–50.

Richard, J. H. (1997). After the diagnosis: Supporting Alzheimer's patients and their families. *Postgraduate Medicine, 101,* 6–8.

Richards, L. (2007). *The management of behavioral problems in persons with dementia: The role of the occupational therapist.* The University of Kansas Medical Center. Retrieved September 2007, from http://coa.kumc.edu/GEC/modules/BehavDisorder/OccupationalTherapy/OT_Frame-ModContent.htm

Ripich, D. N. (1994). Functional communication with AD patients: A caregiver training program. *Alzheimer Disease and Associated Disorders, 8,* 95–109.

Ripich, D. N., Kercher, K., Wykle, M., Sloan, D. M., & Ziol, E. (1998). Effects of communication training on African American and White caregivers of persons with Alzheimer's disease. *Journal of Aging and Ethnicity, 1,* 163–178.

Ripich, D. N., Ziol, E., Fritsch, T., & Durand, E. J. (1999). Training Alzheimer's disease caregivers for successful communication. *Clinical Gerontologist, 21,* 37–56.

Ripich, D. N., Ziol, E., & Lee, M. M. (1998). Longitudinal effects of communication training on caregivers of persons with Alzheimer's disease. *Clinical Gerontologist, 19,* 37–55.

Rishton, G. M. (2005). *Alzheimer's disease science.* California State University Channel Islands. Retrieved July 2007, from http://www.csuci.edu/alzheimer/science.htm

Rogers, C. R. (1961). *On becoming a person: A distinguished psychologist's guide to personal growth and creativity.* Boston: Houghton Mifflin.

Rogers, S., & Komisar, H. (2003, May). *Who needs long-term care?* (Fact sheet.) Washington, DC: Georgetown University Long-Term-Care Financing Project.

Rolland, Y., Pillard, F., Klapouszczak, A., Reynish, E., Thomas, D., Andrieu, S., et al. (2007). Exercise program for nursing home residents with Alzheimer's disease: A 1-Year randomized, controlled trial. *Journal of the American Geriatric Society, 55,* 158–165.

Rosenfeld, I. (2000). *Live now age later: Proven ways to slow down the clock.* New York: Grand Central Publishing.

Rossor, M. (2003). The ABCs of neurodegenerative dementias. In L. Radin & G. Radin (Eds.), *What if it's not Alzheimer's?* (pp. 29–40). Amherst, NY: Prometheus Books.

Rubenstein, L. Z. (1997). Preventing falls in the nursing home. *Journal of the American Medical Association, 278,* 595–596.

Rubenstein, L. Z., Josephson, K. R., & Robbins, A. S. (1994). Falls in the nursing home. *Annals of Internal Medicine, 121,* 442–451.

Rubenstein, L. Z., Robbins, A. S., Josephson, K. R., Schulman, B. L., & Osterweil, D. (1990). The value of assessing falls in an elderly population: A randomized clinical trial. *Annals of Internal Medicine, 113,* 308–316.

Runyan, C. W. (1988). Using the Haddon matrix: Introducing the third dimension. *Injury Prevention, 4,* 302–307.

Rush University Medical Center. (2004). *The Rush manual for caregivers* (6th ed.). Chicago: Rush Alzheimer's Disease Center.

Russell, D., Benedictis, T. D., & Segal, J. (2007). *Alzheimer's caregivers support: Support for caregivers of people with Alzheimer's or other dementias.* Helpguide.com. Retrieved July 2007, from http://www.helpguide.org/elder/alzheimers_disease_dementia_support_caregiver.htm

Rydell, C. (2002, December). *Medical groups agree: Resources for treating people with Alzheimer's are available but underutilized.* Retrieved April 2007, from http://www.scienceblog.com/community/older/2002/G/2002104.html

Sabra, L., & Katz-Wise, R. P. (2006). *Should I put my relative with Alzheimer's or other dementia in a nursing home?* Healthwise, Incorporated. Retrieved October 2007, from www.healthwise.org

Salk Institute. (2002). *Salk scientists demonstrate for the first time that newly born brain cells are functional in the adult brain.* Retrieved April 2007, from http://www.salk.edu/news/releases/details.php?id=10

Schneiderman, L. J., Jecker, N. S., & Jonsen, A. R. (1990). Medical futility: Its meaning and ethical implications. *Annals of Internal Medicine, 112,* 949–954.

Schulz, R., Belle, S. H., Czaja, S. J., McGinnis, K. A., Stevens, A., & Zhang, S. (2004). Long-term care placement of dementia patients and caregiver health and well-being. *Journal of the American Medical Association, 292,* 961–967.

Sclan, S. G., & Reisberg, B. (1992). Functional Assessment Staging (FAST) in Alzheimer's disease: Reliability, validity, and ordinality. *International Psychogeriatrics, 4,* 55–69.

Shaw, F. E. (2002). Falls and syncope in elderly patients. *Clinics in Geriatric Medicine, 18,* 159–173.

Shaw, F. E., & Kenny, R. A. (1998). Can falls in patients with dementia be prevented? *Age and Ageing, 27,* 7–9.

Shega, J. W., Levin, A., Hougham, G. W., Cox-Hayley, D., Luchins, D., Hanrahan, P., et al. (2003). Palliative excellence in Alzheimer care efforts (PEACE): A program description. *Journal of Palliative Medicine, 6,* 315–320.

Shelkey, M., & Wallace, M. (1999). Katz Index of Independence in Activities of Daily Living. *Journal of Gerontological Nursing, 25,* 8–9.

Shumaker, S. A., Legault, C., Kuller, L., Rapp, S. R., Thal, L., Lane, D. S., et al. (2004). Conjugated equine estrogens and incidence of probable dementia and mild cognitive impairment in postmenopausal women: Women's Health Initiative Memory Study. *Journal of the American Medical Association, 291,* 2947–2958.

Shumaker, S. A., Legault, C., Rapp, S. R., Thal, L., Wallace, R. B., Ockene, J. K., et al. (2003). Estrogen plus progestin and the incidence of dementia and mild cognitive impairment in postmenopausal women: The Women's Health Initiative Memory

Study: A randomized controlled trial. *Journal of the American Medical Association, 289,* 2651–2662.

Silverman, D. H. S., & Thompson, P. M. (2006, June). Neuroimaging sharpens focus on mild cognitive impairment. *Psychiatric Times.* Retrieved August 2007, from http://www.psychiatrictimes.com/topic/Alzheimer%20and%20Dementia/showArticle.jhtml;jsessionid=3IZ1PAL2YI14QQSNDLQSKHSCJUNN2JVN?articleID=188701396&topic=Alzheimer+and+Dementia

Simon, M. (2000, September). Some conditions mimic Alzheimer's disease. *Genetic Health.* Retrieved August 2007, from http://www.genetichealth.com/ALZ_When_it_Isnt_Alzheimers_Disease.shtml

Sink, K. M., Covinsky, K. E., Barnes, D. E., Newcomer, R. J., & Yaffe, K. (2006). Caregiver characteristics are associated with neuropsychiatric symptoms of dementia. *Journal of the American Geriatrics Society, 54,* 796–803.

Sink, K. M., Covinsky, K. E., Newcomer, R., & Yaffe, K. (2004). Ethnic differences in the prevalence and pattern of dementia-related behaviors. *Journal of the American Geriatrics Society, 52,* 1277–1283.

Sloane, P. D. (1998). Advances in the treatment of Alzheimer's disease. *American Family Physician, 58,* 1577–1586.

Smirnov, I. V. (2006). Mechanism of possible biological effect of activated water on patients suffering from Alzheimer's disease. *Explore, 15,* 53–56.

Smith, C. D., Chebrolu, H., Wekstein, D. R., Schmitt, F. A., Jicha, G. A., Cooper, G., et al. (2007). Brain structural alterations before mild cognitive impairment. *Neurology, 68,* 1268–1273.

Smith, M. (2005). Pain assessment in nonverbal older adults with advanced dementia. *Perspectives in Psychiatric Care, 41,* 99–113.

Sobel, E., Dunn, M., Davanipour, Z., Qian, Z., & Chui, H. C. (1996). Elevated risk of Alzheimer's disease among workers with likely electromagnetic field exposure. *Neurology, 47,* 1477–1481.

Solovitch, S. (2008, January 18). Avantis moves ahead with a look back at colonoscopy. *Silicon Valley/San Jose Business Journal,* 1–3.

Sterling, D. A., O'Connor, J. A., & Bonadies, J. (2001). Geriatric falls: Injury severity is high and disproportionate to mechanism. *Journal of Trauma, Injury, Infection, and Critical Care, 50,* 116–119.

Sullivan, D. (2005). Euthanasia versus letting die: Christian decision-making in terminal patients. *Ethics & Medicine, 21,* 109–118.

Swartz, K. P., Hantz, E. C., Crummer, G. C., Walton, J. P., & Frisina, R. D. (1989). Does the melody linger on? Music cognition in Alzheimer's disease. *Seminars in Neurology, 9,* 152–158.

Tang, M.-X., Cross, P., Andrews, H., Jacobs, D. M., Small, S., Small, S., et al. (2001). Incidence of AD in African-Americans, Caribbean Hispanics and Caucasians in northern Manhattan. *Neurology, 56,* 49–56.

Tangalos, E. G. (2003). *Transforming long-term care for Alzheimer's disease.* Medscape. Retrieved August 2007, from http://www.medscape.com/viewprogram/2410

Tangalos, E. G., Smith, G. E., Ivnik, R. J., Peterson, R. C., Kokmen, E., Kurland, L. T., et al. (1996). The Mini-Mental State Examination in general medical practice: Clinical utility and acceptance. *Mayo Clinic Proceedings, 71,* 829–837.

Tarapchak, P. (1998). *Shining light into the dark. Advance for long-term management.* Retrieved April 2007, from http://long-term-care.advanceweb.com/editorial/content/editorial.aspx?cc=250

Tavee, J., & Sweeney, P. J. (2003). *Alzheimer's disease.* Cleveland Clinic. Retrieved August 2007, from http://www.clevelandclinicmeded.com/medicalpubs/diseasemanagement/neurology/alzheimers/alzheimers.htm#ref15

Taylor, A. H., Cable, N. T., Faulkner, G., Hillsdon, M., Narici, M., & Van Der Bij, A. K. (2004). Physical activity and older adults: A review of health benefits and the effectiveness of interventions. *Journal of Sports & Science, 22,* 703–725.

Teno, J., Mor, V., DeSilva, D., Kabumoto, G., & Roy, J., & Wetle, T. (2002). Use of feeding tubes in nursing home residents with severe cognitive impairment. *Journal of the American Medical Association, 287,* 3211–3212.

Teri, L., Gibbons, L. E., McCurrym, S. M., Logsdon, R. G., Buchner, D. M., Barlow, W. E., et al. (2003). Exercise plus behavioral management in patients with Alzheimer disease: A randomized controlled trial. *Journal of American Medical Association, 290,* 2015–2022.

Teri, L., & Logsdon, R. G. (1991). Identifying pleasant activities for Alzheimer's disease patients: The pleasant events schedule-AD. *Gerontologist, 31,* 124–127.

Thapa, P. B., Brockman, K. G., Gideon, P., Fought, R. L., & Ray, W. A. (1996). Injurious falls in nonambulatory nursing home residents: A comparative study of circumstances, incidence and risk factors. *Journal of the American Geriatrics Society, 44,* 273–278.

Thomas, V. S., & Hageman, P. A. (2003). Can neuromuscular strength and function in people with dementia be rehabilitated using resistance-exercise training? Results from a preliminary intervention study. *Journals of Gerontology Series A: Biological Sciences and Medical Sciences, 58,* M746–M751.

Tideiksaar, R. (2007). Fall risk and Alzheimer's disease: Part 1. *ECPN Journal, 119,* 32–35.

Truog, R. D., Brett, A. S., & Frader, J. (1988). The problem with futility. *New England Journal of Medicine, 326,* 1560–1563.

Tyas, S. L., Manfreda, J., Strain, L. A., & Montgomery, P. R. (2001). Risk factors for Alzheimer's disease: A population-based, longitudinal study in Manitoba, Canada. *International Journal of Epidemiology, 30,* 598–599.

University of California Davis, Alzheimer's Disease Center. (2007). Mild cognitive impairment. Retrieved May 2007, from http://alzheimer.ucdavis.edu/faq/mci.php

U.S. Census Bureau, Department of Commerce. (2000, January 13). *Methodology and assumptions for the population projections of the United States: 1999 to 2100.* Washington, D.C.: Author.

U.S. Congress Office of Technology Assessment. (1987). *Losing a million minds: Confronting the tragedy of Alzheimer's disease and other dementias.* Washington, DC: U.S. Government Printing Office.

U.S. Congress, Office of Technology Assessment. (1990). *Confused minds, burdened families: Finding help for people with Alzheimer's and other dementias.* Retrieved May 2007, from http://www.eric.ed.gov/ERICDocs/data/ericdocs2sql/content_storage_01/0000019b/80/23/15/9e.pdf

U.S. Department of Commerce, Economics and Statistics Administration, U.S. Census Bureau. (2006, August). *Income, earnings, and poverty data from the 2005 American Community Survey.* Retrieved October 2007, from http://www.census.gov/prod/2006pubs/acs-02.pdf

U.S. Department of Health and Human Services. (2000, November). *High service or high privacy assisted living facilities, their residents and staff: Results from a national survey.* Retrieved October 2007, from http://aspe.hhs.gov/daltcp/reports/hshp.htm

U.S. Department of Health and Human Services. (2003). *Falls prevention interventions in the Medicare population: Evidence report and evidence-based recommendations.* Retrieved October 2007, from http://www.cms.hhs.gov/PrevntionGenInfo/Downloads/Falls%20Evidence%20Report.pdf

U.S. Department of Health and Human Services. (2008). *National clearinghouse for long-term care information.* Retrieved February 2008, from http://www.longtermcare.gov/LTC/Main_Site/Paying_LTC/Costs_Of_Care/Costs_Of_Care.aspx

U.S. Department of Health and Human Services, U.S. Administration on Aging. (2005, June). *Long-term care systems change for the aged and Americans with disabilities: State profiles.* Retrieved October 2007, from http://www.aoa.gov/press/fact/pdf/ib_ltc.pdf

U.S. Food & Drug Administration. (2005a). *Medicines and you: A guide for older adults.* Retrieved September 2007, from http://www.fda.gov/cder/consumerinfo/medAndYouEng.htm

U.S. Food & Drug Administration. (2005b). *Menopause and hormones.* Retrieved September 2007, from http://www.fda.gov/womens/menopause/mht-FS.html

U.S. News & World Report. (2007). *Alzheimer's disease.* Retrieved July 2007, from http://health.usnews.com/usnews/health/brain/alzheimers/alz.manage.drive.htm

van Leeuwen, F. W., de Kleijn, D. P., van den Hurk, H., Neubauer, A., Sonnemans, M. A., Sluijs, J. A., et al. (1998). Frameshift mutants of beta amyloid precursor protein and ubiquitin-B in Alzheimer's and Down patients. *Science, 279,* 242–247.

Veld, B. A., Ruitenberg, A., Hofman, A., Launer, L. J., van Duijn, C. M., Stijnen, T., et al. (2001). Nonsteroidal antiinflammatory drugs and the risk of Alzheimer's disease. *New England Journal of Medicine, 345,* 1515–1521.

Volicer, L. (2005). *End-of-life care for people with dementia in residential care settings.* Alzheimer's Association. Retrieved November 2007, from http://www.alz.org/national/documents/endoflifelitreview.pdf

Volicer, L., Rheaume, Y., Brown, J., Fabiszewski, K., & Brady, R. (1986). Hospice approach to the treatment of patients with advanced dementia of the Alzheimer type. *Journal of the American Medical Association, 256,* 2210–2213.

Vu, M. Q., Weintraub, N., & Rubenstein, L. Z. (2005). Falls in the nursing home: Are they preventable? *Journal of the American Medical Directors Association, 6,* S82–S87.

Wallace, M., & Shelkey, M. (2007). *Katz Index of Independence in Activities of Daily Living (ADL).* The Hartford Institute for Geriatric Nursing. Retrieved August 2007, from http://www.hartfordign.org/publications/trythis/issue02.pdf

Wang, R., & Tang, X. C. (2005). Neuroprotective effects of huperzine A: A natural cholinesterase inhibitor for the treatment of Alzheimer's disease. *Neurosignals, 14,* 71–82.

Wanzer, S. H., Adelstein, S. J., Cranford, R. E., Federman, D. D., Hook, E. D., Moertel, C. G., et al. (1984). The physician's responsibility toward hopelessly ill patients. *New England Journal of Medicine, 310,* 955–959.

Warden, V., Hurley, A. C., & Volicer, L. (2003). Development and psychometric evaluation of the PAINAD (Pain Assessment in Advanced Dementia) scale. *Journal of the American Medical Directors Association, 4,* 9–15.

Waters, G. S., Rochon, E., & Caplan, D. (1998). Task demands and sentence comprehension in patients with dementia of the Alzheimer's type. *Brain and Language, 62,* 361–397.

WebMD. (2005, March). *Alzheimer's diagnosis often delayed Survey: Symptoms typically start nearly 3 years before diagnosis.* Retrieved August 2007, from http://www.webmd.com/alzheimers/news/20070314/alzheimers-diagnosis-often-delayed

WebMD. (2005, August). *Seven Alzheimer's warning signs.* Retrieved June 2007, from http://www.webmd.com/alzheimers/guide/7-alzheimers-warning-signs

WebMD. (2007a). *Alzheimer's disease: Daily care of the Alzheimer's patient.* Retrieved September 2007, from http://www.webmd.com/alzheimers/guide/daily-care-alzheimers

WebMD. (2007b). *Alzheimer's disease: Improving communication with Alzheimer's patients.* Retrieved July 2007, from http://www.webmd.com/alzheimers/guide/improving-communication

WebMD. (2007c). *Alzheimer's disease: Making the diagnosis.* Retrieved August 2007, from http://www.webmd.com/alzheimers/guide/making-diagnosis

WebMD. (2007d). *Alzheimer's disease: Types of Alzheimer's disease.* Retrieved July 2007, from http://www.webmd.com/alzheimers/guide/alzheimers-types

Welton, E. P. (2002). *How to choose a residence.* The Assisted Living Federation of America. Retrieved October 2007, from http://www.longtermcarelink.net/eldercare/assisted_living.htm

White, H., Pieper, C., Schmader, K., & Fillenbaum, G. (1997). A longitudinal analysis of weight change in Alzheimer's disease. *Journal of the American Geriatric Society, 45,* 531–532.

White, H. K. (2004). Weight loss in advanced Alzheimer's disease, Part I: Contributing factors and evaluation. *Annals of Long-Term Care: Clinical Care and Aging, 12,* 33–37.

Williams-Gray, C. H. Foltynie, T., Lewis, S. J. G., & Barker, R. A. (2006). Cognitive deficits and psychosis in Parkinson's disease: A review of pathophysiology and therapeutic options. *CNS Drugs, 20,* 477–505.

Wilson, R. S., McCann, J. J., Li, Y., Aggarwal, N. T., & Gilley, D. W. (2007). Nursing home placement, day care use, and cognitive decline in Alzheimer's disease. *American Journal of Psychiatry, 164,* 910–915.

Wolf-Klein, G. P., Silverstone, F. A., Levy, A. P., & Brod, M. S. (1989). Screening for Alzheimer's disease by clock drawing. *Journal of the American Geriatrics Society, 37,* 730–736.

Wong, J. G., Clare, I. C., Gunn, M. J., & Holland, A. J. (1999). Capacity to make health care decisions: Its importance in clinical practice. *Psychological Medicine, 29,* 437–446.

Wong, R. Y. M. (2005). A practical approach to late Alzheimer disease. *British Columbia Medical Journal, 47,* 494–498.

World Health Organization Expert Committee. (1990). *Report. Cancer pain relief and palliative care.* Geneva, Switzerland: Author.

Wynne, C. (2000). Comparison of pain assessment instruments in cognitively intact and cognitively impaired nursing home residents. *Geriatric Nursing, 21,* 20–23.

Yaffe, K., Fox, P., Newcomer, R., Sands, L., Lindquist, K., Dane, K., et al. (2002). Patient and caregiver characteristics and nursing home placement in patients with dementia. *Journal of the American Medical Association, 287,* 2090–2097.

Yan, Q., Zhang, J., Liu, H., Babu-Khan, S., Vassar, R., Biere, A. L., et al. (2003). Anti-inflammatory drug therapy alters beta-amyloid processing and deposition in an animal model of Alzheimer's disease. *Journal of Neuroscience, 23,* 7504–7509.

Yang, F., Lim, G. P., Begum, A. N., Ubeda, O. J., & Simmons, M. R. (2005). Curcumin inhibits formation of amyloid beta oligomers and fibrils, binds plaques, and reduces amyloid in vivo. *Journal of Biological Chemistry, 280,* 5892–5901.

Yellowitz, J. (2005). Cognitive function, aging, and ethical decisions: Recognizing change. *Dental Clinics of North America, 49,* 389–410.

Youngner, S. J. (1988). Who defines futility? *Journal of the American Medical Association, 260,* 2094–2095.

Zandi, P. P., Carlson, M. C., Plassman, B. L., Welsh-Bohmer, K. A., Mayer, L. S., Steffens, D. C., et al. (2002). Hormone replacement therapy and incidence of Alzheimer disease in older women: The Cache County study. *Journal of the American Medical Association, 288,* 2123–21299.

Zanetti, O., Frisoni, G. B., De Leo, D., Della Buono, M., Bianchetti, A., & Trabucchi, M. (1995). Reality Orientation Therapy in Alzheimer's disease: Useful or not? A controlled study. *Alzheimer's Disease and Associated Disorders, 9,* 132–138.

Additional Resources

Alzheimer's Association
225 North Michigan, 17th Floor
Chicago, IL 60601
(312) 335–8700
(800) 272–3900
www.alz.org

Alzheimer's Disease Education and Referral Center (ADEAR)
P.O. Box 8250
Silver Spring, MD 20907–8250
(301) 495–3311
(800) 438–4380
www.alzheimers.org

Alzheimer's Disease International
45/46 Lower Marsh
London
SE1 7RG
United Kingdom
020 7981 0880
www.alz.co.uk

Alzheimer's Disease Research and the American Health Assistance Foundation
15825 Shady Grove Road, Suite 140
Rockville, MD 20850
(301) 948–3244
(800) 437–2423

Alzheimer's Foundation of America
322 Eighth Avenue
7th Floor
New York, NY 10001
866-AFA-8484 (232–8484)
www.alzfdn.org

Alzheimer Support
2040 Alameda Padre Serra, Suite 101
Santa Barbara, CA 93103
(800) 366–5924

AARP
601 E St., NW
Washington, DC 20049
(202) 434–2277

American Geriatrics Society
The Empire State Building
350 Fifth Ave., Suite 801
New York, NY 10118
(212) 308–1414

American Psychiatric Association
1400 K St., NW
Washington, DC 20005
(888) 357–7924

Children of Aging Parents
1609 Woodbourne Road, Suite 302A
Levittown, PA 19057
(800) 227–7294
www.caps4caregivers.org

Clearinghouse on Aging and Developmental Disabilities
RRTC on Aging and Developmental Disabilities (M/C 626)
The University of Illinois at Chicago
1640 West Roosevelt Road
Chicago, IL 60608–6904
(800) 996–8845

The Cognitive Neurology and Alzheimer's Disease Center
320 East Superior St.
Searle 11–450
Chicago, IL 60611–3008
(312) 908–9339

Eldercare Locator
(800) 677–1116
www.eldercare.gov

Elder Care Online
www.ec-online.net

Family Caregiver Alliance
690 Market Street, Suite 600
San Francisco, CA 94104
415–434–3388
www.caregiver.org

National Council on Aging
409 Third St., SW
Suite 200
Washington, DC 20024
(202) 479–1200

National Council of Senior Citizens
8403 Colesville Road
Suite 1200
Silver Spring, MD 20910
(301) 578–8800

National Family Caregivers Association
10400 Connecticut Ave., #500
Kensington, MD 20895–3944
(800) 896–3650

National Hospice and Palliative Care Organization/National Hospice Foundation
1700 Diagonal Road
Suite 625
Alexandria, VA 22314
(800) 658–8898
www.nhpco.org

National Institute on Aging
Building 31, Room 5C27
31 Center Drive, MSC 2292
Bethesda, MD 20892
(301) 496–1752
www.nia.nih.gov

National Institute of Neurological Disorders and Stroke
NIH Neurological Institute
Attn: NINDS
P.O. Box 5801
Bethesda, MD 20824
(800) 352–9424

National Respite Network and Resource Center
800 Eastowne Drive
Suite 105
Chapel Hill, NC 27514
(919) 490–5577 x222
www.archrespite.org

The Simon Foundation for Continence
P.O. Box 815
Wilmette, IL 60091
(800) 237–4666
www.simonfoundation.org

U.S. Department of Health and Human Services
Administration on Aging
330 Independence Ave., SW,
    Room 4759
Washington, DC 20201
(202) 619–0724

Well Spouse Foundation
63 West Main Street, Suite H
Freehold, NJ 07728
(800) 838–0879
www.wellspouse.org

Index